HYPERTENSION AND
THE HEART

ADVANCES IN EXPERIMENTAL MEDICINE AND BIOLOGY

Recent Volumes in this Series

Volume 424
THE FATE OF THE MALE GERM CELL
Edited by Richard Ivell and Adolf-Friedrich Holstein

Volume 425
CHEMISTRY AND BIOLOGY OF SERPINS
Edited by Frank C. Church, Dennis D. Cunningham, David Ginsburg,
Maureane Hoffman, Stuart R. Stone, and Douglas M. Tollefsen

Volume 426
PHYSIOLOGY AND PATHOPHYSIOLOGY OF THE ISLETS OF LANGERHANS
Edited by Bernat Soria

Volume 427
DIETARY FIBER IN HEALTH AND DISEASE
Edited by David Kritchevsky and Charles Bonfield

Volume 428
OXYGEN TRANSPORT TO TISSUE XIX
Edited by David K. Harrison and David T. Delpy

Volume 429
BRAIN PLASTICITY: Development and Aging
Edited by Guido Filogamo, Antonia Vernadakis, Fulvia Gremo, Alain M. Privat,
and Paola S. Timiras

Volume 430
ANALYTICAL AND QUANTITATIVE CARDIOLOGY
Edited by Samuel Sideman and Rafael Beyar

Volume 431
PURINE AND PYRIMIDINE METABOLISM IN MAN IX
Edited by Andrea Griesmacher, Peter Chiba, and Mathias M. Müller

Volume 432
HYPERTENSION AND THE HEART
Edited by Alberto Zanchetti, Richard B. Devereux, Lennart Hansson, and Sergio Gorini

Volume 433
RECENT ADVANCES IN PROSTAGLANDIN, THROMBOXANE, AND
LEUKOTRIENE RESEARCH
Edited by Helmut Sinzinger, Bengt Samuelsson, John R. Vane, Rodolfo Paoletti,
Peter Ramwell, and Patrick Y-K Wong

HYPERTENSION AND THE HEART

Edited by

Alberto Zanchetti

University of Milan
Milan, Italy

Richard B. Devereux

Cornell University Medical College
New York, New York

Lennart Hansson

University of Uppsala
Uppsala, Sweden

and

Sergio Gorini

International Menarini Foundation
Milan, Italy

SPRINGER SCIENCE+BUSINESS MEDIA, LLC

Library of Congress Cataloging-in-Publication Data

Hypertension and the heart / edited by Alberto Zanchetti ... [et al.].
        p.   cm. -- (Advances in experimental medicine and biology ; v.
    432)
        "Proceedings of an International Congress on Hypertension and the
    Heart, held as part of the Menarini series on cardiovascular
    diseases, held February 27-28, 1997, in Berlin, Germany"--T.p.
    verso.
        Includes bibliographical references and index.
        ISBN 978-0-306-45774-6   ISBN 978-1-4615-5385-4 (eBook)
        DOI 10.1007/978-1-4615-5385-4
        1. Heart--Hypertrophy--Congresses.   2. Hypertension-
    -Complications--Congresses.   3. Coronary heart disease--Congresses.
    I. Zanchetti, Alberto.   II. Fondazione internazionale Menarini.
    III. International Congress on Hypertension and the Heart (1997 :
    Berlin, Germany)   IV. Series.
        [DNLM: 1. Hypertension--complications--congresses.
    2. Hypertrophy, Left Ventricular--physiopathology.   W1 AD559 v.432
    1997]
    RC685.H9H953   1997
    616.1'207--dc21
    DNLM/DLC
    for Library of Congress   97-45693
                                                                   CIP

Proceedings of an International Congress on Hypertension and the Heart, held as part of The Menarini
Series on Cardiovascular Diseases, held February 27 – 28, 1997, in Berlin, Germany

ISBN 978-0-306-45774-6

© 1997 Springer Science+Business Media New York
Originally published by Plenum Press, New York in 1997

http://www.plenum.com

10 9 8 7 6 5 4 3 2 1

PREFACE

Left ventricular hypertrophy represents one of the most common complications of the hypertensive state. Indeed, since the Framigham Heart Study, several epidemiological studies have provided clearcut evidence that cardiac hypertrophy represents an important and independent risk factor for the hypertensive patient.

Since the introduction of quantitative ultrasound techniques to evaluate cardiac function and state, the research in the field of left ventricular hypertrophy has been particularly active and fruitful, allowing us to gain new information on the pathophysiology of this condition and on its diagnostic and therapeutic approach.

The international symposium "Hypertension and the Heart," one of the most important meetings held on this issue in recent years, promoted by Fondazione Internazionale Menarini, dealt with cardiac hypertrophy in its structural, molecular, pathophysiological, and clinical aspects, and with related complications, such as myocardial ischemia, arrhythmias, and congestive heart failure.

Prof. A. Zanchetti

CONTENTS

Session I: Left Ventricular Hypertrophy: Structural Aspects and Mechanisms

1. Relations of Left Ventricular Geometry and Function to Prognosis
   in Hypertension 1
   Richard B. Devereux, Giovanni de Simone, and Mary J. Roman

2. Left Ventricular Hypertrophy, Arterial Compliance, and Aging 13
   Mary J. Roman, Antonello Ganau, Pier Sergio Saba, and Richard B. Devereux

3. Left Ventricular Hypertrophy and Arterial Blood Pressure in
   Experimental Models of Hypertension 23
   A. F. Dominiczak, A. M. Devlin, M. J. Brosnan, N. H. Anderson, D. Graham,
   J. S. Clark, A. McPhaden, C. A. Hamilton, and J. L. Reid

4. Regulation and Role of Myocardial Collagen Matrix Remodeling in
   Hypertensive Heart Disease 35
   Reinhard C. Funck, Andreas Wilke, Heinz Rupp, and Christian G. Brilla

5. Ultrasonic Reflectivity of the Heart: A Measure of Fibrosis? 45
   Michele Ciulla, Roberta Paliotti, and Fabio Magrini

6. Local Angiotensin II and Myocardial Fibrosis 55
   Yao Sun

7. Left Ventricular Anatomy and Function in Primary Aldosteronism and
   Renovascular Hypertension 63
   Achille C. Pessina, Alfredo Sacchetto, and Gian Paolo Rossi

Session II: Pathophysiological and Molecular Aspects

8. Hypertension Differentially Affects the Expression of the Gap Junction Protein
   Connexin43 in Cardiac Myocytes and Aortic Smooth Muscle Cells 71
   Jacques-Antoine Haefliger, Einar Castillo, Gérard Waeber,
   Jean-François Aubert, Pascal Nicod, Bernard Waeber,
   and Paolo Meda

 9. Modulation of Cardiac Hypertrophy by Estrogens 83
     Theo Pelzer, Asiya Shamim, Simone Wölfges, Michael Schumann, and
     Ludwig Neyses

10. Salt Sensitivity and Left Ventricular Hypertrophy 91
     Antonio Coca and Alejandro De la Sierra

11. Volume Overload, Atrial Natriuretic Peptide, and
     Left Ventricular Hypertrophy 103
     M. Luque Otero, N. Martell, A. L. Aubele, J. L. Rodrigo, M. Herrero,
     J. Moya, I. Egocheaga, A. Fernández-Cruz, and C. Fernandez Pinilla

12. The Renin-Angiotensin System Gene Polymorphism and
     Left Ventricular Hypertrophy 111
     Laurence Tiret

13. Renin-Angiotensin System Gene Polymorphisms and Left Ventricular
     Hypertrophy: The Case against an Association 117
     M. J. West, K. M. Summers, K. K. Wong, and D. J. Burstow

Session III: Pathophysiological and Therapeutic Aspects

14. Left Ventricular Hypertrophy and Arterial Hypertrophy 123
     Jean-Michel Mallion, Jean-Philippe Baguet, Jean-Philippe Siché, F. Tremel,
     and R. De Gaudemaris

15. Relationship between Cardiac Hypertrophy and Microalbuminuria 135
     Luis M. Ruilope

16. Physiological versus Pathological Hypertrophy:
     The Athlete and the Hypertensive 145
     Cesare Cuspidi, Laura Lonati, Lorena Sampieri, Gastone Leonetti, and
     Alberto Zanchetti

17. Bradykinin and Cardiac Protection 159
     Peter Gohlke, Carsten Tschöpe, and Thomas Unger

18. Left Ventricular Hypertrophy and Sympathetic Activity 173
     Guido Grassi, Gino Seravalle, and Giuseppe Mancia

19. Hypertension, Left Ventricular Hypertrophy, and Heart Rate Variability 181
     Federico Lombardi and Cesare Fiorentini

20. Comparison of Meta-Analyses of Therapeutic Studies on Regression of
     Left Ventricular Hypertrophy 189
     Lennart Hansson

21. Comparison of Therapeutic Studies on Regression of
     Left Ventricular Hypertrophy 191
     Roland E. Schmieder and Markus P. Schlaich

22. Prognostic Significance of Left Ventricular Hypertrophy Regression   199
    Enrico Agabiti-Rosei and Maria Lorenza Muiesan

Session IV: Myocardial Ischemia

23. Hypertension and Coronary Microvascular Disease   207
    B. E. Strauer and B. Schwartzkopff

24. Myocardial Perfusion in Hypertensive Patients with Normal Coronary Arteries . .   215
    Carlo Palombo, Michaela Kozàkovà, Giovanni Bigalli, Danilo Neglia,
       Alessandro Distante, Oberdan Parodi, and Antonio L'Abbate

25. Endothelial Dysfunction in Hypertension   235
    Stefano Taddei and Antonio Salvetti

26. Endothelial Dysfunction in Hypertensives: An Uncertain Association   247
    P. A. van Zwieten

27. Hypertension, Left Ventricular Hypertrophy, and Coronary Flow Reserve   253
    Edward D. Frohlich

28. Hypertensive Heart Disease, Ventricular Dysrhythmias, and Sudden Death   263
    Franz H. Messerli and Leszek Michalewicz

29. Hypertension and Heart Failure   273
    M. Gary Nicholls, A. Mark Richards, and Evan J. Begg

Speakers   281

Index   285

HYPERTENSION AND
THE HEART

RELATIONS OF LEFT VENTRICULAR GEOMETRY AND FUNCTION TO PROGNOSIS IN HYPERTENSION[*]

Richard B. Devereux,[†] Giovanni de Simone, and Mary J. Roman

Department of Medicine
New York Hospital, Cornell Medical Center
New York, New York

The heart plays a central role in systemic hypertension, since it both generates the increased force needed to sustain elevated arterial blood pressure and suffers the morbid consequences thereof. The importance of left ventricular (LV) hypertrophy as a cardinal manifestation of hypertensive target organ damage was first suspected based on the ability of ECG LV hypertrophy to predict morbidity and mortality in patients with hypertension,[1-3] in the general population,[4-5] and in catheterized patients with or without coronary artery obstruction.[6] However, it was uncertain whether these patterns derived their significance from cardiac hypertrophy or from ECG manifestations of myocardial ischemia. This uncertainty has been resolved by the demonstration that increased LV mass is a potent predictor of cardiovascular morbidity and mortality, independent of age, gender, blood pressure or other risk factors.[7-19] It is the purpose of this chapter to review available evidence concerning: 1) the relation of LV hypertrophy to prognosis; 2) whether additional consideration of LV geometric patterns further aids risk stratification; 3) the relation between LV myocardial function and prognosis; 4) potential mechanisms of observed relations between LV muscle mass and function on, the one hand, and morbid events due to vascular thrombosis, on the other; and 5) available evidence concerning the possible prognostic benefit of LV hypertrophy regression.

1. THE RELATION BETWEEN LEFT VENTRICULAR HYPERTROPHY AND AN ADVERSE PROGNOSIS

A large number of studies have reported on the relation between ECG or echocardiographic measures of LV hypertrophy at a baseline examination and the risk of sub-

[*] Supported in part by grants HL 18323 and HL 47540 from the National Heart, Lung and Blood Institute, Bethesda, MD, and grants CDSP 964-0A from Merck and Co., Inc., Whitehouse Station, NJ.
[†] Address for correspondence: Richard B. Devereux, M.D., Division of Cardiology, Box 222, The New York Hospital–Cornell Medical Center, 525 East 68th Street, New York, NY 10021. Phone: (212) 746-4655, Fax: (212) 746-8451, E-mail: rbdevere@mail.med.cornell.edu

Hypertension and the Heart, edited by Zanchetti et al.
Plenum Press, New York, 1997

1

sequent morbid or mortal events in clinical or epidemiological populations As may be seen in Table 1, individuals with LV hypertrophy consistently have from 2 to 4 or more fold higher rates of different adverse events, as indicated by the odds ratios. Not unexpectedly, the absolute differences in the rates of morbid events between individuals with and without LV hypertrophy (the attributable risks) vary with the endpoint and with the overall level of risk in the population under study.

In the first study to relate direct measurements of LV mass to prognosis in hypertension,[7] we followed 140 men with initially uncomplicated essential hypertension for five years to determine the incidence of "hard" cardiovascular morbid events (cardiac death, myocardial infarction, stroke or angina pectoris requiring coronary bypass surgery). The 29 or 20% of the patients in whom baseline LV mass exceeded $125g/m^2$, a partition value for LVH chosen on the basis of previous findings in employed adults, had a roughly 4-fold higher rate of morbid events (7 of 29 or 24%) than the men without LVH (7 of 111 or 6%, p<0.01).

We subsequently extended this study to more than 10-year follow-up of 280 women and men with initially uncomplicated essential hypertension.[13] LV mass index $>125g/m^2$ strongly predicted all-cause mortality and cardiac death as well as myocardial infarction or need for coronary revascularization. Considered as a continuous variable, LV mass index eliminated all conventional risk factors except age from multivariate models; after age adjustment LV mass remained a strong predictor of adverse cardiovascular events. Further analyses during up to 15 year follow-up revealed an especially adverse prognosis in patients with LV mass index $>175g/m^2$.[15]

Other studies have confirmed and extended these findings by demonstrating that LV mass is a strong predictor, independent of blood pressure or other risk factors, of cardiac and cerebrovascular morbidity and mortality among middle-aged and elderly women and men in the general population,[11-12,16] in patients with diverse forms of heart disease including hypertension[6-10,22,24] and in catheterized patients with and without coronary artery disease.[14,19-20] A report from the Framingham Heart Study documented that LV mass strongly predicted of all-cause and cardiac death and coronary heart disease events in adults over age 40, and noted that "only LV mass index and age were strong and consistent predictors of all three outcome events in all age and sex subgroups" in analyses that included conventional risk factors.[12] Of note, the same level of indexed LV mass (140g/m of height) identified high-risk status in both women and men,[12] similar to our finding that LV mass $>125g/m^2$ predicted death or morbid events equally in both genders.[13] In another important study, Ghali et al[14] documented that increased as opposed to normal LV mass predicted subsequent mortality more strongly (odds ratio=3.7) in catheterized patients without obstructive coronary artery disease than in those with stenosis of large coronary arteries (odds ratio=1.9). In a subsequent study using death as the end-point,[19] this group of investigators found that the attributable risk of LV hypertrophy was greater than that of multiple coronary stenoses or a low LV ejection fraction at catheterization.

2. RELATION OF LEFT VENTRICULAR GEOMETRIC PATTERNS TO CARDIOVASCULAR RISK

Recent studies have established that the LV may respond to hypertension by developing a variety of geometric patterns. In fact, the "classic" hypertensive pattern of concentric LV hypertrophy, characterized by increases in both LV mass and relative wall thickness (the ratio of LV wall thickness to chamber radius) has been observed in only a minority (6 to 15 %) of several series of relatively unselected, asymptomatic hypertensive

Table 1. Incidence of cardiovascular events in subjects with and without left ventricular hypertrophy

Reference	Method	Number	LVH criterion	End-point	With pre-clinical disease[a]	Without pre-clinical disease[a]	Odds ratio
Breslin et al (2)	ECG	631	T-wave inversion	Death	4.7	3.7	4.8
Sokolow et al (1)	ECG	439	Sokolow-Lyon	Death	14.0	2.0	8.0
Casale et al (7)	Echo	140	LV mass >125g/m²	Death, MI, CVA, severe angina	4.6	1.2	4.0
Levy et al (11)	Echo	1,141	LV mass >150gm/m	Angina;	2.8[b]	0.6[b]	4.8
				CHD other than angina	3.2[b]	0.7[b]	4.7
Levy et al (12)	Echo	3,220	LV mass >140g/m (>116g/m²)	All cause mortality;	2.0[b]	0.8[b]	2.5
				all cardiovascular events	3.3[b]	1.4[b]	2.4
Koren et al (13)	Echo	280	LV mass >125g/m²	C-V death;	1.4	0.1	14.2
				All C-V events	6.3	2.2	3.0
Sullivan et al (6)	ECG	4,824	Varied by age, leads I, aVL, V1, V5, V6	MI	2.8[c]	0.8[c]	3.6
MacMahon et al (21)	ECG	8,012	Minnesota code	C-V death			2.3
Liao et al (19)	Echo	1,089	LV mass >131g/m² (men), >100g/m² (women)	Death: patients with CAD;	5.8	2.4	2.0
				patients without CAD	3.2	1.8	3.0
Bolgonese et al (17)	Echo	76	LV mass >135g/m² (men), >112g/m² (women)	Cardiac death, MI, unstable angina	2.0	5.6	5.4
Quinones et al (22)	Echo	1,172	LV mass (per 1.5 SD)	Death			1.37
Levy et al (23)	ECG	524	Cornell voltage	C-V events	3.0	8.5	3.2
Silverberg et al (10)	Echo	119	LV mass >125g/m²	Death	15.2	9.6	3.7
Kannel et al (5)	ECG	5,055	Voltage and repolarization	C-V events	5.4	2.2	2.5
Isles (3)	ECG	3,783	"Abnormal ECG"	Death	4.0	2.0	2.0
Parfrey et al (24)	Echo	104	Wall thickness >1.4cm	Death	15.3	4.8	3.6
Aronow et al (9)	Echo	554	LV mass >134g/m² (men), >110g/m² (women)	Ventricular fibrillation or sudden death	11.5	2.7	4.7

[a]Incidence of morbid events per 100 patients years.

[b]Age-adjusted rate.

[c]Percent of subjects with events over 1- to 30-month follow-up period.

Abbreviations: CHD, coronary heart disease; C-V, cardiovascular; CVA, cerebrovascular accident; LV, left ventricular; MI, myocardial infarction.

patients.[13,25-28] In these studies, larger proportions of hypertensive patients have had either eccentric LV hypertrophy (increased LV mass with normal relative wall thickness), concentric LV remodelling (increased LV relative wall thickness with normal overall muscle mass) or normal LV geometry than have had concentric hypertrophy.[13,25-28]

The several LV geometric patterns are associated with, and potentially caused by, different profiles of systemic hemodynamics and cardiac function. Blood pressure in hypertensive patients with concentric LVH is principally elevated by increased peripheral resistance with slightly above average normal cardiac output.[25-28] The concentrically hypertrophied heart derives the increased work capacity needed to sustain moderately elevated blood pressure from increased LV mass and the mechanical advantage bestowed by high relative wall thickness despite decreased myocardial contractility.[25,29] In patients with eccentric hypertrophy increased cardiac output with minimal or no elevation of peripheral resistance support blood pressure elevation that is milder during normal activity than in the clinic.[25-26] Increased LV mass with normal relative wall thicknesses and roughly normal contractility but increased preload due to plasma volume expansion sustain LV ejection phase performance that is normal at rest but may be subnormal during exercise.[25,30] Patients with concentric LV remodelling have relatively mild hypertension despite markedly elevated peripheral resistance because cardiac output is subnormal.[25] The mechanical advantage associated with high relative wall thickness sustains the pressure load at rest and during activity despite normal LV mass and reduced preload due to diminished plasma volume. Patients with normal LV geometry tend to have mild hypertension with above average normal peripheral resistances and/or cardiac outputs.[25] The mild overload is offset by slightly above average normal LV mass with normal contractility.[25,29]

Several studies have suggested that a stepwise increase in the risk of cardiovascular morbidity and mortality occurs from a low event rate in hypertensive patients with normal LV geometry, through intermediate rates in those with concentric LV remodelling or eccentric hypertrophy, to the highest level of risk in patients with concentric LV hypertrophy.[13,31-33] As may be seen in Table 2, this pattern has been observed in hypertensive patients from New York City[13] and from Perugia, Italy[31,33] and in members of the Framingham general population sample.[32] Of note, on average, incident cardiovascular events were suffered each year by about one percent of individuals with normal LV geometry and in three percent or more of those with concentric LV hypertrophy in each population, with intermediate event rates in the subjects with concentric LV remodelling or eccentric LV hypertrophy. While the consistency of these findings in quite different populations from two continents is impressive, it still remains uncertain to what extent the gradient in cardiovascular risk among patients with different LV geometric patterns is independent of

Table 2. Incidence of morbid events in subjects classified by pattern of left ventricular geometry

| | | Proportion of subjects with events (percent/year) | | | |
Study	Event	Normal LV geometry	Concentric remodelling	Eccentric hypertrophy	Concentric hypertrophy
Koren (13)	C-V events	1.1	1.5	2.3	3.1
Koren (13)	C-V death	0	0.3	1.0	2.1
Verdecchia (31)	C-V events	1.1	2.4	Not studied	Not studied
Verdecchia (33)	C-V events	Not studied	Not studied	2.2	3.3
Krumholz (32)	C-V events	1.2	2.0	2.1	3.6
Krumholz (32)	All-cause mortality	0.7	1.6	1.4	2.7

Abbreviation: C-V=cardiovascular

differences among groups in blood pressure, other conventional risk factors and the level of LV mass itself.[32-33]

3. RELATION OF LEFT VENTRICULAR CHAMBER AND MYOCARDIAL FUNCTION TO PROGNOSIS IN HYPERTENSION

In most mildly to moderately hypertensive patients, LV systolic performance at rest is normal or mildly increased. Supernormal LV ejection fraction or fractional shortening in patients with mild hypertension and little or no LVH has been interpreted as reflecting enhanced myocardial contractility, whereas marked concentric LVH in severely hypertensive patients facilitates LV contraction by reducing wall stress. However, a conceptual mismatch exists in analyses relating chamber size or shortening at the endocardium to the mean level of end-systolic wall stress, which is applied approximately at the LV midwall.[34] When midwall shortening-end-systolic stress relations were analyzed in relatively unselected hypertensive patients, patients with concentric LV hypertrophy had decreased myocardial contractility and no significant hypercontractility was observed in patients without hypertrophy.[25]

To determine whether depressed LV midwall performance in hypertensive patients has prognostic implications, we analyzed baseline midwall LV fractional shortening/circumferential end-systolic stress relations in 294 hypertensive patients as predictors of cardiovascular events that occurred in 50 patients (including 14 deaths) during a 10-year mean follow-up.[35] Patients with initially lower midwall, but not endocardial, shortening, either in absolute terms or as a percentage of the value predicted for observed end-systolic stress, were significantly (p<0.004) more likely to suffer morbid events than those with initially normal values. The combination of relatively low midwall fractional shortening and relatively high LV mass increased the likelihood of all cardiovascular events 3.4-fold (95% confidence interval 1.8 to 6.3) and of cardiovascular death 5.3 (95% CI 1.6 to 17.3). Survival analysis controlling for age confirmed that low midwall shortening independently predicted cardiac morbidity or death, especially in the subgroup of patients with LV hypertrophy.[35]

4. POSSIBLE MECHANISMS OF THE RELATION BETWEEN LEFT VENTRICULAR ABNORMALITIES AND VASCULAR EVENTS

The most widely accepted mechanism for this association is the occurrence in LV hypertrophy of increased total myocardial oxygen demand due to the combination of increased pressure load and increased myocardial mass, a situation that would reduce the heart's ability to withstand either further increases in demand or decreases in flow without developing ischemia or suffering infarction. As discussed below, reduced coronary flow reserve secondary to increased basal demand and/or altered microvascular function has been documented in patients with hypertensive LV hypertrophy, whereas flow reserve may be reduced on a microvascular basis in some patients without hypertrophy. In addition to this now traditional concept, recent evidence documents parallisms between abnormalities in the heart and arterial tree that appear to be independent of age, gender, body size or blood pressure.

The availability of accurate non-invasive ultrasound imaging of large arteries and the heart has allowed *in vivo* comparison of human cardiac and vascular structure[36] and of the impact of altered vascular properties on ventricular adaptation.[37-38] Pulse wave velocity, an index of vascular stiffness, and brachial artery compliance have been related to the LV mass-volume ratio. In addition, the pulsatile component of blood pressure, evidenced either by higher pulse pressure or a greater augmentation index, appears to induce less favorable LV geometric adaptation — characterized by higher LV relative wall thickness — independent of mean arterial pressure.

Direct ultrasound measurement of LV and carotid artery anatomy in untreated, asymptomatic hypertensive patients studied in our laboratory demonstrated greater absolute (0.89 ± 0.21 vs 0.71 ± 0.15 mm, $p < 0.00005$) and relative (0.30 ± 0.07 vs 0.26 ± 0.06, $p < 0.005$) wall thicknesses than in matched controls.[37] The significant univariate relation between carotid and LV wall thicknesses ($r = 0.40$, $p < 0.005$) remained independent in multivariate analyses taking age and blood pressure into account, an observation that has been confirmed in a subsequent study in which age, ambulatory blood pressure and the level of Doppler stroke volume were considered as covariates.[39] Vascular hypertrophy was more common than LV hypertrophy (28 vs 14%) among the hypertensive patients in this series; however, in a larger population in which the potentially confounding effects of age and blood pressure could be taken into account, arterial and LV hypertrophy were equally common.[40] Significant increases have also been found in intimal-medial thickness of carotid and femoral[41] arteries in hypertensive patients.

More recent studies have documented strong parallelisms between LV geometric abnormalities and additional manifestations of arterial disease. In a series of 486 normotensive or generally mildly hypertensive subjects, we found that LV hypertrophy was positively related to the presence of systemic atherosclerosis detected by carotid ultrasound, independently of age, gender, blood pressure or other conventional risk factors.[42] In this study, the proportion of subjects with discrete carotid atherosclerotic plaques rose from less than 10% in the subjects with the lowest 20% of values of LV mass indexed for body size to more than 30% in the highest quintile of LV mass. A parallel association between LV mass and the presence and severity of coronary artery stenoses has previously been documented in selected groups of patients undergoing coronary arteriography.[43–44]

To explore further the relationship between LV and arterial status, we subsequently undertook an analysis of arterial structure and function in hypertensive patients grouped into the four previously-discussed LV geometric patterns based on echocardiographic findings.[28] We evaluated arterial structure and function by carotid ultrasonography and applanation tonometry in 271 unmedicated hypertensive patients classified by echocardiography as having normal ventricular geometry (n=176), concentric remodelling (n=54), concentric hypertrophy (n=16) or eccentric hypertrophy (n=25). All groups were similar in age, gender distribution and body size. Patients with concentric and eccentric hypertrophy had similar blood pressures (mean=173/100 and 171/99 mmHg, respectively) and LV mass. However, as may be seen in Table 3, only the patients with concentric hypertrophy had increased arterial wall thickness, end-diastolic diameter and cross-sectional area compared to those with normal LV geometry. Similarly (Table 4), compared to the patients with normal LV geometry, only those with concentric hypertrophy had reduced arterial strain and an elevated elastic modulus as evidence of stiffer arterial walls. Patients with concentric remodelling and eccentric hypertrophy had similar values for these arterial wall thickness, lumenal diameter, arterial cross-sectional area, arterial strain and elastic modulus despite lower systolic blood pressure in the former group (156/94 mmHg, $p < 0.001$). The prevalence of plaque was highest in subjects with concentric (56%) or eccentric (42%) hypertrophy and significantly greater than in those with normal geometry (21%). Thus, among patients with uncomplicated systemic hypertension, arterial structure and function are most abnormal when concentric left ventricular hypertrophy is present and may contribute to the more adverse

Table 3. Carotid artery structure in unmedicated hypertensive patients
grouped by left ventricular geometric pattern

Variable	Normal geometry (n=176)	Concentric remodelling (n=54)	Eccentric hypertrophy (n=25)	Concentric hypertrophy (n=16)
End-diastolic diameter (mm)	5.76±0.87	5.67±0.77	6.04±0.44	6.38±0.97*[†]
Intimal-medial thickness (mm)	0.80±0.18	0.85±0.22	0.89±0.21	0.96±0.20*
Relative wall thickness	0.28±0.06	0.30±0.08	0.30±0.07	0.31±0.11
Cross-sectional area (mm²)	16.64±5.41	17.20±5.44	19.65±5.88	22.10±5.71*[†]
Plaque (%)	21	31	44*	56*

*$p<0.05$ vs. Normal geometry
[†]$p<0.05$ vs. Concentric remodelling

outcome associated with this geometric pattern. Other investigators have identified parallel abnormalities of coronary blood flow patterns in hypertensive patients LV hypertrophy documented by echocardiography.[45–47] These abnormalities reduce the flow reserve of hypertrophied LV myocardium, increasing its vulnerability to ischemia and infarction under conditions of either reduced blood supply due to coronary thrombosis or to hypotension or of heightened demand due to tachycardia, hypertensive emergencies, etc. Intriguing and potentially important evidence of an ability of repeated intermittent coronary artery occlusions in experimental animals to induce segmental hypertrophy of the LV wall supplied by the affected artery[48] suggests that large-vessel coronary disease could actually promote LV hypertrophy, thus exaggerating myocardial oxygen demand at the same time as it reduces the potential blood supply.

5. DOES CHANGE IN LEFT VENTRICULAR MASS PREDICT SUBSEQUENT PROGNOSIS?

Before considering the available evidence, it is worthwhile to consider the characteristics of optimal studies of the relation between change in LV mass and subsequent prognosis. As recently reviewed,[49] sound studies of this question need to use methods of LVH assessment that have been validated by comparison with actual anatomic increases in LV mass. At present, available studies have relied on echocardiographic or ECG methods that have been validated by comparison with necropsy LV weight, but other methods such as magnetic resonance imaging or cine computed tomography could also be useful if they were

Table 4. Carotid artery function in unmedicated hypertensive patients
grouped by left ventricular geometric pattern

Variable	Normal geometry (n=176)	Concentric remodelling (n=54)	Eccentric hypertrophy (n=25)	Concentric hypertrophy (n=16)
Vascular strain (%)	12.4±3.7	12.0±4.7	10.8±3.8	9.5±2.2*
Elastic modulus (dynes/cm²×10⁻⁶)	471±241	558±263	614±257	713±265*
Young's modulus (dynes/cm²/mm×10⁻⁶)	601±296	699±373	683±262	777±219
Stiffness index (b)	5.79±3.44	6.75±3.23	6.80±3.55	6.38±1.40

*$p<0.05$ versus patients with normal LV geometry

Table 5. Left ventricular hypertrophy regression and prognosis: Available data

| | Proportion of patients suffering morbid events | | | |
| | LV mass increase | | LVH on 2nd study | |
	Yes	No	Yes	No
Koren (50)	20%	9%	29%	9%
Yurenev (52)	39%	12%	35%	9%
Levy* (23)	13.2%	6.7%	—	—
Muiesan** (55)	59%	9%	37%	7%

*Change in ECG measure of LVH; other studies used echocardiographic LV mass.
**No increase = at least 10% decrease in LV mass.

applied serially in large enough populations. For results to be generalizable, studies should at the least include both women and men; the applicability of findings is further enhanced if more than one ethnic group is represented. Valuable information can be gained both from observational studies — which may assess relatively representative samples of the population because entry criteria are not too rigid, but which often do not obtain complete information about antihypertensive or other treatments — and from treatment trials — which by definition take treatment into account, often with random assignment, but usually enroll highly selected subjects drawn from a much larger source population.

To date, four studies provide information that bear directly on the relation between LVH regression and subsequent morbidity and mortality. The initial study, presented in abstract form by Koren et al[50-51] involved follow-up of a group of clinical patients with essential hypertension who had not suffered complications at baseline or at the time of follow-up echocardiography a mean of more than five years later. Of the 166 patients 37% were women and more than 90% were white. This observational study followed the patients for an average of nearly 6 years after the interim echocardiogram. Echocardiographic LV mass was measured by an anatomically-validated method. Blood pressure and weight at the time of the interim echocardiogram as well as self-reported use of antihypertensive medications were taken into account. As may be seen in Table 5, individuals who failed to have LVH regression or in whom LVH developed during follow-up were much more likely to suffer morbid events than those in whom LVH regressed or never developed; a more conservative analysis comparing patients with even minimal increases in LV mass to those with even minimal decreases showed a greater likelihood of cardiovascular events in the former group.

A second relevant study, by Yurenev et al[52] was a therapeutic trial that enrolled a total of 304 men, most or all of whom were white, from Moscow, Berlin, Prague, Riga and Tbilisi, and followed them for four years. All patients had WHO Stage II hypertension based on clinical evaluation and all had LVH or high normal LV mass at baseline echocardiographic examination. Patients were randomized to non-blinded treatments with either of two treatment regimens, based on a diuretic *or* a beta-blocker to which one or more other drugs could be added as needed to control blood pressure. Baseline and annual follow-up echocardiograms were performed, with measurements performed in the individual centers. Echocardiographic LV mass was measured by the Teichholz formula, which has been shown to underestimate anatomic LV mass in necropsy validation studies.[53-54] Blood pressure, weight, lipids and assigned treatment arm were all known. Retrospective comparison of groups with (n=54) or without (n=250) complications was performed; the greatest difference between groups was the change in LV mass (mean = +0.3 vs −30.1g).

LVH regression or progression was strongly associated with the likelihood of morbid events (Table 5).

The third published study related to this question, by Levy et al,[23] assessed a total of 524 participants in the Framingham study, of whom 48% were women, with few if any minority group members included. Subjects were included if they had LVH recognized by one or more of multiple ECG criteria; Cornell voltage (RaVL+SV3) at baseline and its change over two-year inter-examination intervals were related to cardiovascular events over up to 18 2-year follow-up periods (mean = 5.1). The Cornell voltage combination (RaVL+SV3) was used as the measure of LVH on both baseline and follow-up studies. Age, blood pressure, serum cholesterol level, diabetes, smoking and baseline ECG voltage and repolarization were considered as confounders. Analyses compared groups that increased or decreased by a quartile of Cornell voltage — each about 25% of subjects — using logistic regression of pooled biennial data, a technique considered to approximate Cox proportional hazards models. As may be seen in Table 5, individuals with increases in Cornell voltage were approximately twice as likely to suffer morbid events during a single two-year follow-up period than those in whom Cornell voltage decreased.

The fourth relevant study, by Muiesan et al,[55] followed a total of 151 white patients, of whom 42% were women, who had initially uncomplicated hypertension. Patients were recalled after 7–13 years. Baseline and follow-up echocardiograms were read blindly, and echocardiograms that had been performed for clinical purposes at intervening intervals were also assessed. Patients were grouped by the presence or absence of LVH at baseline and follow-up; echocardiographic LV mass, measured at baseline and mostly before, but sometimes early after morbid events, was used as the measure of LVH. Other confounders were taken into consideration, such as age, gender, body mass index, diabetes, blood lipids and blood pressure at baseline and the end of the study. Analyses relied on Cox models in groups defined partially retrospectively as having persistently normal LV mass, having regression of LVH or having LVH that did not regress. Similar to the other studies, Cox survival analysis showed that presence of LVH at the end of the study was the factor most strongly related to morbid events; in addition, similarly low rates of morbid events were observed in the group of patients in whom baseline LVH had regressed and in the group who had normal LV mass on both baseline and end of study echocardiograms (Table 5).

The data considered above suggest but do not prove that LV hypertrophy regression in hypertensive patients predicts an improved prognosis independently of the type of treatment used. One source of additional data concerning this question are ongoing therapeutic trials in which the comparative effects of either different treatments or different goal blood pressures on both morbidity/mortality and LVH regression are being assessed. Definitive testing of the hypothesis that two antihypertensive agents differ with regard to their ability to regress hypertensive LVH requires a large-scale randomized trial involving at least 150–200 patients per treatment arm — including women and men, non-whites and whites — with a study duration of one year or more.[56] As reviewed in more detail elsewhere,[49] several such trials have begun in hypertensive patients or in patients with clinically evident atherosclerosis who might or might not have elevated arterial pressure. In addition, the Treatment of Mild Hypertension Study[57] performed serial echocardiograms over a four-year period on patients randomized to either placebo or one of five active treatments in addition to a nutritional-hygienic regimen. These studies have recruited or plan to enroll nearly 12,000 patients, and will have variable lengths of follow-up for morbid events following an initial in-study assessment of LVH by echocardiogram or ECG. When these studies are completed, the results will increase more than 10-fold the available information on the relation between serial change in quantitative measures of LVH and subsequent prognosis.

Because the populations enrolled in therapeutic trials are often highly selected, and frequently healthier than the source population from which they are drawn, it is also important that the relation between change in LV mass and subsequent prognosis also be assessed in observational studies of populations with varied characteristics. Several large studies of this type have had echocardiograms performed on two or more occasions, providing data on the change in LV mass that can be related to the subsequent risk of morbid events. These include the Framingham Heart Study (n > 3,000 with serial echocardiograms)[11–12] the Cardiovascular Health Study (n > 3,000)[58] and the CARDIA study (nearly 2,000).[59]

6. CONCLUSIONS

A large number of studies have established that baseline LVH consistently predicts adverse events in a wide variety of populations and disease states. A smaller number of studies, summarized in Table 3, indicate that the change in LV mass during treatment of hypertension or observation of populations predicts the likelihood of subsequent complications. However, this point cannot yet be considered conclusively proven because of limitations of available studies with regard to the knowledge and control of blood pressure, treatment type and other potentially important covariates, the relatively small size of most of the studies, under-representation of non-white patients and lack of concordant studies with several different types of antihypertensive agents. Future studies of the relation between LV mass change and prognosis will need analyses with full consideration of induced changes in blood pressure, treatment type and other relevant covariates that might confound results.

REFERENCES

1. Sokolow M, Perloff D: The prognosis of essential hypertension treated conservatively. *Circulation 23*:697 (1961)
2. Breslin DJ, Gifford RW Jr, Fairbairn JF II: Essential hypertension: a twenty-year follow-up study. *Circulation 33*:87 (1966)
3. Isles CG, Walker LV, Beevers DG et al: Mortality in the Glasgow blood pressure clinic. *J Hypertens 4*:141 (1987)
4. Kannel WB, Castelli WP, McNamara PM, McKee PA, Feinleib M: Role of blood pressure in the development of congestive heart failure: the Framingham study. *N Engl J Med 287*:781 (1972)
5. Kannel WB, Abbott RD: A prognostic comparison of asymptomatic left ventricular hypertrophy and unrecognized myocardial infarction: The Framingham Study. *Am Heart J 111*:391 (1986)
6. Sullivan JM, Vander Zwaag R, El-Zeky F, Ramanathan KB, Mirvis DM: Left ventricular hypertrophy: Effect on survival. *J Am Coll Cardiol 22*:508 (1993)
7. Casale PN, Devereux RB, Milner M, Zullo G, Harshfield GA, Pickering TG, Laragh JH: Value of echocardiographic measurement of left ventricular mass in predicting cardiovascular morbid events in hypertensive men. *Ann Intern Med 105*:173 (1986)
8. Nestrova AL, Novikov ID, Yurenev AP: Prognostic significance of blood pressure and left ventricular hypertrophy in systematic and non-systematic treatment of essential hypertension. *Kardiologia 8*:89 (1986)
9. Aronow WS, Epstein S, Koenigsberg M, Schwartz KS: Usefulness of echocardiographic left ventricular hypertrophy, ventricular tachycardia and complex ventricular arrhythmias in predicting ventricular fibrillation or sudden death in elderly patients. *Am J Cardiol 62*:1124 (1988)
10. Silberberg JS, Barre PE, Prichard SS, Sniderman AD: Impact of left ventricular hypertrophy on survival in end-stage renal disease. *Kidney Int 36*:286 (1989)
11. Levy D, Garrison RJ, Savage DD, Kannel WB, Castelli WP: Left ventricular mass and incidence of coronary heart disease in an elderly cohort: The Framingham Study. *Ann Intern Med 110*:101 (1989)
12. Levy D, Garrison RJ, Savage DD, Kannel WB, Castelli WP: Prognostic implications of echocardiographically determined left ventricular mass in the Framingham Heart Study. *N Engl J Med 322*:1561 (1990)

13. Koren MJ, Devereux RB, Casale PN, Savage DD, Laragh JH: Relation of left ventricular mass and geometry to morbidity and mortality in uncomplicated essential hypertension. *Ann Intern Med 114*:345 (1991)
14. Ghali JK, Liao Y, Simmons B, Castaner A, Cao G, Cooper RS: The prognostic role of left ventricular hypertrophy in patients with or without coronary artery disease. *Ann Intern Med 117*:831 (1992)
15. Mensah GA, Pappas TW, Koren MJ, Ulin RJ, Laragh JH, Devereux RB: Comparison of classification of hypertension severity by blood pressure level and World Health Organization criteria for prediction of concurrent cardiac abnormalities and subsequent complications in essential hypertension. *J Hypertens 11*:1433 (1993)
16. Bikkina M, Levy D, Evans JC et al: Left ventricular mass and the risk of stroke in an elderly cohort. The Framingham Heart Study. *JAMA 272*:33 (1994)
17. Bolognese L, Dellavese P, Rossi L, Sarasso G, Bongo AS, Scianaro MC: Prognostic value of left ventricular mass in uncomplicated acute myocardial infarction and one-vessel coronary artery disease. *Am J Cardiol 73*:1 (1994)
18. de Simone G, Devereux RB, Daniels SR, Koren MJ, Meyer RA, Laragh JH: Effect of growth on variability of left ventricular mass: assessment of allometric signals in adults and children and of their capacity to predict cardiovascular risk. *J Am Coll Cardiol 25*:1056 (1995)
19. Liao Y, Cooper RS, McGee DL, Mensah GA, Ghali JK: The relative effects of left ventricular hypertrophy, coronary artery disease, and ventricular dysfunction on survival among black adults. *JAMA 273*:1592 (1995)
20. Liao Y, Cooper RS, Durazo-Arvizu R, Mensah GA, Ghali JK: Prediction of mortality risk by different methods of indexing for left ventricular mass. *J Am Coll Cardiol 29*:(1 March 1997 issue).
21. MacMahon S, Collins G, Rautaharju P, Cutler J, Neaton J, Prineas R, Crow R, Stamler J for the Multiple Risk Factor Intervention Trial Research Group. Electrocardiographic left ventricular hypertrophy and effects of drug therapy in the Multiple Risk Factor Intervention Trial. *Am J Cardiol 63*:202 (1989)
22. Quinones MA, Weiner DH, Shelton BJ, Greenberg BH, Limacher MC, Kollpillai C, Shindler DM, Yusuf S for the SOLVD Investigators: Echocardiographic predictors of one-year clinical outcome in the Study of Left Ventricular Dysfunction (SOLVD) Trial and Registry: A study of 1,172 patients. (abstr) *Circulation 90* (Suppl I):I-304 (1993)
23. Levy D, Salomon M, D'Agostino RB, Belanger AJ, Kannel WB: Prognostic implications of baseline electrocardiographic features and their serial changes in subjects with left ventricular hypertrophy. *Circulation 90*:1786 (1994)
24. Parfrey PS, Harnett JD, Griffiths SM et al: The clinical course of left ventricular hypertrophy in dialysis patients. *Nephron 55*:114 (1990)
25. Ganau A, Devereux RB, Roman MJ et al: Patterns of left ventricular hypertrophy and geometric remodeling in essential hypertension. *J Am Coll Cardiol 19*:1550 (1992)
26. Devereux RB, James GD, Pickering TG: What is normal blood pressure? comparison of ambulatory pressure level and variability in patients with normal or abnormal left ventricular geometry. *Am J Hypertens 6*:211s (1993)
27. de Simone G, Devereux RB, Roman MJ, Alderman MH, Laragh JH: Relation of obesity and gender to left ventricular hypertrophy in normotensive and hypertensive adults. *Hypertension 23*:600 (1994)
28. Roman MJ, Pickering TG, Schwartz JE, Pini R, Devereux RB: Relation of arterial structure and function to left ventricular geometric patterns in hypertensive adults. *J Am Coll Cardiol 28*:751 (1996)
29. de Simone G, Devereux RB, Roman MJ, Ganau A, Saba PS, Alderman MH, Laragh JH: Assessment of left ventricular function by the mid-wall fractional shortening-end-systolic stress relation in human hypertension. *J Am Coll Cardiol 23*:1444 (1994)
30. Blake J, Devereux RB, Borer JS, Szulc M, Pappas TW, Laragh JH: Relation of obesity, high sodium intake and eccentric left ventricular hypertrophy to left ventricular exercise dysfunction in essential hypertension. *Am J Med 88*:477 (1990)
31. Verdecchia P, Schillaci G, Borgioni C, Ciucci A, Battistelli M, Bartoccini C, Santucci A, Santucci C, Reboldi G, Porcellati C: Adverse prognostic significance of concentric remodelling of the left ventricle in hypertensive patients with normal left ventricular mass. *J Am Coll Cardiol 25*:871 (1995)
32. Krumholz H M, Larson M, Levy D: Prognosis of left ventricular geometric patterns in the Framingham Heart Study. *J Am Coll Cardiol 25*:879 (1995)
33. Verdecchia P, Schillaci G, Borgioni C, Ciucci A, Gattobiggio R, Zampi I, Santucci A, Santucci C, Reboldi G, Porcellati C: Prognostic value of left ventricular mass and geometry in systemic hypertension with left ventricular hypertrophy. *Am J Cardiol 78*:197 (1996)
34. Shimuzu G, Hirota Y, Kita Y, Kawamura K, Saito T, Gaasch WH: Left ventricular midwall mechanics in systemic arterial hypertension. Myocardial function is depressed in pressure-overload hypertrophy. *Circulation 83*:1676 (1991)

35. de Simone G, Devereux RB, Koren MJ, Mensah GA, Casale PN, Laragh JH: Midwall left ventricular mechanics: an independent predictor of cardiovascular risk in arterial hypertension. *Circulation 93*:259 (1996)

36. Roman MJ, Saba PS, Pini R, Spitzer M, Pickering TG, Rosen S, Alderman MH, Devereux RB: Parallel cardiac and vascular adaptation in hypertension. *Circulation 86*:1909 (1992)

37. Saba PS, Roman MJ, Pini R, Ganau A, Devereux RB: Relation of arterial pressure waveforms to left ventricular and carotid anatomy in normotensive subjects. *J Am Coll Cardiol 22*:1873 (1993)

38. Asmar RG, Pannier B, Santoni JP et al: Reversion of cardiac hypertrophy and reduced arterial compliance after converting enzyme inhibition in essential hypertension. *Circulation 88*:941 (1988)

39. Jones EC, Devereux RB, O'Grady MJ, Schwartz JE, Liu JE, Pickering TG, Roman MJ: Relation of hemodynamic volume load to arterial and cardiac size. *J Am Coll Cardiol 29*:1303–1310 (1997).

40. Roman MJ, Pickering TG, Schwartz JE, Devereux RB: Prevalence and determinants of cardiac and vascular hypertrophy in hypertension. *Hypertension 26*:369 (1995)

41. Gariepy J, Massonneau M, Levenson J, Heudes D, Simon A: Evidence for in vivo carotid and femoral wall thickening in human hypertension. *Hypertension 22*:111 (1993)

42. Roman MJ, Pickering TG, Schwartz JE, Pini R, Devereux RB: The association of carotid atherosclerosis and left ventricular hypertrophy. *J Am Coll Cardiol 25*:83 (1995)

43. Pech HJ, Witte R, Romaniuk R, Parsi RA, Porstmann W: Left ventricular mass in coronary artery disease without hypertension. *Br Heart J 36*:362 (1974)

44. Gould KL, Lipsomb K, Hamilton GW, Kennedy JW: Relation of left ventricular shape, function and wall stress in man. *Am J Cardiol 34*:627 (1974)

45. Houghton JL, Frank MJ, Carr AA, von Dohlen TW, Prisant LM: Relations among impaired coronary flow reserve, left ventricular hypertrophy and thallium perfusion defects in hypertensive patients without obstructive coronary artery disease. *J Am Coll Cardiol 15*:43 (1990)

46. Polese A, DeCesare N, Montorsi P et al: Upward shift of the lower range of coronary flow autoregulation in hypertensive patients with hypertrophy of the left ventricle. *Circulation 83*:845 (1991)

47. Antony I, Nitenberg A, Foult J-M, Aptecar E: Coronary vasodilator reserve in untreated and treated hypertensive patients with and without left ventricular hypertrophy. *J Am Coll Cardiol 22*:514 (1993)

48. Fujita M, Mikuniya A, McKown DP, McKown MD, Franklin D: Regional myocardial volume alterations induced by brief repeated coronary occlusion in conscious dogs. *J Am Coll Cardiol 12*:1048 (1988)

49. Devereux RB, Agabiti-Rosei E, Dahlof B. Gosse P, Hahn RT, Okin PM, Roman MJ: Regression of left ventricular hypertrophy as a surrogate end-point for morbid events in hypertension treatment trials. *J Hypertens 14*(Suppl 2):s95 (1996)

50. Koren MJ, Ulin RJ, Laragh JH, Devereux RB: Reduction of left ventricular mass during treatment of essential hypertension is associated with improved prognosis. *Am J Hypertens 4*:1A (1991)

51. Koren MJ, Savage DD, Casale PN, Laragh JH, Devereux RB: Changes in left ventricular mass predict risk in essential hypertension. *Circulation 82*(Suppl III):III-29 (1990)

52. Yurenev AP, Dyakonova HG, Novikov ID, Vitols A, Pahl L, Haynemann G, Wallrabe D, et al: Management of essential hypertension in patients with different degrees of left ventricular hypertrophy. Multicenter trial. *Am J Hypertens 5*:182s (1992)

53. Devereux RB, Alonso DR, Lutas EM, et al: Echocardiographic assessment of left ventricular hypertrophy: comparison to necropsy findings. *Am J Cardiol 57*:450 (1986)

54. Yurenev AP, de Quattro V, Devereux RB: Hypertensive heart disease: Relationship of silent ischemia to coronary artery disease and left ventricular hypertrophy. *Am Heart J 120*:928 (1990)

55. Muiesan ML, Salvetti M, Rizzoni D, Castellano M, Donato F, Agabiti-Rosei E: Association of change in left ventricular mass with prognosis during long-term antihypertensive treatment. *J Hypertens 13*:1091 (1995)

56. Devereux RB, Dahlof B: Requirements for an informative trial of left ventricular hypertrophy regression. *J Hum Hypertens 8*:735 (1994)

57. Liebson PR, Grandits GA, Dianzumba S, Prineas RJ, Grimm RH Jr, Neaton JD et al: Comparison of five antihypertensive monotherapies and placebo for change in left ventricular mass in patients receiving nutritional-hygienic therapy in the Treatment of Mild Hypertension Study (TOMHS). *Circulation 91*:698 (1995)

58. Gardin JM, Siscovick D, Anton-Culver H, Lynch JC, Smith VE, Klopfenstein HS, et al: Sex, age and disease affect echocardiographic left ventricular mass and systolic function in the free-living elderly: the Cardiovascular Health Study. *Circulation 91*:1739 (1995)

59. Gardin JM, Wagenknecht LE, Anton-Culver H, Flack J, Gidding S, Kurosaki T, Wong ND, Manolio TA: Relationship of cardiovascular risk factors to left ventricular mass in healthy young black and white adult men and women. The CARDIA study. Coronary Artery Risk Development in Young Adults. *Circulation 92*:380 (1995)

LEFT VENTRICULAR HYPERTROPHY, ARTERIAL COMPLIANCE, AND AGING

Mary J. Roman,[1] Antonello Ganau,[2] Pier Sergio Saba,[2] and
Richard B. Devereux[1]

[1]Division of Cardiology
Cornell University Medical College
525 East 68th Street
New York, New York 10021
[2]Istituto di Clinica Medica
Universita di Sassari
Viale San Pietro 8
07100 Sassari, Italy

1. INTRODUCTION

An increase in arterial stiffness (or decrease in compliance) is a common feature of both the aging process[1,2] and of hypertension[3,4]. The increase in vascular stiffness associated with aging is due to structural changes within the capacitance arteries resulting in an increase in pulse wave velocity, an alteration in arterial pressure waveform and the age-associated increase in systolic blood pressure[1,5,6]. In hypertension, the increase in vascular stiffness may simply reflect the increase in distending pressure, particularly when arterial stiffness is estimated using pressure-dependent indices[3,7–9], but may also indicate an alteration in the physical properties of the vasculature due to structural changes attributable to hypertension *per se*[10]. Although both hypertension and the aging process are associated with characteristic changes in left ventricular structure[11,12], the extent to which vascular structural and functional alterations contribute, independently of blood pressure, to left ventricular remodelling is not well understood.

2. ARTERIAL COMPLIANCE

2.1. Measurement of Arterial Compliance

Arterial compliance is defined as the relation between changes in arterial pressure and volume or dimension. Because this relation is curvilinear, an increase in distending pressure will result in a reduction in arterial compliance (due to a change in the slope) unrelated to

Hypertension and the Heart, edited by Zanchetti et al.
Plenum Press, New York, 1997

13

intrinsic changes in the physical properties of the vessel (a shift in the curve). This phenomenon partially confounds the interpretation of studies wherein arterial compliance has
been measured using methods which are not independent of distending pressure. One of the
earliest and most common methods of estimating arterial compliance involves measurement
of the pulse wave velocity, or the time delay between the feet of two simultaneously-re-
corded pressure or flow waves[1,2]. Newer methods, utilizing advances in non-invasive technology, provide pressure-independent, or isobaric, measurement of arterial compliance[8,9].

2.2. Relation of Arterial Compliance to Aging in Normal Subjects

Systematic measurement of arterial compliance using pulse wave velocity in a large
number of normotensive subjects over a wide age range was reported by Hallock in 1934[1].
He found a strong linear relation between pulse wave velocity and age in both men and
women with a greater velocity in men than in women following adolescence. In an
attempt to determine the extent to which the decrease in pulse wave velocity was related
to degenerative changes within the vessel wall as opposed to atherosclerosis, Avolio et al.
measured pulse wave velocity in 480 Chinese subjects (16% hypertensive) with a low
prevalence of atherosclerosis[2]. Pulse wave velocity rose with age (figure 1) and appeared
to be higher than that reported in Occidental populations wherein the prevalence of
atherosclerosis is higher, suggesting that age-related vascular changes rather than atherosclerosis were the predominant cause of the reduction in arterial compliance.

Although these authors also detected a significant relation of pulse wave velocity to
mean arterial pressure (r=0.55, p<0.001), emphasizing the pressure-dependence of this
measure of arterial compliance, the relation between pulse wave velocity and age did not
appear to differ when the population was stratified according to mean blood pressure, suggesting that the rises in blood pressure and pulse wave velocity were occuring independently. In support of this observation, arterial stiffness has been shown to be related to
aging[8,13] (figure 2) using a method which takes distending pressure into account[14,15].

2.3. Arterial Compliance in Hypertensive Patients

By definition, distending pressure is increased in hypertension, resulting in a decrease
in arterial compliance or an increase in arterial stiffness when pressure-dependent methods
are used. The pressure-dimension relation can be refined by adjusting for vessel diameter
with Peterson's elastic modulus or by adjusting for vessel diameter and wall thickness using
Young's modulus[8]. Figure 3 examines age-adjusted mean values of various estimates of
common carotid artery function in normotensive subjects and hypertensive patients. Vascular strain, or pulsatility, is significantly reduced in hypertensive patients. Both Peterson's
and Young's moduli are increased in hypertensive patients, the latter to a lesser extent
because of the greater increase in wall thickness in hypertensive patients[10]. In contrast, the
arterial stiffness index or beta, does not significantly differ between the two groups, indicating that although arterial compliance is reduced at the operating level of blood pressure, differences are significantly lessened when distending pressure is considered[8]. Similar results
have been obtained by other investigators measuring isobaric compliance of the radial
artery in normotensive and hypertensive subjects[9,16].

2.4. Relation of Arterial Compliance to Aging in Hypertension

The aging process is likewise associated with a reduction in arterial compliance in
hypertensive patients (figure 4). Using the pressure-independent measure of arterial stiff-

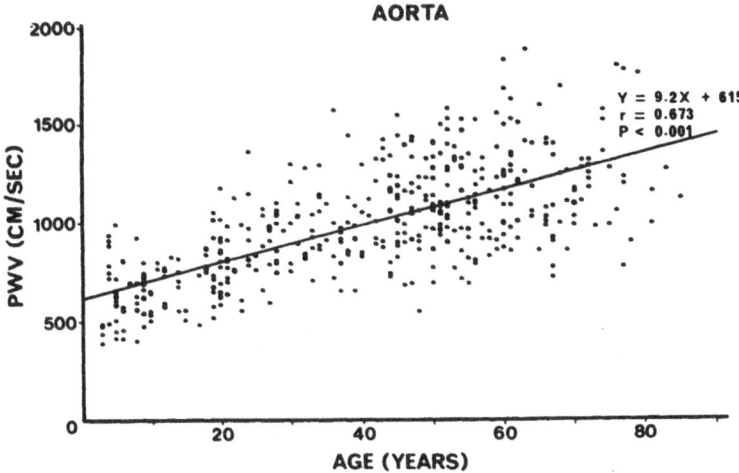

Figure 1. The relation of aortic pulse wave velocity to age in 480 normal Chinese subjects. Reproduced with permission from reference 1.

ness (beta) in 144 hypertensive patients, common carotid artery stiffness was directly related to age (r=0.41, p<0.0001) and arterial diameter (r=0.25, p<0.005) and inversely to height (r=−0.19, p<0.05), with age and arterial diameter as the most important independent determinants of arterial stiffness[17].

3. ALTERATIONS IN LEFT VENTRICULAR STRUCTURE ASSOCIATED WITH HYPERTENSION, AGING, AND THEIR COMBINATION

3.1. Impact of Hypertension on Left Ventricular Structure

The chronic pressure overload of essential hypertension does not invariably result in concentric left ventricular hypertrophy. A substantial proportion of otherwise healthy

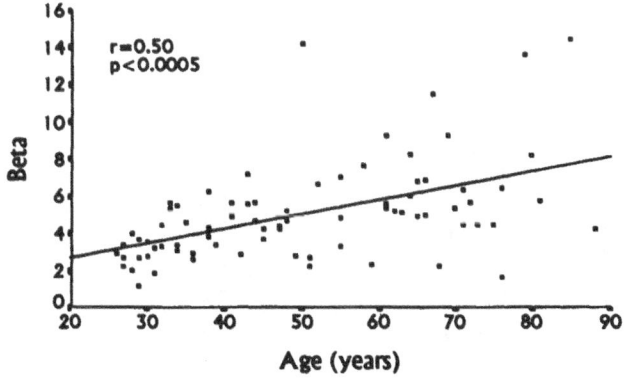

Figure 2. Relation of arterial stiffness (beta) to aging in normotensive subjects.

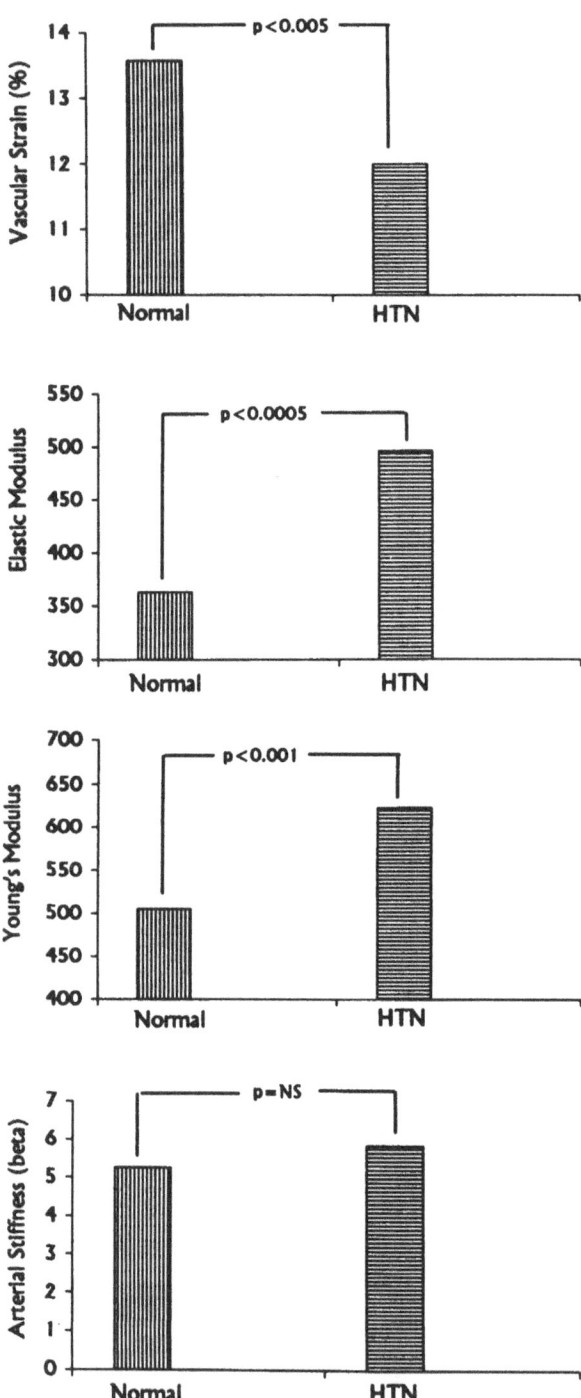

Figure 3. Comparison of measures of arterial function in normotensive and hypertensive individuals. Abbreviation: HTN=hypertension.

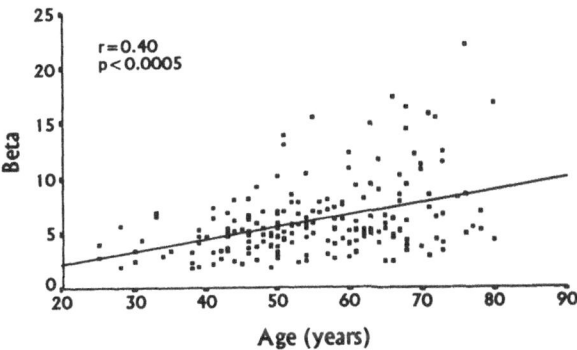

Figure 4. Relation of arterial stiffness (beta) to aging in hypertensive patients.

hypertensive individuals have normal left ventricular mass and, among those with an increase in left ventricular mass, eccentric hypertrophy may be more common than concentric hypertrophy. Among 165 hypertensive patients, Ganau et al. found eccentric hypertrophy in 27% of patients whereas concentric hypertrophy was present in only 8%[11]. Furthermore, relative wall thickness (the ratio of wall thickness to chamber diameter) may be increased even in the absence of left ventricular hypertrophy, a geometric pattern termed concentric remodelling[11,18]. These different left ventricular geometric patterns do not appear to reflect a continuum but rather correspond to different profiles of hemodynamic parameters, including cardiac output and peripheral resistance[11], underscoring the contribution of factors other than blood pressure to changes in left ventricular structure[19].

3.2. Impact of Aging on Left Ventricular Structure

In the absence of clinically apparent disease, including hypertension, aging results in little, if any, increase in overall left ventricular mass (figure 5), despite the significant increase in systolic pressure (albeit within the normal range) and pulse pressure[12]. However aging does alter left ventricular geometry. There is a direct association between age and both absolute and relative left ventricular wall thicknesses and an inverse association with end-diastolic diameter. Thus, aging results in concentric remodelling of the left ventricle[12].

3.3 Age-Related Changes in Left Ventricular Structure in Hypertension

The superimposition of the aging process on hypertension does not appear to result in further increases in left ventricular mass in the absence of concurrent disease[20,21]. However, as in the case of normotension but to a lesser extent, aging is associated among hypertensive patients with a slight but significant increase in absolute and relative wall thicknesses and a tendency for chamber diameter to decrease[22] (figure 6). Thus, although normotensive and hypertensive individuals differ on average in overall left ventricular mass and relative wall thickness, the aging process appears to affect both groups similarly, i.e., causing an increase in relative wall thickness consistent with the process of concentric remodelling. Interestingly, the most common left ventricular geometric pattern in elderly patients with isolated systolic hypertension has recently been reported to be concentric remodelling[23]. The unifying feature in this process appears to be the age-associated increase in vascular stiffness.

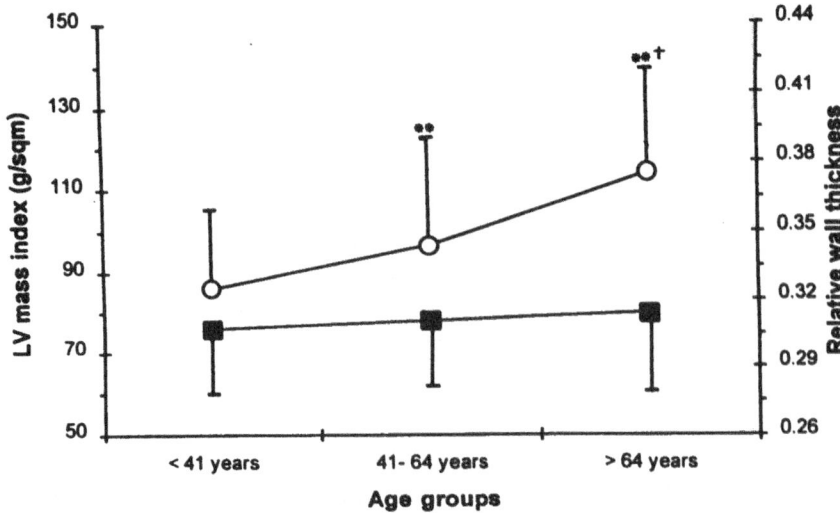

Figure 5. Impact of age on left ventricular mass and relative wall thickness in 430 normal subjects. Reproduced with permission from reference 12.

4. ARTERIAL COMPLIANCE AND LEFT VENTRICULAR STRUCTURE

4.1. Relation of Arterial Compliance to Left Ventricular Structure

The most important determinant of vascular stiffness in both normotensive and hypertensive individuals is the aging process[17]. Since, as indicated above, the aging process *per se* does not result in significant increases in left ventricular mass in normotensive or hypertensive adults, it is not surprising that measures of vascular stiffness likewise do not correlate with left ventricular mass, independently of age and the mean level of arterial pressure[24]. However, like the aging process, vascular stiffness is related to left ventricular geometry (Table 1). Among normotensive individuals, vascular stiffness is directly related to relative wall thickness and inversely to chamber diameter. Similar relationships exist in hypertensive individuals although the strengths of association are less strong[22].

4.2. Arterial Compliance and the Pressure Waveform

The mechanism whereby vascular stiffness alters left ventricular geometry may relate more to its impact on the arterial pressure waveform than on actual level of blood pressure[13]. Vascular stiffening results in an increase in pulse wave velocity and an earlier return of the major reflected wave to the central aorta, thereby resulting in late-systolic rather than early diastolic augmentation of arterial pressure[25,26]. Thus, the potential for a more sustained increase throughout systole in ventricular afterload appears to be a stimulus for an increase in left ventricular wall thicknesses, independent of the actual peak systolic blood pressure. The augmentation of late-systolic pressure as a proportion of the pulse pressure may be quantified as the augmentation index[5] (figure 7). A compliant vessel, as found in a young and normotensive individual, will result in a slow pulse wave velocity with augmentation occuring during diastole (negative augmentation index). In

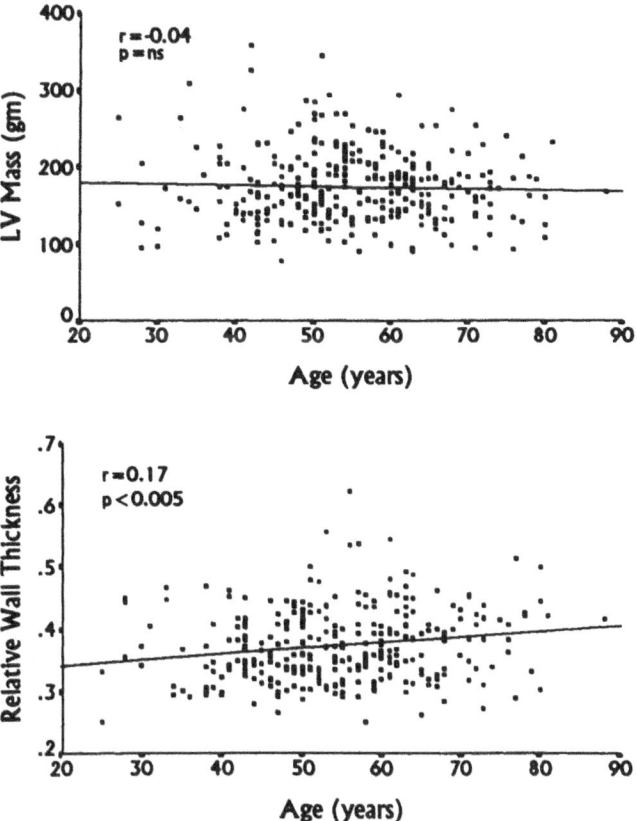

Figure 6. Relation of aging to left ventricular mass (top panel) and relative wall thickness (bottom panel) in 334 healthy hypertensive patients.

contrast, a stiff vessel, as encountered in an older or hypertensive individual, will result in a more rapid pulse wave velocity with a shift of the major reflected wave from diastole into systole resulting in late-systolic augmentation of the waveform (postitive augmentation index). Similar to other measures of vascular stiffness, the augmentation index has been shown to increase with aging[6,13].

Table 1. Relation of arterial stiffness (beta) to left ventricular structure in normotensive and hypertensive subjects

Variable	r	p value
LV mass	−0.02	ns
LV mass index	0.06	ns
Posterior wall	0.11	ns (0.06)
Diastolic diameter	−0.16	0.01
Relative wall thickness	0.21	0.001

Abbreviation: LV=left ventricular

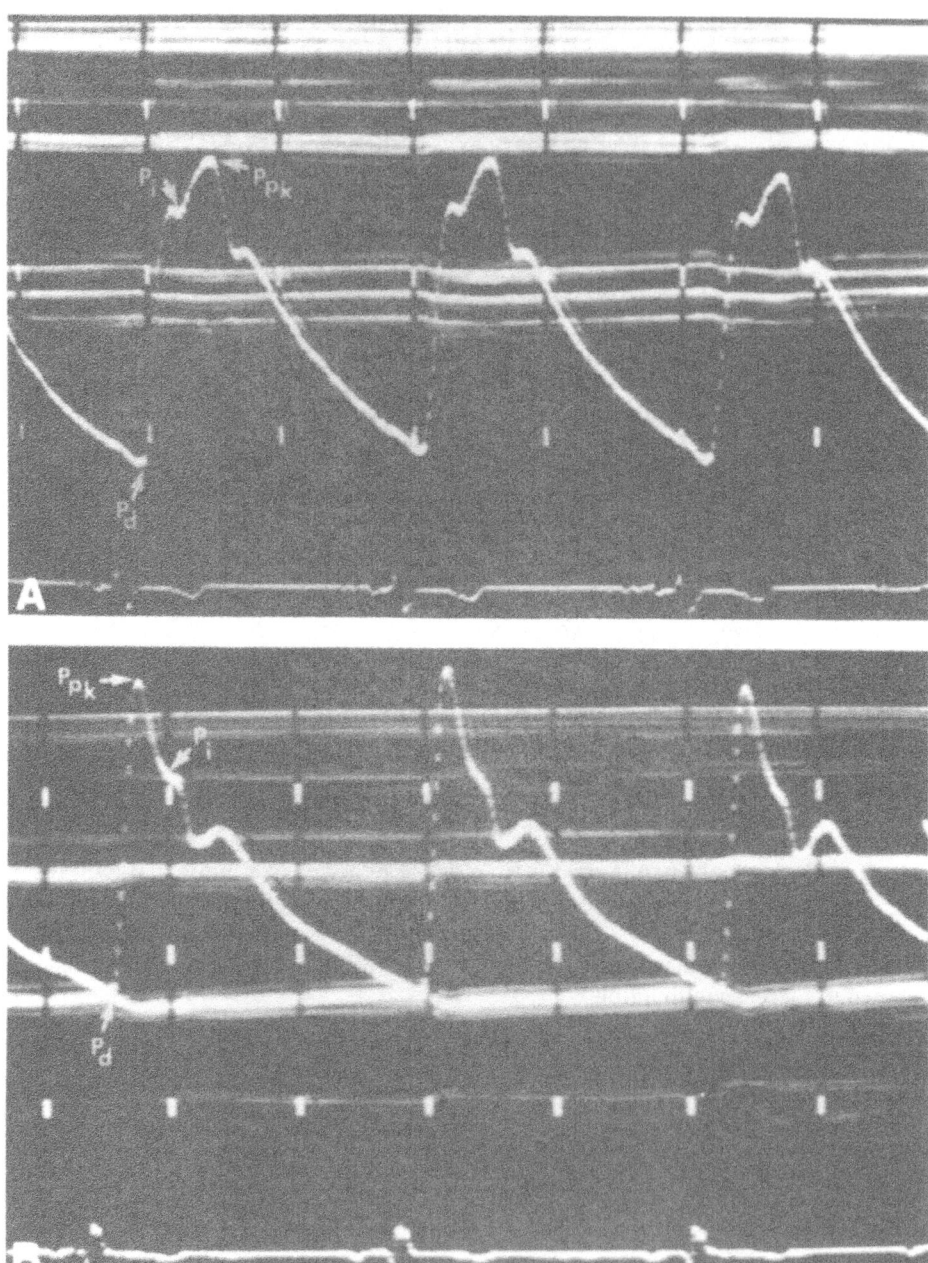

Figure 7. Simultaneous recording of M-mode tracing of the distal common carotid artery with superimposed pressure waveform of the contralateral carotid artery demonstrating late-systolic augmentation (panel A) in a 51 year-old man and diastolic augmentation (panel B) in a 27 year-old man with similar peak systolic blood pressures (118 and 120 mmHg, respectively). Reproduced with permission from reference 13.

4.3. Arterial Pressure Waveform and Left Ventricular Structure

The relation of the arterial pressure waveform to chronic changes in vascular and left ventricular structure and function has only recently been evaluable. Saba et al. studied 67 normotensive individuals and found late-systolic pressure wave augmentation in the common carotid artery to be associated with older age, higher systolic blood pressure and significant increases in left ventricular mass index and relative wall thickness due to an increase in ventricular wall thicknesses. Late-systolic augmentation was also associated with an increase in carotid artery absolute and relative wall thicknesses and in vascular stiffness[13]. The changes in left ventricular wall thicknesses and mass were independent of age and mean arterial blood pressure whereas those in carotid artery structure and function were not, suggesting that the vascular changes might be related to the aging process, anteceding and possibly influencing alterations in left ventricular structure. These findings have recently been confirmed in an experimental preparation involving surgical induction of either proximal or distal aortic coarctation in Wistar rats[27]. Distal coarctation, proximal to the renal arteries, resulted in late-systolic loading of the left ventricle whereas banding of the aortic arch resulted in early-systolic loading. Although peak systolic pressure was similarly increased in both groups in comparison to control rats, the group with distal coarctation and late-systolic loading experienced significantly greater increases in the ratio of left ventricular weight to body weight. Wall volume was greater in the group with distal banding and the ratio of chamber volume to wall volume was significantly lower consistent with an increase in relative wall thickness as has been observed in the aging human ventricle. Interestingly, there were no differences between the two groups in the extent to which angiotensin II levels were increased.

5. CONCLUSION

In summary, chronic changes in left ventricular anatomy in the setting of essential hypertension are variable and relate to a variety of hemodynamic (and non-hemodynamic) factors. Vascular stiffening, unrelated to distending pressure, primarily results from structural changes in the capacitance vessels associated with the aging process and appears to predominantly influence left ventricular geometry as opposed to overall left ventricular mass, both in the presence and absence of hypertension, resulting in concentric remodelling.

REFERENCES

1. Hallock P. Arterial elasticity in man in relation to age as evaluated by the pulse wave velocity method. *Arch Int Med* 54:770 (1934)
2. Avolio AP, Chen S, Wang R, Zhang C, Li M, O'Rourke MF. Effects of aging on changing arterial compliance and left ventricular load in a northern Chinese urban community. *Circulation* 68:50 (1983)
3. Nichols WW, O'Rourke MF, Avolio AP, Yaginuma T, Pepine CJ, Conti CR. Ventricular/vascular interaction in patients with mild systemic hypertension and normal peripheral resistance. *Circulation* 74:455 (1986)
4. Ting CT, Brin KP, Lin SJ, Wang SP, Chang MS, Chiang BN, Yin FCP. Arterial hemodynamics in human hypertension. *J Clin Invest* 78:1462 (1986)
5. Murgo JP, Westerhof N, Giolma JP, Altobelli SA. Aortic input impedance in normal man: relationship to pressure wave forms. *Circulation* 62:105 (1980)
6. Kelly R, Hayward C, Avolio A, O'Rourke M. Noninvasive determination of age-related changes in the human arterial pulse. *Circulation* 80:1652 (1989)
7. Gribbin B, Pickering TG, Sleight P. Arterial distensibility in normal and hypertensive man. *Clin Sci* 56:413 (1979)

8. Roman MJ, Pini R, Pickering TG, Devereux RB: Non-invasive measurements of arterial compliance in hypertensive compared with normotensive adults. *J Hypertens* 10 (Suppl 6):S115 (1992)

9. Hayoz D, Rutschmann B, Perret F, Niederberger M, Trady Y, Mooser V, Nussberger J, Waeber B, Brunner HR. Conduit artery compliance and distensibility are not necessarily reduced in hypertension *Hypertension* 20:1 (1992)

10. Roman MJ, Saba PS, Pini R, Spitzer M, Pickering TG, Rosen S, Alderman MH, Devereux RB. Parallel cardiac and vascular adaptation in hypertension. *Circulation* 86:1909 (1992)

11. Ganau A, Devereux RB, Roman MJ, de Simone G, Pickering TG, Saba PS, Vargiu P, Simongini I, Laragh JH. Patterns of left ventricular hypertrophy and geometric remodelling in essential hypertension. *J Am Coll Cardiol* 19:1550 (1992)

12. Ganau A, Saba PS, Roman MJ, de Simone G, Realdi G, Devereux RB. Ageing induces left ventricular concentric remodelling in normotensive subjects. *J Hypertens* 13:1818 (1995)

13. Saba PS, Roman MJ, Pini R, Ganau A, Devereux RB. Relation of carotid pressure waveform to left ventricular anatomy in normotensive subjects. *J Am Coll Cardiol* 22:1873 (1993)

14. Hayashi K, Handa H, Nagasawa S, Okumura A, Moritaki K. Stiffness and elastic behavior of human intracranial and extracranial arteries. *J Biomechanics* 13:175 (1980)

15. Hirai T, Sasayma S, Kawasaki T, Yagi S. Stiffness of systemic arteries in patients with myocardial infarction. A noninvasive method to predict severity of coronary atherosclerosis. *Circulation* 80:78 (1989)

16. Laurent S, Hayoz D, Trazzi S, Boutouyrie P, Waeber B, Omboni S, Brunner HR, Mancia G, Safar M. Isobaric compliance of the radial artery is increased in patients with essential hypertension *J Hypertens* 11:89 (1993)

17. Roman MJ, Pini R, Pickering TG, Devereux RB. Determinants of arterial stiffness in normotensive and hypertensive individuals. *Circulation* 90:I-506 (1994)

18. Verdecchia P, Schillaci G, Borgioni C, Ciucci A, Battistelli M, Bartoccini C, Santucci A, Santucci C, Reboldi G, Porcellati C. Adverse prognostic significance of concentric remodeling of the left ventricle in hypertensive subjects with normal left ventricular mass. *J Am Coll Cardiol* 25:871 (1995)

19. Ganau A, Devereux RB, Pickering TG, Roman MJ, Schnall PL, Santucci S, Spitzer MC, Laragh JH. Relation of left ventricular hemodynamic load and contractile performance to left ventriuclar mass in hypertension. *Circulation* 81:25 (1990)

20. Roman MJ, Pickering TG, Pini R, Schwartz JE, Devereux RB. Prevalence and determinants of cardiac and vascular hypertrophy in hypertension. *Hypertension* 26:369 (1995)

21. Hammond IW, Devereux RB, Alderman MH, Laragh JH. Relation of blood pressure and body build to left ventricular mass in normotensive and hypertensive employed adults. *J Am Coll Cardiol* 12:996 (1988)

22. Roman MJ, Pickering TG, Schwartz JE, Pini R, Devereux RB. Differential impact of aging and hypertension on cardiac and vascular structure. *Circulation* 92:I-746 (1995)

23. Heesen WF, Beltman FW, May JF, Smit AJ, de Graeff PA, Havinga TK, Schuurman FH, van der Veur E, Hamer JPM, Meyboom de-Jong B, Lie KI. High prevalence of concentric remodeling in elderly individuals with isolated systolic hypertension from a population survey. *Hypertension* 29:539 (1997)

24. Roman MJ, Pickering TG, Schwartz JE, Pini R, Devereux RB. Relation of arterial structure and function to left ventricular geometric patterns in hypertensive adults. *J Am Coll Cardiol* 28:751 (1996)

25. Westerhof N, Sipkema P, van den Bos GC, Elzinga G. Forward and backward waves in the arterial system. *Cardiovasc Res* 6:648 (1972)

26. O'Rourke MF, Yaginuma T. Wave reflection and the arterial pulse. *Arch Intern Med* 144:366 (1984)

27. Kobayashi S, Yano M, Kohno M, Obayashi M, Hisamatsu Y, Ryoke T, Ohkusa T, Yamakawa K, Matsuzaki M. Influence of aortic impedance on the development of pressure-overload left ventricular hypertrophy in rats. *Circulation* 94:3362 (1996)

3

LEFT VENTRICULAR HYPERTROPHY AND ARTERIAL BLOOD PRESSURE IN EXPERIMENTAL MODELS OF HYPERTENSION

A. F. Dominiczak,[*] A. M. Devlin, M. J. Brosnan, N. H. Anderson, D. Graham, J. S. Clark, A. McPhaden, C. A. Hamilton, and J. L. Reid

Department of Medicine and Therapeutics, Gardiner Institute
Western Infirmary, Glasgow G11 6NT

1. INTRODUCTION

Hypertensive left ventricular hypertrophy (LVH) is a major independent risk factor for cardiovascular morbidity and mortality in human essential hypertension. It has been shown that LVH is a better predictor of coronary artery disease and stroke than high blood pressure itself, hyperlipidaemia and cigarette smoking[1,2]. The spontaneously hypertensive rat (SHR) and its close relative stroke-prone SHR (SHRSP) have been used as models of hypertensive LVH and have allowed us to develop a number of mechanistic and genetic studies which would not have been feasible in human essential hypertension.

This brief review aims to describe some chosen strategies in this area of research, which have resulted in a new or better understanding of the widely disputed issue of inter-relationship between blood pressure and LVH.

2. STUDIES ON REGRESSION AND PREVENTION OF CARDIAC AND VASCULAR HYPERTROPHY

Several groups including ourselves studied reversal of cardiac and vascular hypertrophy in the SHR or SHRSP using various pharmacological interventions[3-6]. Our early studies compared treatment with perindopril (2mg/kg/day), losartan (10mg/kg/day) and a combination of hydralazine and hydrochlorothiazide (4mg/day of each) administered to mature (16–20 weeks old) SHRSP rats for 30 days in their drinking water. The three treatment regimens resulted in a comparable blood pressure control[3,4]. However, a complete regression of cardiac hypertrophy as measured by heart weight to body weight or left

---

[*] Correspondence: Dr. A.F. Dominiczak, Department of Medicine and Therapeutics, Western Infirmary, Glasgow G11 6NT, Tel.: +44 141 211 2688, Fax.: +44 141 211 1763

Hypertension and the Heart, edited by Zanchetti et al.
Plenum Press, New York, 1997

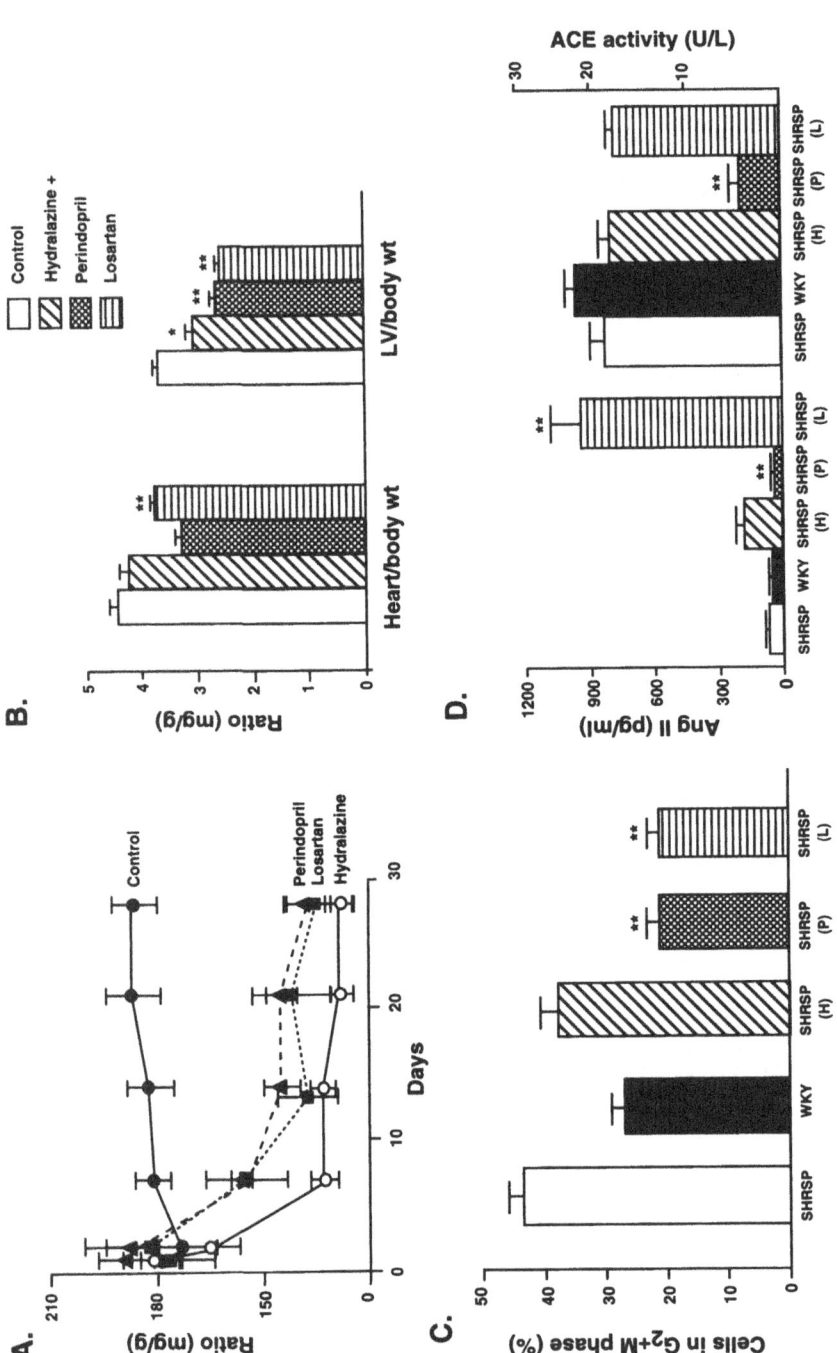

Figure 1. **A.** Effects of treatment of the SHRSP with hydralazine/hydrochlorothiazide (n=16), perindopril (n=12) and losartan (n=5) on systolic blood pressure measured with tail cuff plethysmography. **B.** Heart weight to body weight and left ventricle to body weight ratios in the SHRSP (n=17), SHRSP (H) treated with hydralazine/hydrochlorothiazide (n=16), SHRSP (P) treated with perindopril (n=12) and SHRSP (L) treated with losartan (n=5). **C.** Percentage of cells in G_2+M phase of the cell cycle in the SHRSP controls and SHRSP treated with three types of pharmacological interventions. Symbols and n values as in B. **D.** Concentrations of circulating plasma angiotensin II in four groups of rats; symbols and n values as in B. All data are means ± s.e.m.; ** $P<0.01$. Modified from reference 3 with permission from Stockton Press.

ventricle weight to body weight ratio was present only in perindopril and losartan treated groups (Fig. 1)[3,4]. In line with these findings, vascular smooth muscle polyploidy which is used as an index of aortic hypertrophy, showed a highly significant regression in perindopril treated and losartan treated SHRSP whereas the group treated with a combination of hydralazine/hydrochloro thiazide did not differ from untreated SHRSP rats (Fig. 1)[3,4]. These experiments may be interpreted as suggesting a direct role for angiotensin II in cardiac and vascular hypertrophy. This is supported by the high concentrations of circulating and perhaps also tissue angiotensin II in hydralazine/hydrochlorothiazide group.

The analysis of the processes involved in cardiac and vascular smooth muscle growth at the cellular level implies that angiotensin II is a growth factor which acts via induction of c-fos and other proto-oncogenes[7,8]. It has been suggested that under some conditions, angiotensin II may act as a an incomplete growth factor whereby the cell receives signals for the increased cell mass and DNA replication associated with cell cycle progression but not for cell division[7]. DNA endoreduplication and resulting polyploidy often accompany cellular hypertrophy, occurring in terminally differentiated cardiac myocytes[9] as well as in nonterminally differentiated hepatocytes[10] and smooth muscle cells[3,11]. Moreover, a study by Black et al[12] confirms that angiotensin II might stimulate cardiac and vascular hypertrophy directly in the SHR, independent of its effect on blood pressure.

Further studies performed in our laboratory were designed to test the hypothesis that ACE inhibitor or AT_1 receptor antagonist treatment of young SHRSP rats, before hypertension is fully developed, would prevent vascular and cardiac hypertrophy. We also wished to test the contribution of NO to the effects of ACE inhibitor and AT_1 receptor antagonists. Treatment consisted of perindopril (2mg/kg/day) or losartan (20mg/kg/day) either alone or in combination with L-NAME (20mg/kg/day) given for 7 weeks, starting at 8 weeks of age. The measurements of heart weight and left ventricular weight were again expressed as ratios to body weight (Fig 2)[13]. Similarly to regression experiments, we were able to demonstrate prevention of both cardiac and vascular hypertrophy in the SHRSP treated with either perindopril or losartan. The most puzzling observation in this series of experiments was that heart weight to body weight and left ventricle weight to body weight ratios were the lowest in perindopril + L-NAME treated group despite blood pressure being higher than in the group treated with perindopril alone[13]. These data are in agreement with previous studies which showed that a nonspecific NO synthase inhibitor, such as L-NAME, when given alone causes lesser cardiac hypertrophy than would be expected from blood pressure elevation[14,15]. It has been suggested that L-NAME may compete with ribosomal enzymes involved in the incorporation of L-arginine into protein[15]. This effect combined with reduced coronary blood flow may contribute to reduced protein synthesis in cardiomyocytes[13].

The analysis of vascular polyploidy in the same experiment contrasts with cardiac hypertrophy data (Fig 2). All four treatment regimens resulted in significant prevention of vascular hypertrophy with the magnitude of difference comparable to those differences observed in previous regression studies[3-5,16]. These results suggest the existence of different regulatory mechanisms for cardiac and vascular hypertrophy.

3. STUDIES ON INDUCTION OF CARDIAC AND VASCULAR HYPERTROPHY BY CHRONIC INHIBITION OF NITRIC OXIDE SYNTHASE

The studies described above suggested that the basal nitric oxide (NO) production *in vivo* may play an important counter-regulatory role to the pressor and trophic actions of

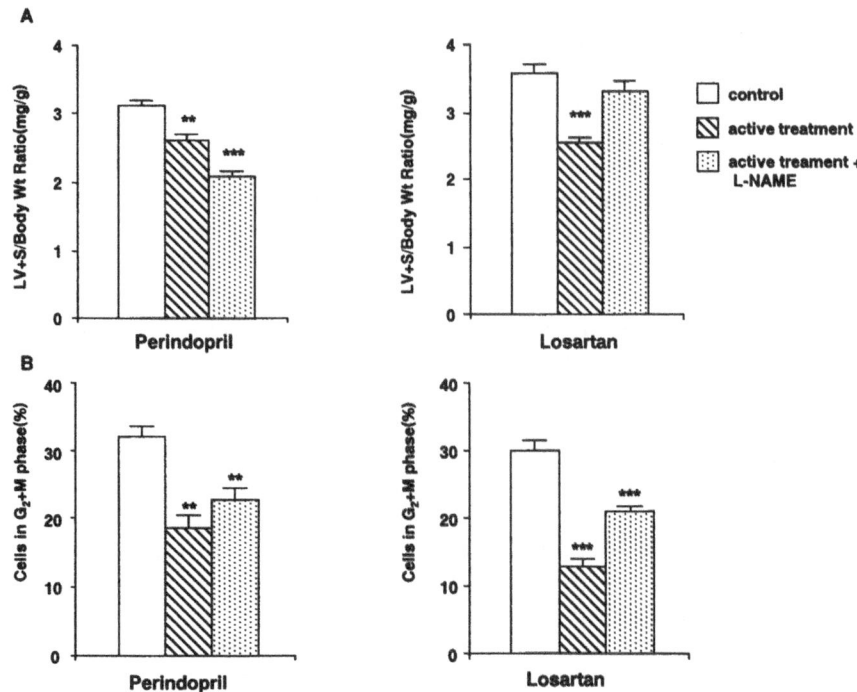

Figure 2. **A. Left panel** — ratios of left ventricle weight to body weight in SHRSP (n=6), SHRSP treated with perindopril (n=6) and SHRSP treated with a combination of perindopril and L-NAME (n=6). **Right panel** — ratios of left ventricle weight to body weight in SHRSP (n=6), SHRSP treated with losartan (n=8) and SHRSP treated with a combination of losartan and L-NAME (n=6). Statistical analysis by a one-way ANOVA with Tukey's pairwise comparisons. Values are means ± s.e.m. **P=0.02 and ***P<<0.001. **B. Left panel** — percentage of cells in the G_2+M phase of the cell cycle in SHRSP (n=6), SHRSP treated with perindopril (n=6) and SHRSP treated with a combination of perindopril and L-NAME (n=6). **Right panel** — percentage of cells in G_2+M phase of the cell cycle in SHRSP (n=6), SHRSP treated with losartan (n=8) and SHRSP treated with a combination of losartan and L-NAME (n=6). Statistical analysis and symbols as in A. Modified from reference 13 with permission from the American Heart Association.

angiotensin II. One of the interesting strategies to study these relationships is the chronic administration of L-arginine analogues such as N^G-nitro-L-arginine methyl ester (L-NAME) *in vivo*. These studies showed divergent effects on blood pressure and cardiac and vascular hypertrophy. For example, Arnal et al[14] found that L-NAME treatment in the WKY (50mg/kg/day) for 8 weeks, caused hypertension but no cardiac hypertrophy. In a recent study carried out in the SHR, treatment with L-NAME for 4 weeks, resulted in malignant hypertension and vascular hypertrophy but there was no evidence of cardiac hypertrophy[17]. We have therefore designed a series of experiments to study in detail vascular and cardiac hypertrophy in L-NAME induced hypertension using cellular and molecular biology techniques. It is of interest that L-NAME treatment in either young or mature SHRSP results in death within 24–48 hours (unpublished observations). However, inbred WKY rats tolerate this treatment well. We administered L-NAME (10mg/kg/day) for 3 weeks in the animals' drinking water, starting at 8 weeks of age[18]. This treatment resulted in a significant increase of systolic blood pressure (Fig 3; ANOVA F=62.1, P<<0.0001). The heart weight to body weight and left ventricle weight to body weight ratios were significantly higher in the L-NAME treated group than in the control group (Fig 3).

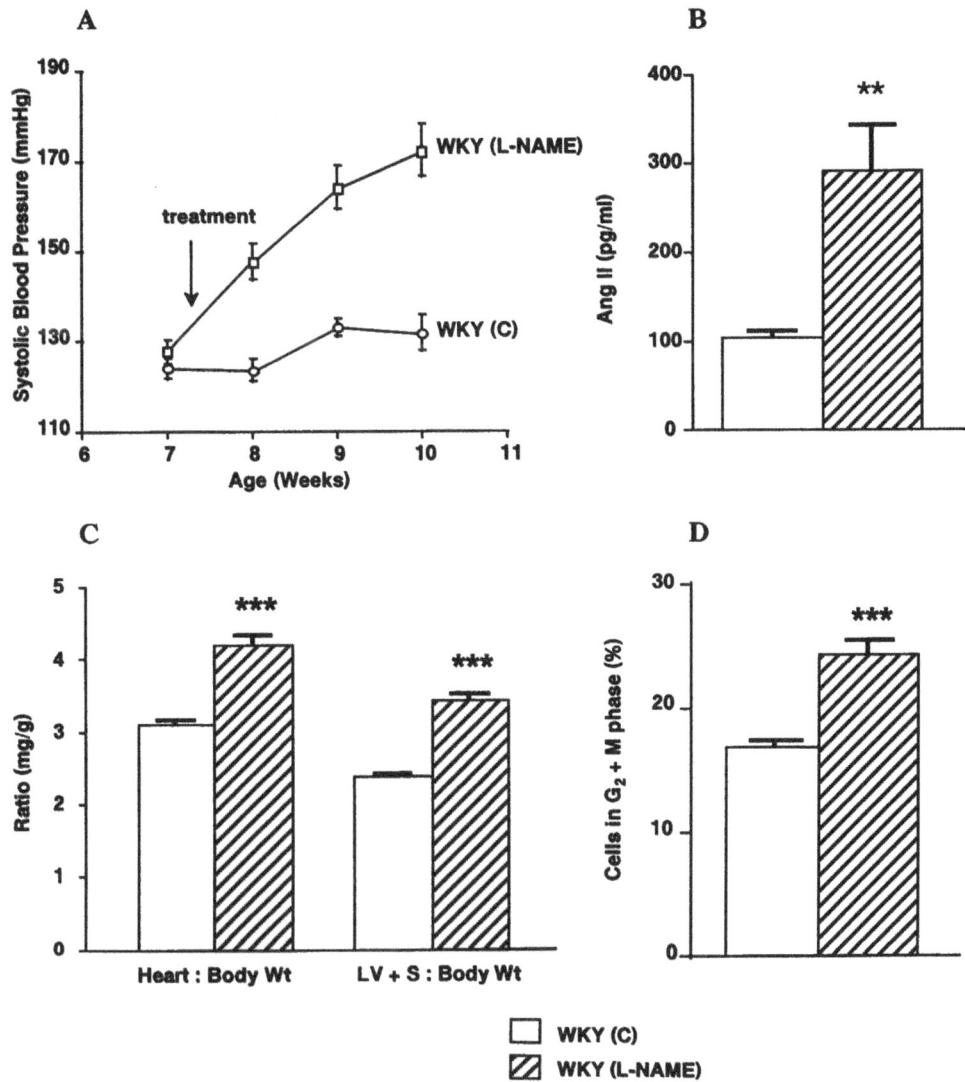

Figure 3. **A.** Systolic blood pressure in control WKY (C); n=16 and in L-NAME treated WKY (L-NAME); n=15. One-way ANOVA; F=62.1, P<<0.0001. Values are means ± s.e.m. **B.** Plasma angiotensin II concentration in WKY (C); n=8 and WKY (L-NAME); n=7. **P<< 0.01. **C.** Ratios of heart weight to body weight and left ventricle weight to body weight in WKY (C); n=16, WKY (L-NAME); n=15. ***P<<0.0001 by unpaired t-test. **D.** Percentage of cells in the G_2+M phase of the cell cycle in WKY(C); n=16 and WKY (L-NAME); n=14. ***P<<0.0001 by unpaired t-test. All values are means ± s.e.m. Modified from reference 18 with permission from the American Heart Association.

In several experimental models, the development of cardiac hypertrophy is accompanied by the altered expression of myosin heavy chain and α-actin genes in cardiac myocytes and collagen genes in cardiac fibroblasts[19,20]. We therefore investigated the expression of collagen type I mRNA and skeletal α-actin mRNA, the latter being a fetal form of sarcomeric actin which is re-expressed in the hypertrophied myocardium. Chronic administration of L-NAME increased the expression ratio of skeletal to cardiac α-actin mRNA but cardiac collagen type I expression was unchanged (Fig 4). These results dem-

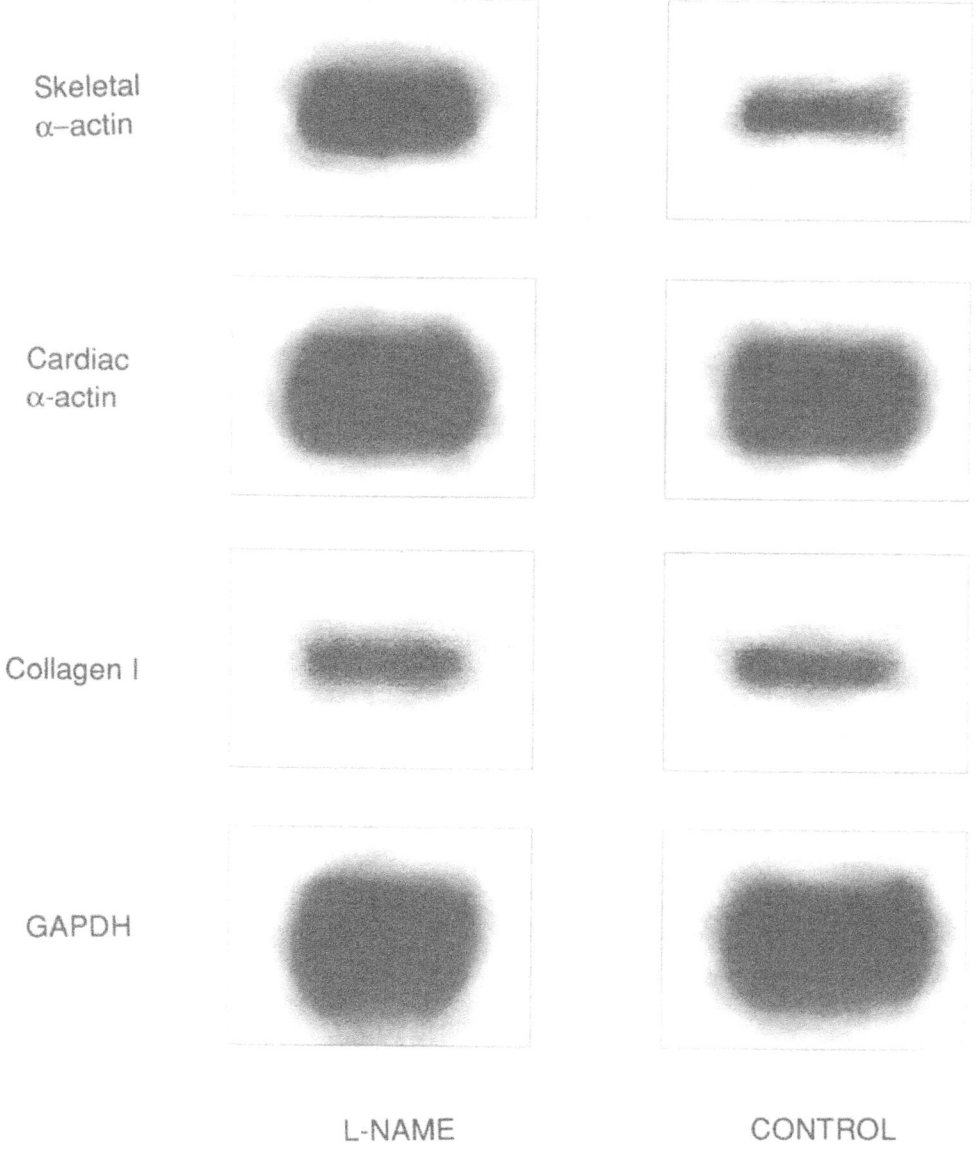

Skeletal
α–actin

Cardiac
α-actin

Collagen I

GAPDH

L-NAME   CONTROL

Figure 4. L-NAME administration enhanced the expression of skeletal α-actin mRNA. Representative bands from Northern blots are presented for ventricles from the L-NAME treated WKY and from the WKY control group. The upper band corresponds to skeletal α-actin, the second band corresponds to cardiac α-actin, the third band corresponds to collagen type I and the lower band corresponds to the housekeeping gene GAPDH. Expression ratio of skeletal to cardiac α-actin mRNA was 0.463±0.07 for WKY (L-NAME) and 0.173±0.04 for WKY (C); P=0.03, 95% CI −0.54 to −0.05. From reference 18 with permission from the American Heart Association.

onstrate true cardiac myocyte hypertrophy in L-NAME induced hypertension, a characteristic shared with the SHRSP but not necessarily with the SHR[21]. These molecular studies were confirmed further by histopathological evidence of cardiomyocyte hypertrophy in sections of the myocardium from L-NAME treated WKY. There were also regions of myocardial necrosis with an associated focal reparative response; these features were not present in sections from control WKY (Fig 5).

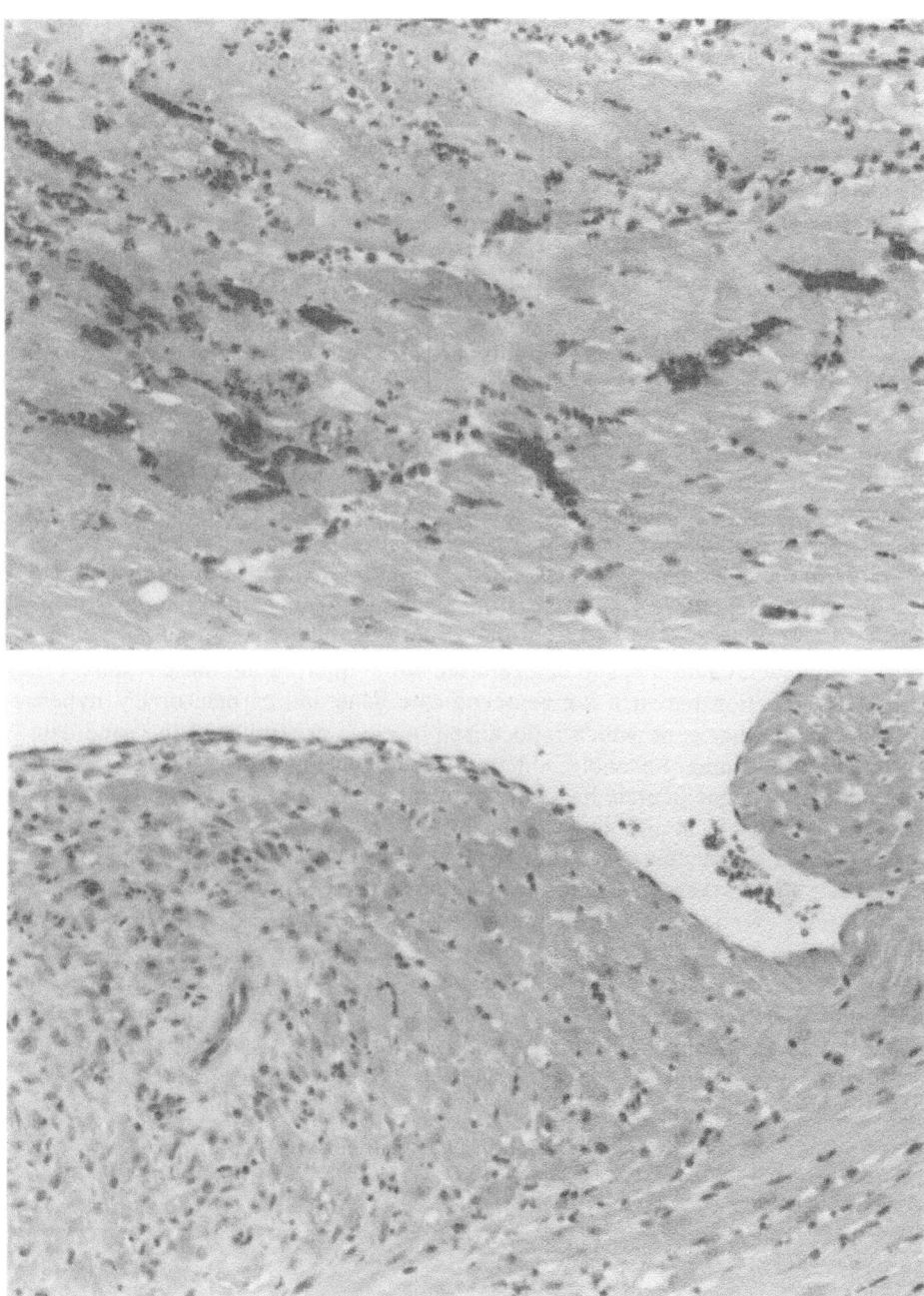

Figure 5. **A** and **B** represent photomicrographs of the left ventricular myocardium from L-NAME treated WKY rats. In **A** the myocardium occupying the upper two thirds of the photograph has undergone very recent necrosis with focal haemorrhage and an early acute inflammatory infiltrate. Viable myocardium is present at the bottom of the photograph. **B** demonstrates an area of resolving subendocardial necrosis with early scar formation in the left half of the field. Viable myocardium is present on the right. Haematoxylin and eosin × 250.

Moreover, we showed increased aortic polyploidy in L-NAME treated WKY thus providing evidence for parallel cardiac and vascular hypertrophy in this model. These changes were associated with significantly increased concentrations of circulating angiotensin II, suggesting yet again that stimulation of the renin-angiotensin system may have a permissive effect for cardiac and vascular hypertrophy.

4. GENETIC SUSCEPTIBILITY TO LEFT VENTRICULAR HYPERTROPHY — A SEARCH FOR THE BEST PARADIGM TO DISSOCIATE BLOOD PRESSURE AND LV MASS

Early studies by Tanase et al[22] have examined the relationship between blood pressure and cardiac mass in 23 strains of normotensive and hypertensive rats. They found that heart weight increased in proportion to blood pressure only in the hypertensive strains and that genetic variance accounted for 65–75% of the total variability of cardiac mass. The authors concluded that heart weight was a highly heritable trait; the effect of genetic factors on cardiac mass being greater than that of blood pressure[22]. With the advent of novel methods of molecular genetics, it was possible to take these studies further using either a candidate gene or a total genome search strategy. The candidate gene strategy assumes that genes, which encode proteins which have already been shown to play a pathophysiological role in the disease phenotype studied, should be investigated for an association or linkage with this phenotype. Table 1 lists the candidate genes which have been shown to co-segregate with increased heart or LV weight in crosses involving inbred hypertensive rat strains. However, caution has to be exercised while interpreting these results. Firstly, a positive co-segregation between a given candidate gene and cardiac or LV hypertrophy cannot exclude another gene which is localised in close proximity to the candidate gene on the same chromosome. Secondly, although each of the studies[23–27] tried to exclude the situation where the same genetic locus is responsible for blood pressure and LV variance, this has proven less than straightforward in some of these studies[25,26].

The alternative genetic strategy, a genome search or scan, uses a panel of polymorphic microsatellite markers to detect quantitative trait loci (QTLs) which contain a gene responsible for a given phenotype. This strategy has been used extensively to study blood pressure QTLs in several experimental crosses[28–31]. Two of these studies[30,31] included a search for potential LV mass QTLs in their analysis. Pravanec et al[30] studied recombinant inbred strains and found that a QTL around Drd 1a, a microsatellite marker within the dopamine 1A receptor on rat chromosome 17, is linked to LV weight and that this rela-

Table 1. Candidate genes for left ventricular hypertrophy

Chromosome	Locus	Strains (cross)	Reference
3	ET-3	Dahl S x Dahl R	Cicila 1994 (22)
10	ACE	NGH x BN	Harris 1995 (23)
10	ACE	SHR x WKY	Zhang 1996 (24)
12	HSP27	RIS & SHRxWKY	Hamet 1996 (26)
13	Renin	Dahl S x Dahl R	Rapp 1989 (25)

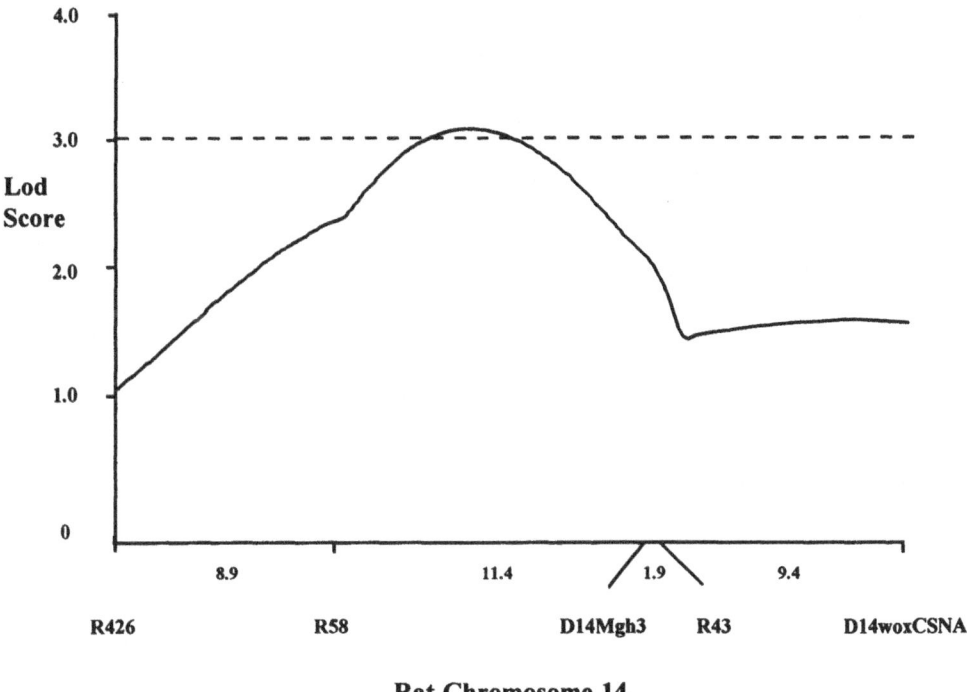

4.0

3.0

Lod
Score

2.0

1.0

0

8.9   11.4   1.9   9.4

R426   R58   D14Mgh3   R43   D14woxCSNA

Rat Chromosome 14

Figure 6. Rat chromosome 14 linkage map and left ventricular mass QTL localisation for an F_2 population derived from crossing SHRSP and WKY (n=140). Distances between markers are in cM, with Haldane correction. The following are anonymous microsatellite markers; R426, R58, D14Mgh 3 and R43. The marker D14 wox CSNA is within a casean alpha gene. From reference 31 with permission from the American Heart Association.

tionship is blood pressure independent. The animals homozygous for the SHR allele at this locus had the lowest LV weight to body weight ratios whereas those homozygous for the BN allele had the highest LV weight. This suggests that the identified QTL plays an inhibitory or protective role during the development of LV hypertrophy in the SHR[30]. The second QTL for LV mass was recently identified by ourselves in a genome scan performed in the Glasgow SHRSP×WKY cross[31]. We found a suggestive linkage (LOD score 3.1) for LV weight to body weight ratio localised to a relatively wide region around the anonymous microsatellite marker R58 on rat chromosome 14 (Fig. 6). This is a susceptibility locus with rats homozygous for the SHRSP allele having the highest LV mass. We have also shown that this locus is entirely blood pressure idependent[31].

It has to be noted that a detection of QTL represents only the first step in a complex process of positional cloning which requires fine mapping of the QTL of interest using congenic strategies followed by direct cloning and sequencing of the putative candidate region. These strategies are time-consuming and labour-intensive but might result not only in positional cloning of the LV hypertrophy gene(s) in animal models but also in the identification of new candidate genes for human studies.

5. SUMMARY

Cardiac hypertrophy in essential and experimental (genetic) hypertension have been initially attributed to increased pressure load. However, the level of blood pressure does not parallel the degree of cardiac hypertrophy, i.e., a complex relationship rather than a simple dose-response effect has to be suggested. Several non-haemodynamic factors which influence LV mass have been identified with genetic and neuro-hormonal influences playing a major role. The experimental strategies which have been used to highlight one or more of these influences include pharmacological studies of regression or prevention of LVH and studies designed to produce LVH de-novo in normotensive strains. All these studies while confirming an important role of haemodynamic factors also stress the major influence of the renin-angiotensin system and the inter-relationship between angiotensin II and nitric oxide.

In contrast, genetic strategies, from simple co-segregation analysis to most complex genome scan studies, suggest the existence of "susceptibility genes" for LV hypertrophy, a finding which deserves further study in large collections of siblings and family groups with essential hypertension.

ACKNOWLEDGMENTS

These studies have been funded by the British Heart Foundation Grants PG 95123, PG 96175 and FS 93025. AFD is a British Heart Foundation Senior Research Fellow. We thank Mrs. S. Thomson for editorial assistance.

REFERENCES

1. G.A. Mensah, T.W. Pappas, M.J. Koren, R.J. Ulin, J.H. Laragh and R.B. Devereux. Comparison of classification of hypertension severity by blood pressure level and World Health Organization criteria for prediction of conccurrent cardiac abnormalities and subsequent complications in essential hypertension. J Hypertens 1993; 11: 1429–1440.
2. D. Levy, R.J. Garrison, D.D. Savage, W.B. Kannel and W.P. Castelli. Prognostic implications of echocardiographically determined left ventricular mass in the Framingham Heart Study. N Engl J Med 1990; 322: 1561–1566.
3. A.M. Devlin, J.F. Gordon, A.O. Davidson, J.S. Clark, C.A. Hamilton, J.J. Morton, A.M. Campbell, J.L. Reid and A.F. Dominiczak. The effects of perindopril on vascular smooth muscle polyploidy in stroke-prone spontaneously hypertensive rats. J Hypertens 1995; Vol 13 No. 2: 211–218.
4. A.M. Devlin, A.O. Davidson, J.F. Gordon, A.M. Campbell, J.J. Morton, J.L. Reid and A.F. Dominiczak. Vascular smooth muscle polyploidy in genetic hypertension. J Human Hypertens 1995; 9: 497–500.
5. G.K. Owens. Differential effect of antihypertensive drug therapy on vascular smooth muscle cell hypertrophy, hyperploidy and hyperplasia in the spontaneously hypertensive rat. Circ Res 1985; 56: 525–536.
6. J.M. Pfeffer, M.A. Pfeffer, I. Mirsky and E. Braunwald. Regression of left ventricular hypertrophy and prevention of left ventricular dysfunction by captopril in the spontaneously hypertensive rat. Proc Natl Acad Sci USA 1982; 79: 3310–3314.
7. A.A.T. Geisterfer, M.J. Peach and G.K. Owens. Angiotensin II induces hypertrophy, not hyperplasia of cultured rat aortic smooth muscle cells. Circ Res 1988; 62: 749–756.
8. M.B. Taubman, B.C. Berk, S. Izumo, T. Tsudo, R.W. Alexander and B. Nadal-Ginard. Angiotensin II induces c-fos mRNA in aortic smooth muscle. Role of Ca^{2+} mobilization and protein kinase C activation. J Biol Chem 1989; 264: 526–530.
9. G. Engelmann, J. Vitullo and R. Gerrity. Age-related changes in ploidy levels and biochemical parameters in cardiac myocytes isolated from spontaneously hypertensive rats. Circ Res 1986; 58: 137–147.
10. W. Brodsky and I.V. Uryvaeva. Cell polyploidy: its relation to tissue growth and function. Int Rev Cytol 1977; 50: 275–332.
11. G.K. Owens. Control of hypertrophic versus hyperplastic growth of vascular smooth muscle cells. Am J Physiol 1989; 257: H1755–H1765.
12. M.J. Black, J.F. Bertram, J.H. Campbell and G.R. Campbell. Angiotensin II induces cardiovascular hypertrophy in perindopril-treated rats. J Hypertens 1995; 13: 683–692.

13. A.F. Dominiczak, A.M. Devlin, W.K. Lee, N.H. Anderson, D.F. Bohr and J.L. Reid. Vascular smooth muscle polyploidy and cardiac hypertrophy in genetic hypertension. Hypertension 1996; 27: 752–759.

14. J.F. Arnal, A. El Amrani, G. Chatellier, J. Menard and J.B. Michael. Cardiac weight in hypertension induced by nitric oxide synthase blockade. Hypertension 1993; 22: 380–387.

15. N.E. Rhaleb, X.P. Yang, A.G. Scicli and A.O. Carretero. Role of kinins and nitric oxide in the antihypertensive effect of ramipril. Hypertension 1994; 23: 865–868.

16. M.J. Black, M.A. Adams, A. Bobik, J.H. Campbell and G.R. Campbell. Effect of enalapril on aortic smooth muscle polyploidy in the spontaneously hypertensive rat. J Hypertens 1989; 7: 997–1003.

17. P. Sventek, J-S. Li, K. Grove, C.F. Deschepper and E.L. Schiffrin. Vascular structure and expression of endothelin-1 gene in L-NAME-treated spontaneously hypertensive rats. Hypertension 1996; 27: 49–55.

18. A.M. Devlin, J.M. Brosnan, D. Graham, J.J. Morton, A. McPhaden, M. McIntyre, C.A. Hamilton, J.L. Reid, A.F. Dominiczak. Cellular and molecular mechanisms of aortic and cardiac hypertrophy due to chronic inhibition of nitric oxide synthase. Hypertension 1997 (submitted).

19. C.G. Brilla, B. Maisch and W.T. Weber. Renin-angiotensin system and myocardial collagen matrix remodelling in hypertensive heart disease: *in vivo* and *in vitro* studies on collagen matrix regulation. J Clin Invest 1993; 71: S35–S41.

20. N.H. Bishopric, P.C. Simpson and C.P. Ordahl. Induction of the skeletal alpha-actin gene in alpha$_1$-adrenoceptor-mediated hypertrophy of rat cardiac myocytes. J Clin Invest 1987; 80: 1194–1199.

21. H. Tanase, Y. Yamori, C.T. Hansen and W. Lovenberg. Heart size in inbred strains of rats. Part 2. Cardiovascular DNA and RNA contents during the development of cardiac enlargement in rats. Hypertension 1982; 4: 872–880.

22. H. Tanase, Y. Yamori, C.T. Hansen and Lovenberg W. Heart size in inbred strains of rats. Part 1. Genetic determination of the development of cardiovascular enlargement in rats. Hypertension 1982; 4: 864–872.

23. G.T. Cicila, J.P. Rapp, K.D. Bloch, T.W. Kurtz, M. Pravenac, V. Kren et al. Cosegregation of the endothelin-3 locus with blood pressure and relative heart weight in inbred Dahl rats. J Hypertens 1994; 12: 643–651.

24. E.L. Harris, E.L. Phelan, C.M. Thomson, J.A. Millar and M.R. Grigor. Heart mass and blood pressure have separate genetic determinants in the New Zealand genetically hypertensive (GH) rat. J Hypertens 1995; 13: 397–404.

25. L. Zhang, K.M. Summers and M.J. West. Angiotensin I converting enzyme gene polymorphism on chromosome 10 cosegregates with blood pressure and heart weight in F$_2$ progeny derived from spontaneously hypertensive and normotensive Wistar-Kyoto rats. Clin Exp Hypertens 1996; 8: 753–771.

26. J.P. Rapp, S.M. Wang and H Dene. A genetic polymorphism in the renin gene of Dahl rats cosegregates with blood pressure. Science 1989; 243: 542–544.

27. P. Hamet, M.A. Kaiser, Y. Sun, V. Page, M. Vincent and V. Kren et al. HSP 27 locus cosegregates with left ventricular mass independently of blood pressure. Hypertension 1996; 28: 1112–1117.

28. P. Hilbert, K. Lindpaintner, J.S. Beckmann, T. Serikawa, Soubrier F and C. Dubay et al. Chromosomal mapping of two genetic loci associated with blood pressure regulation in hereditary hypertensive rats. Nature 1991; 353: 521–529.

29. H.L. Jacob, K. Lindpaintner, S.E. Lincoln, K. Kusumi, R.K. Bunker and Y.P. Mao et al. Genetic mapping of a gene causing hypertension in the stroke-prone spontaneously hypertensive rat. Cell 1996; 67: 213–224.

30. M. Pravanec, D. Gauguier, J.J. Schott, J. Buard, V. Kren and V. Bila et al. Mapping of quantitative trait loci for blood pressure and cardiac mass in the rat by genome scanning of recombinant inbred strains. J Clin Invest 1995; 96: 1973–1978.

31. J. Clark, B. Jeffs, A.O. Davidson, W.K. Lee, N.H. Anderson and M.T. Bihoreau et al. Quantitative trait loci in genetically hypertensive rats: possible sex specificity. Hypertension 1996; 28: 898–906.

4

REGULATION AND ROLE OF MYOCARDIAL COLLAGEN MATRIX REMODELING IN HYPERTENSIVE HEART DISEASE[*]

Reinhard C. Funck, Andreas Wilke, Heinz Rupp, and Christian G. Brilla[†]

Molecular Cardiology Laboratory
Division of Cardiology
Philipps-University of Marburg
Marburg, Germany

1. ABSTRACT

In hypertensive heart disease, reactive myocardial fibrosis represents as an excessive accumulation of fibrillar collagen within the normal connective tissue structures of the myocardium. The fact, that the myocardium of both ventricles is involved, irrespective of ventricular loading conditions, suggests that circulating factors, and not the hemodynamic load are primary responsible for this adverse response of the myocardial fibrous tissue. In various experimental *in vivo* models, it has been shown that myocardial fibrosis is always associated with activation of circulating or local renin-angiotensin-aldosterone systems (RAAS).

Cardiac collagen metabolism is regulated by cardiac fibroblasts which express mRNAs for types I and III collagens, the major fibrillar collagens in the heart, and for interstitial collagenase or matrix metalloproteinase (MMP) 1 which is the key enzyme for interstitial collagen degradation.

In order to elucidate the role of the RAAS effector hormones, angiotensin II (AngII) and aldosterone (ALDO), in the regulation of collagen synthesis or inhibition of MMP 1 production, adult human cardiac fibroblasts were cultured. Collagen synthesis was determined by ^{3}H-proline incorporation, and MMP 1 activity by degradation of ^{14}C-collagen measured under serum-free conditions in confluent fibroblasts after 24 hour-incubation with either AngII or ALDO over a wide range of concentrations (10^{-11}–10^{-6}M). In addition, the effects of the mineralocorticoid, deoxycorticosterone (DOC), and prostaglandin E_2 (PGE_2) on cardiac fibroblast function were determined. Compared with untreated control fibroblasts, collagen synthesis, normalized per total protein synthesis, showed a significant and dose-dependent increase after

* Supported by DFG grant Br-1029/2-1.
† Correspondence to: C. G. Brilla, MD, PhD, Philipps-Universität Marburg, Zentrum Innere Medizin, SP Kardiologie, Baldingerstr., 35033 Marburg, Tel.: 06421-286462, Fax.: 06421-288954

Hypertension and the Heart, edited by Zanchetti et al.
Plenum Press, New York, 1997

35

incubation with either mineralocorticoid hormone, ALDO or DOC, or after incubation with AngII. In contrast, collagen synthesis of cardiac fibroblasts was significantly decreased by PGE$_2$ treatment. AngII type 1 or mineralocorticoid receptor antagonists, respectively, were able to completely inhibit the AngII- or mineralocorticoid-mediated increase of collagen synthesis. Furthermore, AngII significantly decreased MMP 1 activity while ALDO or DOC had no effect on cardiac fibroblast-mediated collagen degradation. In contrast, PGE$_2$ significantly increased MMP 1 activity.

Thus cardiac fibroblast function is modulated by either effector hormone of the RAAS, AngII and ALDO, via specific receptors that lead to progressive myocardial fibrosis in disease states where circulating or local RAAS is activated, i.e., in hypertensive heart disease. In contrast, PGE$_2$, which would be elevated in myocardial tissue after angiotensin-converting enzyme inhibition, counteracts the fibrotic effects of the RAAS on myocardial tissue.

2. INTRODUCTION

Based on their results of *in vivo* studies Weber and Brilla[1,2] suggested that the renin-angiotensin-aldosterone system (RAAS) primarily regulates the development of myocardial fibrosis of the right and left ventricles in hypertensive heart disease. This reactive fibrosis presents as diffuse interstitial and perivascular fibrosis occurring within the normal connective tissue network of the myocardium irrespective of ventricular loading and myocyte necrosis. Cardiac fibroblasts which express types I and III collagen proteins, the major fibrillar collagens of the myocardium[3], and which produce matrix metalloproteinase (MMP) 1, the key enzyme for interstitial collagen degradation, represent the target cells on which the effector hormones of the RAAS, angiotensin II (AngII) and aldosterone (ALDO), would need to act.

Therefore, adult human cardiac fibroblasts derived from endomyocardial biopsies of patients with hypertensive heart disease were cultured. We found that either effector hormone of the RAAS, AngII and ALDO, stimulated collagen synthesis of cardiac fibroblasts in a dose-dependent manner. Likewise, the mineralocorticoid hormone, deoxycorticosterone (DOC), significantly increased collagen synthesis normalized to total protein synthesis, whereas prostaglandin E$_2$ (PGE$_2$) significantly inhibited the production of collagen. While MMP 1 activity in cultured cardiac fibroblasts was not altered by either mineralocorticoid hormone, it was increased by PGE$_2$ and significantly decreased by AngII.

Thus, it appears that ALDO and AngII with their direct effects on collagen turnover of cultured adult human cardiac fibroblasts are responsible for the disproportionate and diffuse deposition of fibrillar collagen in the myocardial interstitium in hypertensive heart disease. The kinin-prostaglandin system may have regulatory effects on the myocardial collagen matrix as well, since PGE$_2$ was seen to counteract the trophic effects of the RAAS on progressive interstitial collagen accumulation.

3. FIBRILLAR COLLAGEN NETWORK OF THE MYOCARDIUM

The fibrillar collagen matrix of the myocardium is a structural continuum including valve leaflets, chordae tendineae, and an interstitial collagen network with various components termed epimysium, perimysium, and endomysium[4] (Fig. 1). The epimysium consists of subendocardial and subepicardial connective tissue weaves.[5] The perimysium surrounds groups of myocytes and forms muscle bundles. Perimysial strands connect adjacent muscle bundles, thereby prevent muscle bundle slippage and facilitate force transmission. Wavy

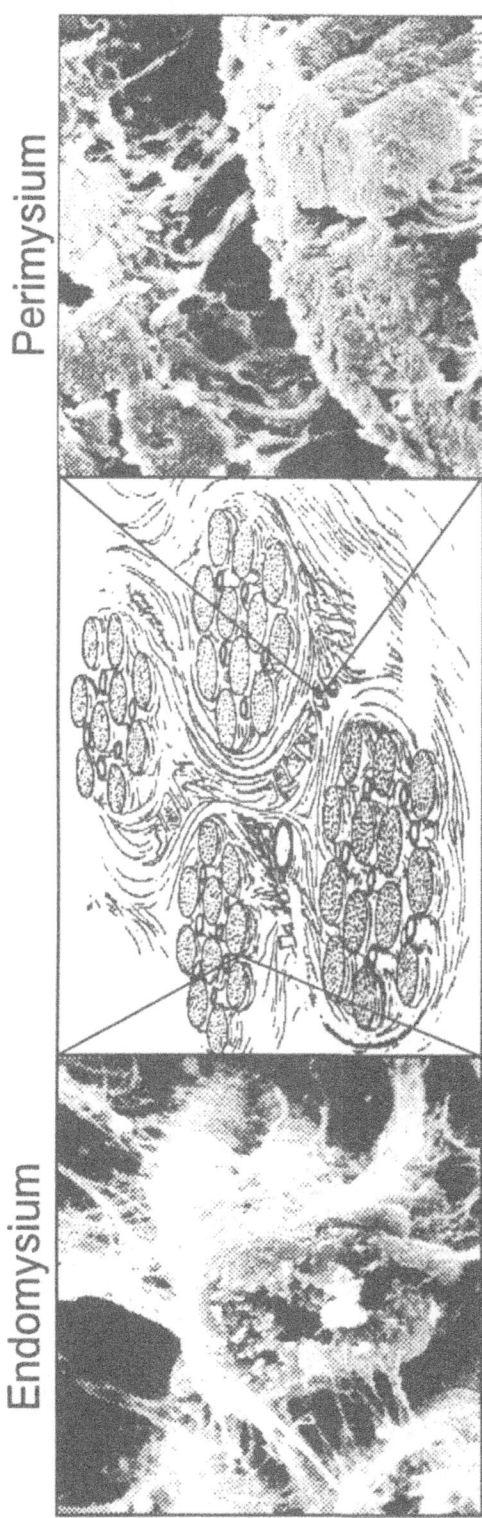

Figure 1. Myocardial collagen network: the endomysium forms a weave of collagen fibers around each individual myocyte connecting myocytes to one another and to their neighboring capillaries (left panel; scanning electron microscopy; × 3000) while the perimysium surrounds groups of myocytes with connective tissue where perimysial collagen strands connect adjacent muscle bundles to prevent muscle bundle slippage throughout the heart cycle (right panel, scanning electron microscopy; × 3000).

perimysial fibers, which are arranged in-parallel to myocytes, markedly increase myocardial stiffness if their slack length has been exceeded.[4] Finally, the endomysium forms a collagen weave around each individual myocyte connecting myocytes to one another and to their neighboring vascular and lymphatic capillaries.[5] Endomysial struts provide myocyte alignment and prevent their slippage, thereby maintaining the architecture of the myocardium throughout the geometric changes of the heart chambers during the cardiac cycle.[6]

Types I and III collagens, which may coexist in common collagen fibers, are the predominant components of the myocardial collagen matrix. These fibers are coated by type VI collagen weaves which appear to determine their thickness. In normal nonhuman primate myocardium the ratio of type I to type III collagen is 7.4:1.[7] Other types of collagen proteins including type IV and type V collagens are represented in small amounts within the myocardium and are mainly associated with cell membranes. The overall mechanical behavior of the myocardium is predominantly determined by type I collagen which has by far the greatest tensile strength of all myocardial tissue components. Therefore, any structural changes within the fibrillar collagen matrix of the myocardium will unequivocally influence myocardial function.

4. REMODELING OF THE MYOCARDIAL COLLAGEN MATRIX

Besides hypertrophy and phenotypical changes of cardiac myocytes, i.e., reduced expression of sarcoplasmic Ca_{2+} ATPase with subsequent impairment of intracellular Ca^{2+} cycling, an increase of types I and III collagen gene expression occurs already at the early stage of the development of left ventricular hypertrophy (LVH) as shown for renovascular hypertension (RHT).[8] A rise in protocollagen proline hydroxylase activity and enhanced proline incorporation into collagen has been found during the first week after suprarenal abdominal aorta banding in the rat.[9] In the same model fibroblast proliferation was observed.[10] In the rat, perivascular fibrosis of intramural coronary arteries is evident after 8 weeks of RHT. In addition, interstitial fibrosis is established by collagen fibers emanating from the adventitia of intramyocardial coronary arteries and radiating outward between neighboring muscle fibers.[11,12] This early phase of hypertrophy is characterized by a two- to threefold increase of left ventricular collagen volume fraction[2,11,12] which is associated with increased diastolic stiffness and occurrence of left ventricular diastolic dysfunction while myocardial contractility is still preserved or even enhanced. This reactive myocardial fibrosis occurs in the absence of myocyte necrosis within the normal connective tissue structures of the myocardium and is of progressive nature.[13,14] After 12 weeks of RHT, collagen volume fraction has increased fourfold above normal with further increase after 20 weeks where diffuse interstitial fibrosis is now established. At 32 weeks, a sixfold increase of collagen volume fraction is evident accounting for almost 25% of the myocardial structural space.[15] At this late stage of LVH, perimuscular fibrosis reduces myocyte generated force leading to progressive myocyte atrophy and subsequent reparative fibrosis due to myocyte cell loss[16] associated with marked increase in diastolic stiffness and impaired contractility of the myocardium[17] (Fig. 2).

5. REGULATION OF MYOCARDIAL COLLAGEN DEPOSITION AT THE TISSUE LEVEL

To examine regulatory systems promoting reactive myocardial fibrosis in hypertensive heart disease, various potential determinants need to be considered: hemodynamic

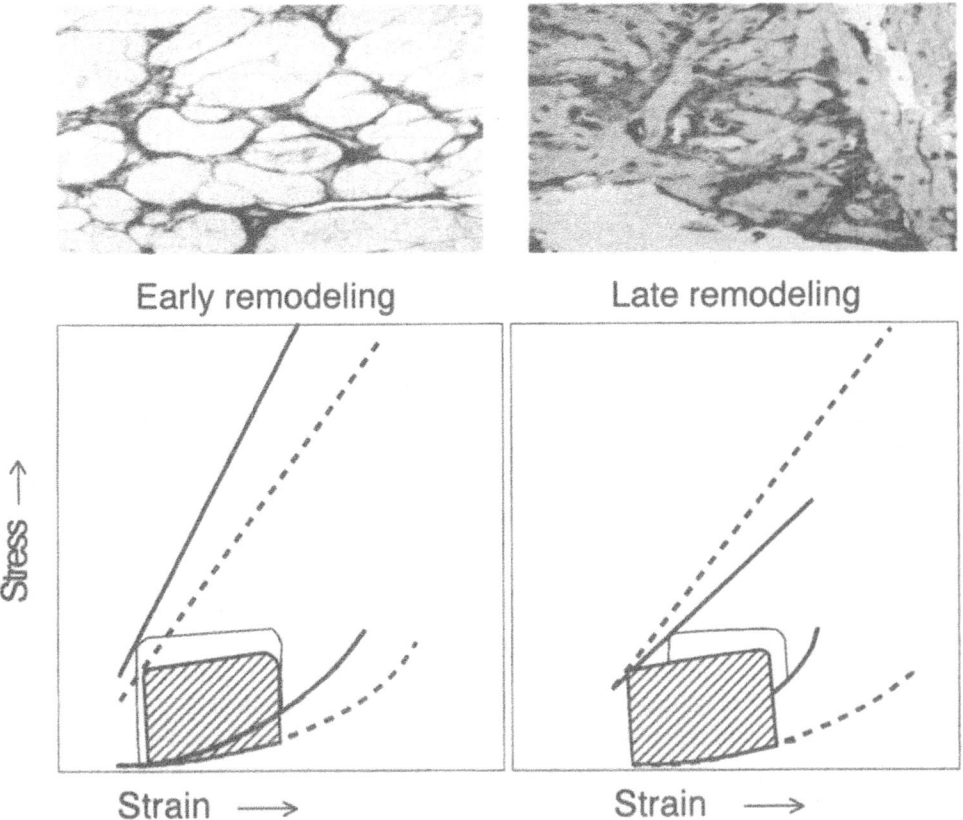

Figure 2. Cardiac structure-function relation in hypertensive heart disease: diastolic (lower curves) and systolic (upper curves) stress-strain relationships in early (left lower panel) and late (right lower panel) remodeling of the left ventricle. During early remodeling both curves are shifted upwards (control curves = dashed lines), that means increased contractility and diastolic myocardial stiffness. Patients being in this stage of their disease with a modest degree of interstitial fibrosis (left upper panel; sirius red stain of left ventricular myocardium obtained by endomyocardial biopsy; collagen fibers are shown with red color; × 100) have diastolic dysfunction and preserved systolic function of the left ventricle. In late stage remodeling of hypertensive heart disease, the systolic stress-strain relation is shifted downwards in addition to a further upward shift of the diastolic function curve revealing combined diastolic and systolic dysfunction of the left ventricle due to marked interstitial fibrosis (right upper panel).

factors, i.e., elevation of left ventricular diastolic or systolic pressures, activation of the RAAS and the influence of local growth factors.

The importance of left ventricular systolic pressure and of the RAAS was evaluated in several rat models of arterial hypertension.[2] The experimental design included RHT (2-kidney/1-clip model) where circulating RAAS was activated, infrarenal aorta banding (IRB) with normal circulating AngII and ALDO levels, and chronic ALDO administration via subcutaneously implanted minipumps (AL) to raise circulating ALDO to the same level as found in RHT. Systolic left ventricular and arterial pressures were increased to an equivalent degree in each model. In all models, there was no right ventricular hypertrophy in the presence of an equivalent degree of LVH. In the hypertrophied left ventricle after RHT and AL, myocyte hypertrophy was accompanied by interstitial and perivascular fibrosis (Table 1). Fibrosis did not occur in LVH in IRB. This data showed that ventricular systolic pressure is not the predominant determinant of fibroblast growth and/or collagen

Table 1. Association of myocardial fibrosis and activation
of the renin-angiotensin-aldosterone system

	Afterload	Preload	LVH	RAAS	LV/RV fibrosis
RHT	↑	–	+	↑	+
AL	↑	↑	+	↑	+
IRB	↑	–	+	-	-
AL + spiro	↑	–	+	↑↓	–
RHT + cap	–	-	-	↑↓	–
1K + Na$^+$	–	-	+	↓	–
RP	–	-	+	↑	

synthesis since there was no fibrosis with IRB despite an equivalent degree of systolic load and LVH compared to RHT and AL models. This conclusion is also supported by the fact that reactive myocardial fibrosis did also occur in the normotensive, nonhypertrophied right ventricle in RHT and AL models.

The above noted models of arterial hypertension coincide with completely different hormonal profiles represented by circulating AngII and ALDO. In contrast to IRB where no fibrosis occurred, circulating AngII and/or ALDO were increased in RHT and AL models where fibrosis occurred in either ventricle irrespective of right and left ventricular afterload. Therefore, the effector hormones of the RAAS, AngII and ALDO, which gain access to either ventricle appear to be involved in the fibrotic response of the myocardial tissue. This hypothesis is further supported by the fact that in RHT plasma AngII and ALDO could be suppressed by the angiotensin-converting enzyme inhibitor captopril and myocardial fibrosis could be prevented in these rats.[18] In rats with hyperaldosteronism, pretreated with low doses of the ALDO antagonist spironolactone, which did not prevent hypertension or LVH, the development of interstitial and perivascular fibrosis could be prevented as well.[19]

The effects of preload are similar. In uninephrectomized rats, in which preload was increased by a high salt diet, LVH was seen to be proportional with the degree of volume overload but neither the overloaded right nor the overloaded left ventricle showed myocardial fibrosis.[2] The RAAS is suppressed in this volume overload model. In low output heart failure models, like rapid pacing in dogs, the RAAS is activated in combination with an elevated preload. Both ventricles showed myocardial fibrosis in these models.[20]

These findings suggest that myocardial fibrosis is associated with RAAS activation irrespective of the hemodynamic load of the left or right ventricle.

6. EFFECTS OF THE RAAS AND PGE$_2$ ON COLLAGEN METABOLISM AT THE CELLULAR LEVEL

In vitro studies were performed to eliminate numerous confounding influences like hemodynamic factors and potential interferences of the RAAS with other hormonal systems which are present *in vivo*, e.g., the adrenergic and bradykinin-prostaglandin systems[21,22], and various growth factors, such as transforming growth factor (TGF) β$_1$ and insulin-like growth factor (IGF)-1 which are known to stimulate collagen synthesis in human lung fibroblasts.[23,24] In these studies, we found a dose-dependent increase of collagen synthesis in confluent adult cardiac fibroblasts incubated with AngII under serum-free conditions, i.e., in the absence of any other hormone or growth factor.[25] The rise in collagen synthesis was determined by ^{3}H-proline incorporation normalized to total protein syn-

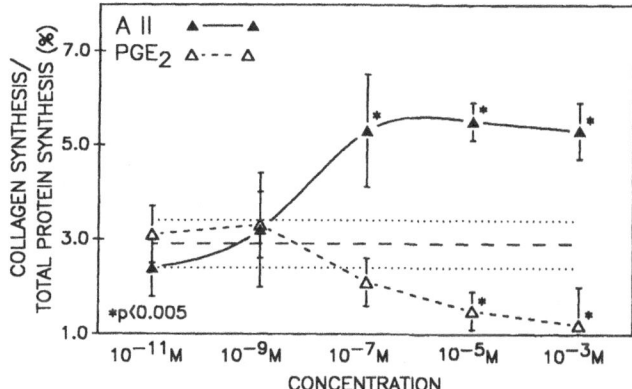

Figure 3. Collagen synthesis normalized per total protein synthesis (percent) of adult human cardiac fibroblasts in culture at passage 1–3 incubated with either angiotensin II (AngII) or prostaglandin E_2 (PGE$_2$) at different concentrations. A dose-dependent rise in collagen synthesis was found for AngII, whereas PGE$_2$ significantly inhibited collagen synthesis compared with untreated control fibroblasts (normal range, mean ± SEM are indicated; with permission).[31]

thesis (Fig. 3). Such direct stimulating effects of AngII on collagen synthesis of cardiac fibroblasts require the presence of specific receptors on these cells.

Five types of specific membrane bound receptors for the RAAS effector hormone AngII are currently known. Of these receptors the AngII type 1 (AT$_1$) receptor appears to be the starting point of the intracellular signal transduction pathway for collagen synthesis.[25,26] The knowledge about the intracellular responses to AT$_1$ receptor activation has been derived particularly from Swiss 3T3 mouse fibroblasts.[27] After attachment of AngII to the ligand binding domain of the AT$_1$ receptor on the cell surface the second messenger pathway is initiated including a G protein representing the effector domain of the receptor and the subsequent activation of phospholipase C (PLC) within the cell membrane. Phosphatidylinositol 4,5-biphosphate (PIP$_2$) is hydrolysed by PLC to water soluble inositol 1,4,5-triphosphate (IP$_3$) and 1,2-diacylglycerol (DAG). IP$_3$ is able to bind to the cytosolic endoplasmic reticulum where three IP$_3$ molecules are necessary to open one calcium channel. Calcium can now be released into the cytosol. Indeed, incubation of cultured cardiac fibroblasts leads to a dose-dependent increase in intracellular Ca^{2+} concentration that can be abolished by simultaneous treatment with the AT$_1$ receptor antagonist CV-11974.[28] The mechanism how calcium-mediated messenger pathways modulate collagen synthesis is unknown. DAG activates proteinkinase C (PKC). The AngII-stimulated biosynthesis of ALDO in the zona glomerulosa of adrenals is initiated by a DAG-mediated rise in PKC. PKC is thought to directly influence the nucleus and the expression of the protoncogenes *c-fos* and *c-myc*. The PKC signal transduction pathway is of utmost importance for the control of cell growth. Further investigations are required for an exact definition of the function of PKC with respect to growth control of cardiac fibroblasts.

The effects of the mineralocorticoid ALDO on collagen synthesis in cultured adult cardiac fibroblasts are similar to that of AngII.[25] Cardiac fibroblasts were incubated with ALDO using a concentration (10^{-9}M) which corresponds to ALDO plasma levels as they are present in patients with renovascular hypertension due to endogenous activation of RAAS. We found a dose-dependent rise in collagen synthesis normalized to total protein synthesis measured by ^{3}H-proline incorporation (Fig. 4). The mineralocorticoid effect

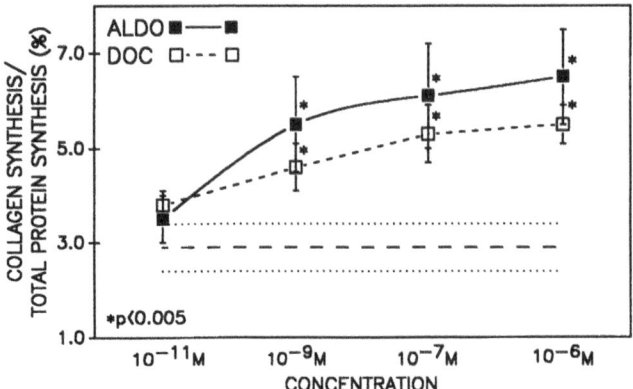

Figure 4. Collagen synthesis normalized per total protein synthesis (%) of adult rat cardiac fibroblasts in culture at passage 6–10 incubated with either aldosterone (ALDO) or deoxycorticosterone (DOC) at different concentrations. A dose-dependent rise in collagen synthesis was found for either mineralocorticoid hormone compared with untreated control fibroblasts (normal range, mean ± SEM, are indicated; with permission).[29]

on fibroblast-mediated collagen synthesis has been confirmed by incubation of cardiac fibroblasts with another mineralocorticoid hormone (DOC) (Fig. 4).[29]

The way of action of the steroid hormones, ALDO and DOC, on cardiac fibroblast-mediated collagen synthesis is completely different compared with AngII. The mineralocorticoids, ALDO and DOC, enter the cell by binding to the cytosolic corticoid type 1 receptor, which is a dimer protein held together by a heat shock protein. The receptor-protein complex dissociates by releasing the heat shock protein and the activated hormone-receptor complex moves from the cytosol to the nucleus with its exposed DNA-binding domain. After DNA binding, the transcriptional rate of specific genes will be changed, and either type I and/or type III collagen genes, or genes which are responsible for the expression of specific membrane bound carriers, e.g., the Ca^{2+}/Na^+ exchanger that might indirectly enhance collagen synthesis, will be activated.[1] In addition, in cultured cardiac fibroblasts ALDO is known to induce the expression of endothelin-1 which may stimulate collagen synthesis in cardiac fibroblasts in an autocrine manner.[30]

Since the development of myocardial fibrosis is also dependent on collagen turnover, i.e., the degradation of interstitial collagen we examined the effects of the RAAS on the collagenolytic system. While the mineralocorticoids, ALDO and DOC, had no effect on collagen degradation in cultured cardiac fibroblasts (no Figure) AngII significantly inhibited MMP 1 activity which is the key enzyme for interstitial degradation of fibrillar collagen (Fig. 5). The mechanism of MMP 1 expression is unknown. Potential interactions between AngII and the AT_2 receptor deserves further studies.[25] This AngII/AT_2 interaction might be similar to an alpha$_1$ receptor concerning the activation of adenylate cyclase and subsequent formation of cAMP which binds to the regulatory subunits of cAMP-dependent protein kinase. Thus, the net effect of the effector hormones of the RAAS, AngII and ALDO, on cardiac fibroblasts leads to a progressive accumulation of collagens.

In addition, we investigated the effects of PGE_2 on myocardial collagen turnover, i.e., collagen synthesis and degradation in serum deprived, cultured adult human cardiac fibroblasts.[31] In contrast to the effects of AngII and ALDO on cardiac fibroblasts, PGE_2 was found to decrease cardiac fibroblast-mediated collagen synthesis in a concentration-dependent manner (Fig. 3). The PGE_2 concentrations required to achieve this effect, however, were larger (10^{-5} M) due to proteinase-mediated degradation of PGE_2 in fibroblast

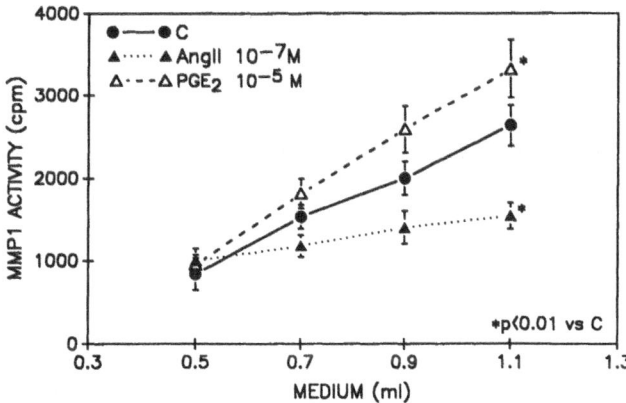

Figure 5. Matrix metalloproteinase (MMP) 1 activity in counts per minute (cpm) of degraded ^{14}C-collagen/ml medium/mg protein/30 min of adult human cardiac fibroblasts incubated with either 10^{-5}M prostaglandin E_2 (PGE$_2$) or 10^{-7}M angiotensin II (AngII), compared with untreated control fibroblasts (C). While PGE$_2$ significantly stimulated collagen degradation, AngII significantly decreased MMP1 activity (mean ± SEM is indicated; with permission).[31]

cultures. Synergistically, MMP1 activity was significantly increased by PGE$_2$ incubation of human cardiac fibroblasts (Fig. 5). Thus, the net effect of PGE$_2$ on cardiac fibroblasts leads to reduced collagen deposition in the myocardium.

7. CLINICAL IMPLICATIONS

Based on these *in vivo* and *in vitro* findings, it can be concluded that the RAAS and the bradykinin-prostaglandin system play important roles in regulating the myocardial collagen matrix by modulating cardiac fibroblast function. In contrast, hemodynamic factors appear to have no effects on excessive collagen deposition in hypertensive heart disease. While the effector hormones of the RAAS, AngII and ALDO, increase fibroblast-mediated collagen synthesis, and AngII synergistically inhibits collagen degradation, that leads to progressive accumulation of fibrillar collagens within the normal connective tissue structures of the myocardium, the effector hormone of the bradykinin-prostaglandin system, PGE$_2$, appear to counteract these fibrotic effects of the RAAS on the myocardium. This is of particular importance in choosing pharmacological agents to treat hypertensive heart disease. Indeed, angiotensin-converting enzyme inhibitors and competitive ALDO receptor antagonists have proven to be effective in regressing or preventing myocardial fibrosis in hypertensive heart disease[19,32] thereby preventing or at least delaying the occurrence of congestive heart failure.[33] The same may be true for AT$_1$ receptor antagonists.

REFERENCES

1. Weber KT, Brilla CG (1991) Pathological hypertrophy and cardiac interstitium: fibrosis and renin-angiotensin-aldosterone system. Circulation 83:1849–1865
2. Brilla CG, Pick R, Tan LB, Janicki JS, Weber KT (1990) Remodeling of the rat right and left ventricle in experimental hypertension. Circ Res 67:1355–1364
3. Weber KT (1989) Cardiac interstitium in health and disease: the fibrillar collagen network. J Am Coll Cardiol 13:1637–1652

4. Factor SM, Robinson TF (1988) Comparative connective tissue structure - function relationships in biologic pumps. Lab Invest 58:150–156
5. Caulfield JB, Borg TK (1979) The collagen network of the heart. Lab Invest 40:364–372
6. Factor SM, Zhao MJ, Eng C, Robinson TF (1988) The effects of acutely increased ventricular cavity pressure on intrinsic myocardial connective tissue. J Am Coll Cardiol 12:1582–1589
7. Weber KT, Janicki JS, Shroff SG, Pick R, Chen RM Bashey RI (1988) Collagen remodeling of the pressure-overloaded, hypertrophied nonhuman primate myocardium. Circ Res 62:757–765
8. Chapman D, Weber KT, Eghbali M (1990) Regulation of fibrillar collagen types I and III and basement membrane type IV collagen gene expression in hypertrophied rat myocardium. Circ Res 67:787–794
9. Lindy S, Turto H, Uitto J (1972) Protocollagen proline hydroxylase activity in rat heart during experimental cardiac hypertrophy. Circ Res 30:205–209
10. Morkin E, Ashford TP (1968) Myocardial DNA synthesis in experimental cardiac hypertrophy. Am J Physiol 215:1409–1413
11. Doering CW, Jalil JE, Janicki JS, Pick R, Aghili S, Abrahams C, Weber KT (1988) Collagen network remodeling and diastolic stiffness of the rat left ventricle with pressure overload hypertrophy. Cardiovasc Res 22:686–695
12. Jalil JE, Janicki JS, Pick R, Shroff SG, Weber KT (1989) Fibrillar collagen and myocardial stiffness in the intact hypertrophied rat left ventricle. Circ Res 64:1041–1050
13. Silver MA, Pick R, Brilla CG, Jalil JE, Janicki JS, Weber KT (1990) Reactive and reparative fibrosis in the hypertrophied rat left ventricle: Two experimental models of myocardial fibrosis. Cardiovasc Res 24:741–747
14. Brilla CG, Weber KT (1992) Reactive and reparative myocardial fibrosis in arterial hypertension. Cardiovasc Res 26:671–677
15. Weber KT, Janicki JS, Pick R, Capasso J, Anversa P (1990) Myocardial fibrosis and pathologic hypertrophy in the rat with renovascular hypertension. Am J Cardiol 65:1G–7G
16. Jalil JE, Janicki JS, Pick R, Abrahams C, Weber KT (1989) Fibrosis-induced reduction of endomyocardium in the rat after isoproterenol treatment. Circ Res 65:258–264
17. Capasso JM, Palackal T, Olivetti G, Anversa P (1990) Left ventricular failure induced by long term hypertension in rats. Circ Res 66:1400–1412
18. Jalil JE, Janicki JS, Pick R, Weber KT (1991) Coronary vascular remodeling and myocardial fibrosis in the rat with renovascular hypertension: response to captopril. Am J Hypertens 4:51–55
19. Brilla CG, Matsubara LS, Weber KT (1993) Anti-aldosterone treatment and the prevention of myocardial fibrosis in primary and secondary hyperaldosteronism. J Mol Cell Cardiol 25:563–575
20. Weber KT, Pick R, Silver MA, Moe GW, Janicki JS, Zucker IH, Armstrong PW (1990) Fibrillar collagen and the remodeling of the dilated canine left ventricle. Circulation 82:1387–1401
21. Berg RA, Moss J, Baum BJ, Crystal RG (1981) Regulation of collagen production by the β-adrenergic system. J Clin Invest 67:1457–1462
22. Fine A, Goldstein RH (1987) The effect of PGE2 on the activation of quiescent lung fibroblasts. Prostaglandins 33:903–913
23. Goldstein RH Poliks CF, Pilch PF, Smith BD, Fine A (1989) Stimulation of collagen formation by insulin and insulin-like growth factor 1 in cultures of human lung fibroblasts. Endocrinology 124:964–970
24. Fine A, Goldstein RH (1987) The effect of transforming growth factor-β on cell proliferation and collagen formation by lung fibroblasts. J Biol Chem 262:3897–3902
25. Brilla CG, Zhou G, Matsubara L, Weber KT (1994) Collagen metabolism in cultured adult rat cardiac fibroblasts: response to angiotensin II and aldosterone. J Mol Cell Cardiol 26:809–820
26. Villareal FJ, Kim NN, Ungab GD, Printz MP, Dillmann WH (1993) Identification of functional angiotensin II receptors on rat cardiac fibroblasts. Circulation 88:2849–2861
27. Rana RS, Hokin LE (1990) Role of phosphoinositides in transmembrane signaling. Physiol Rev 70:115–164
28. Brilla CG, Scheer C, Rupp H (1997) Renin-angiotensin system and myocardial collagen matrix: modulation of cardiac fibroblast function by angiotensin II type 1 receptor antagonism. J Hypertens: in press
29. Brilla CG, Maisch B, Zhou G, Weber KT (1995) Hormonal regulation of cardiac fibroblast function. Europ Heart J 16 (Suppl C):45–50
30. Katwa LC, Weber KT (1996) Aldosterone-induced expression of ET_1, ET_3 and ET_B receptors by cultured adult rat cardiac fibroblasts (abstract). Circulation 94:848
31. Brilla CG, Zhou G, Rupp H, Maisch B, Weber KT (1995) Role of angiotensin II and prostaglandin E_2 in regulating cardiac fibroblast collagen turnover. Am J Cardiol 76:8D–13D
32. Brilla CG, Janicki JS, Weber KT (1991) Cardioreparative effects of lisinopril in rats with genetic hypertension and left ventricular hypertrophy. Circulation 83:1771–1779
33. Brilla CG, Matsubara L, Weber KT (1996) Advanced hypertensive heart disease in spontaneously hypertensive rats: Lisinopril-mediated regression of myocardial fibrosis. Hypertension 28:269–275

5

ULTRASONIC REFLECTIVITY OF THE HEART: A MEASURE OF FIBROSIS?

Michele Ciulla,[1] Roberta Paliotti,[1] and Fabio Magrini[1,2]

[1]Centro di Fisiologia Clinica e Ipertensione
Istituto di Clinica Medica Generale e Terapia Medica
Ospedale Maggiore
Università di Milano, Italy
[2]Cattedra di Medicina Interna, C.L.O.
Università di Cagliari, Italy

1. INTRODUCTION

The conventional echo image depicts at a relative low resolution the echo reflections from the various components of the myocardium, such as muscle fibers, capillaries and collagen strands, acting as diffuse reflectors. In normal conditions the resulting ultrasonic image texture of the myocardium is rather fine and homogeneous, and it is bordered by two thin echolucent lines corresponding to the wide endocardium-blood and epicardium-lung acoustic interfaces[1].

When the myocardium regular tridimensional architecture is altered, the acoustic properties of the tissue are changed and the interactions of echoes within the tissue produce a non-homogeneous pattern that has been observed in several pathological conditions (figure 1).

In the last two decades different methods have been proposed to quantitatively define the state of cardiac muscle with ultrasounds[2] by evaluating the echo image pattern as a marker of tissue structure integrity[3].

The importance of fibrosis in mediating a structural remodelling of the heart in different pathological conditions[4,5] has been demonstrated in several experimental studies. The possibility of evaluating ventricular wall structure by assessing myocardial collagen content has been suggested because the marked acoustic impedance of fibrous tissue (low water content)[6,7] that is responsible for an increase in echoreflectivity.

Various approaches have been used to quantitatively assess collagen content with ultrasounds[2] by analyzing tissue echoreflectivity. Methods have included direct attenuation measurement and gray scale or backscatter analysis of returning echoes[8,9,10]. In this article we review the physical basis and the experimental evidences supporting the possibility of non invasive assessment of myocardial fibrosis using ultrasounds.

Hypertension and the Heart, edited by Zanchetti et al.
Plenum Press, New York, 1997

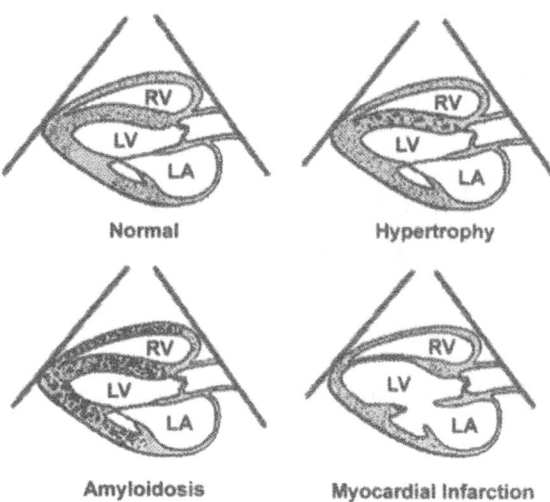

Figure 1.   Echo patterns in different pathologic conditions reflect changes in tissue structure. Modified from (1).

2. PHYSICAL BACKGROUND

The identification of abnormalities in the pathophysiological state of tissues based on the analysis of returning ultrasounds is currently defined ultrasonic tissue characterization. This approach is based on the hypothesis that ultrasounds attenuation is related to the physical properties of individual tissues.

2.1. Ultrasound Beam Characteristics

Clinical ultrasounds are high frequency waves (>2 MHz) transmitted and received as short impulses by a piezoelectric vibrating crystal. The diagnostic potential relies in the behaviour of waves that act according to the Rayleigh's law[11] of reflection and refraction while encountering interfaces of tissues with different acoustic characteristics. The resulting signal is in part redirected to the source and can be visualized, after signal processing, on a video display. The visual pattern obtained provides a mean by which normal conditions can be distinguished from pathologic ones. The ability to distinguish as separate closely lying structures (resolution power), along the main ultrasound axis and laterally, is direclty proportional to the operating frequency of the ultrasound probe, and inversely to the wave length. The linear and the lateral resolution are not equal because of the limited lateral resolution resulting from the finite beam width of echocardiographs[12,13]. On the contrary the ability to reach deep structures (penetration power) is inversely proportional to the frequency and can be set at different distances (focus); off-focus structures are subjected to signal changes. The wave length of the ultrasound beam is defined as:

$$\lambda = V / \Phi\tau \tag{1}$$

where λ is the wave length, V is the speed of ultrasound propagation and $\Phi\tau$ is the frequency of the transducer.

Since a high-frequency beam (short wave length) is unable to penetrate chest wall, lower frequency are used in transthoracic approach with a reduction in the resolution

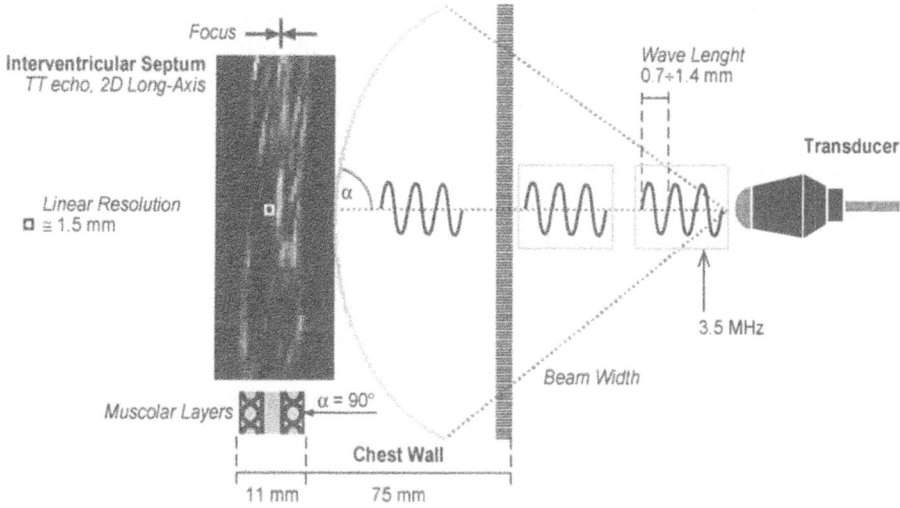

Figure 2.   Relation between ultrasounds characteristics and target distance. Using the 2D long-axis transthoracic approach the interventricular septum can be explored with a correct angle of incidence.

power. The relation between ultrasounds characteristics and target distance are summarized in figure 2.

2.2. Interactions between Ultrasounds and Tissues

The interaction between ultrasounds and a target is markedly influenced by the angle of incidence, showing a characteristic angular dependance that is due to the anisotropic properties of echoes[14]. The signal, depending on the sinus of the angle, is maximal at about 90 degrees; when the sound beam is oriented parallel to the surface of the target the echo returning signal drops out.

The propagation properties of ultrasounds in elastic media, such as biological tissues and organs, depend also on the speed with which the signal propagates, on the attenuation properties and on the impedance of the medium (table 1). These physical variables affect the echographic image, producing a visual pattern that could be considered as an unique signature of each medium[15]. From an acoustic point of view, these patterns may be

Table 1. Propagation properties of ultrasounds in human tissues

Angle of incidence
Speed (1.450–1.640 m/sec)
  energy of the ultrasounds (100 mWatt/cm2)
  density of the tissue (0.92–1.07 g/cm3)
Impedance
  density of the tissue x velocity
Attenuation (0.3–2.0 db/cm/mHz)
  absorption
  scattering properties
    • specular reflections
    • diffuse reflections or back-scattered

regarded as exhibiting typical spacings of acoustically different targets[16]. The resulting signal is, in the "time domain", the Fourier transform of the original one[17]. In a diagnostic setting the energy transferred to the target is originally about 100 mWatt/cm^2; the speed of ultrasound signal propagation is proportional to the tissue density and to the energy that is transferred to the particles of the medium by vibration and finally it is dissipated as heat. The impedance is related to speed and density as follows:

$$I = V \, \delta \qquad (2)$$

where I is the acoustic impedance, V is the speed of ultrasound propagation and δ is the density of the tissue.

The interaction of ultrasounds with tissue produces an attenuation of the original signal as consequence of the absorption of wave energy and of the scattering properties of the tissue. We can describe the scattering behaviour as specular or diffuse, according to the relationship between the pulse length of the frequency utilized and the scatters dimensions. The specular reflection takes place when the target dimension is greater then the pulse length of the ultrasounds and it is perpendicular to the beam. The target, acting as a mirror, returns a maximal signal to the source. When the target is made of little scatters, smaller than a pulse length, such as the myocardium encompassed between the wide endo-cardium-blood and the epicardium-lung acoustic interfaces, the interaction produces a casual diffuse reflection in all directions. The waves, redirected to the source, are defined as back-scattered waves (figure 3). The following formula explains the relationship between the spacing of tissue single elements and the ultrasonic wave length, and it considers also the scattering angle:

$$\lambda = 2d \sin \Theta \qquad (3)$$

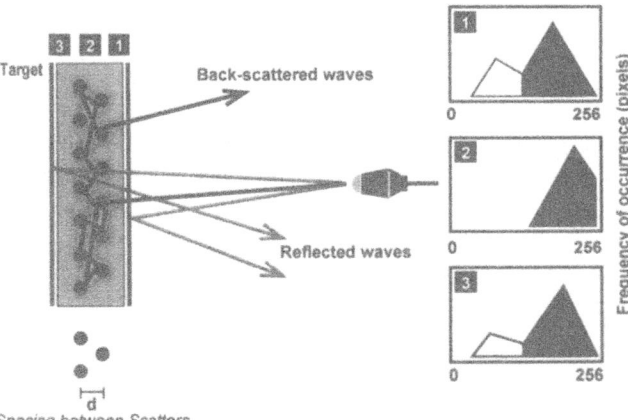

Figure 3. Scheme illustrating returning ultrasounds from ventricular wall. In conventional echocardiography, reflected waves from wide acoustic interfaces are used for linear measurements while tissue characterization approach analyzes quantitatively back-scattered waves to obtain information about tissue structure. The corresponding gray-scale frequency distributions (histograms) are represented in the right portion of the panel. Histogram 1 and 3 are derived from wide acoustic interfaces while histogram 2 is derived from the interaction with little scatters, inside ventricular wall.

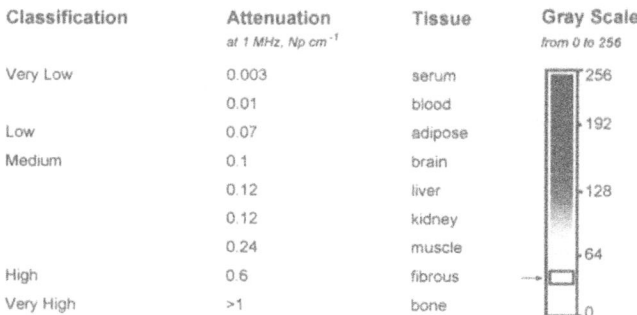

Classification	Attenuation at 1 MHz, Np cm⁻¹	Tissue	Gray Scale from 0 to 256
Very Low	0.003	serum	256
	0.01	blood	192
Low	0.07	adipose	
Medium	0.1	brain	128
	0.12	liver	
	0.12	kidney	
	0.24	muscle	64
High	0.6	fibrous	
Very High	>1	bone	0

Figure 4. Attenuation properties in different tissues. Fibrous tissue shows an attenuation factor that is about 60 times higher than the value of blood. The scale represented on the right corresponds to the conventional echo gray-scale (low echoreflectivity = black, high echoreflectivity = white).

where λ is the wave length, d is the distance between adjacent scatters and Θ is the angle from the horizontal to the scattered signal.

The attenuation process is specific for each tissue with great differences between different ones (figure 4). The intensity of the acoustic wave is attenuated in biological tissues by both, absorption and scattering in a linear fashion with frequency, the greater the frequency the greater the attenuation. For the heart the scattering properties are not fixed, but subject to changes through the cardiac cycle. The changes in the angle of incidence between ultrasounds and myocardial fibers and the local variations in tissue density, as result of contractile performance, are responsible for the so called cycle-dependent acoustic properties of the heart[18,19,20].

3. METHODS FOR TISSUE CHARACTERIZATION

Tissue characterization with ultrasounds represents an extension of conventional echocardiography for the evaluation of myocardial physical properties[21]. The conventional echo image depicts the interaction between ultrasounds and the singular components, or scatters, that constitute the tissue under study. Associated with the hypothesis that alteration in the echo image pattern is due to alterations in tissue structure[3], various approaches have been proposed to quantitatively define the pathophysiological state of cardiac muscle with ultrasound[2]. Methods for ultrasonic characterization have included direct attenuation measurement and gray scale and backscatter analysis of returning echoes, that have been employed in several cardiac disorders[8,9,10,22]. The methods for the ultrasonic tissue characterization are summarized in figure 5.

3.1. Direct Attenuation Measurement

Attenuation properties of a tissue can be evaluated directly in *in vitro* studies, by placing a fresh specimen in a water bath between a transmitter and a receiver transducer; the relative values can be obtained by comparing the attenuation properties of different tissues or by using as reference a perfect reflector such as a metallic surface. This approach provides an ideal set-up to assess the physical properties of tissues, without any limitation in the operating frequency of the probe. This method is however limited because it requires a tissue sample.

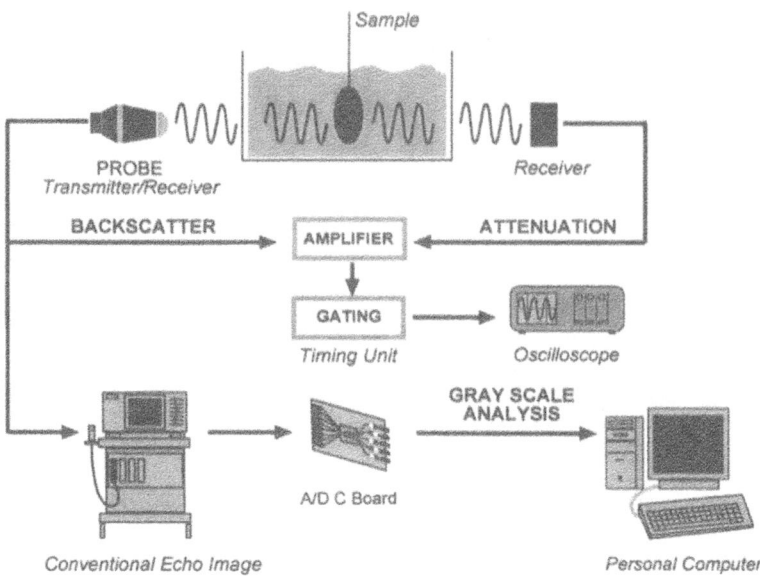

Figure 5. Methods for ultrasonic tissue characterization. Gray-scale approach has the advantage that can be added, in a clinical set-up, to commercially available echocardiographic instruments.

3.2. Backscatter Analysis

Backscatter approach provides a measurement of the structural and functional properties of the myocardium by analysing the unprocessed radiofrequency data. The native signal is obtained direclty from the probe, and does not underwent the standard echo instrument processing steps; the signal is amplified using a specific device and then could be visualized with an oscilloscope. In a clinical set-up a conventional imaging system is required to monitor the structure under analysis.

3.3. Gray Scale Analysis or Videodensitometry

The gray-level approach or videodensitometry analyzes the gray level of individual pixels and its frequency distribution obtained from specific regions of interest inside the ultrasonic image. This technology is relatively simple and has the advantage that can be added to commercially available echocardiographic instruments. The image is acquired and digitized from the echocardiograph in the original clinical configuration, through the video standard output, into a personal computer. By using specific image analysis softwares[23,24] it is possible to derive frequency histogram of reflected echo amplitudes (figure 3) and to measure the spread of echoes about the mean (standard deviation), the asymmetry of the distribution (skewness), the histogram curvature (kurtosis) and the energy (amplitude squared). This method requires a calibration procedure to ensure a more independent approach from the characteristics of the image system and to obtain comparable data between subjects. Some Authors use parietal pericardium as an internal standard for setting the gain of the instrumentation[7]. Another possibility is to indicize all the values obtained using blood echoreflectivity (figure 6)[22]. Although backscatter analysis provides a more independent approach from instrumentation settings, and from the operator in comparison

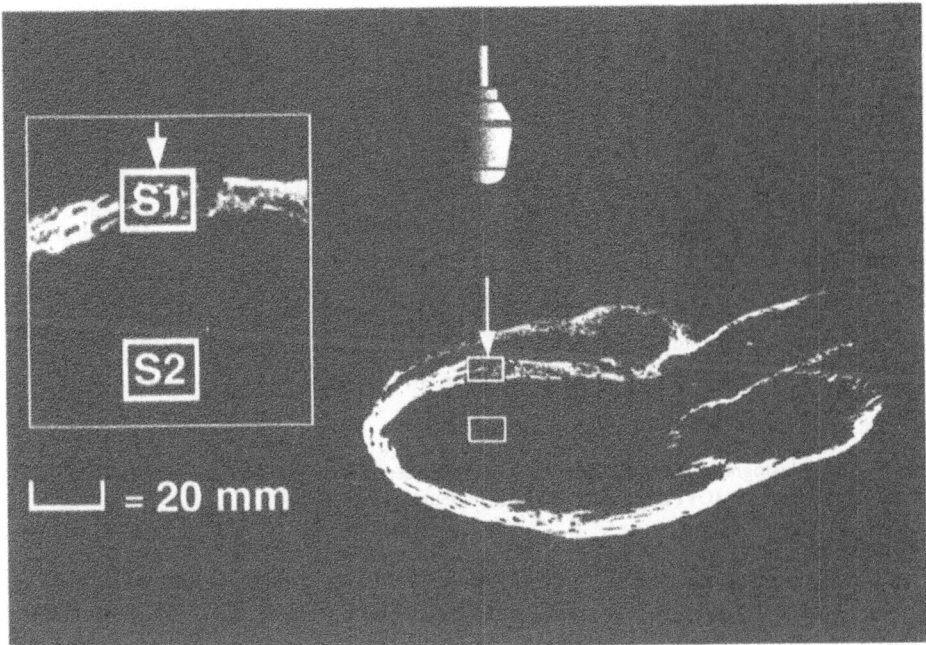

Figure 6. Schematic diagram of a long-axis view of the heart illustrating the region of analysis (S1) in the mid-apex interventricular septum and the scale for blood echoreflectivity (black = 256) assessed along the same axis inside the left ventricle (S2). The main echo beam is carefully kept perpendicular to the interventricular septum.

with gray scale method, it is more complex because requires a system not readily available. In addition the potential of gray-scale analysis has been shown to reproduce the information of backscatter in many conditions[18,21].

4. DETECTION OF MYOCARDIAL FIBROSIS

Experimental and clinical studies have demonstrated the possibility to assess non-invasively the ultrastructural properties of tissues by ultrasounds.

Picano et al. have studied the fibrotic heart during different pathological conditions, involving a structural cardiac remodelling (i.e. hypertension and myocardial infarction)[25], by comparing the backscatter and the hystological assessed collagen content, in vivo and in vitro; the results indicate collagen accumulation is the major determinant of the cardiac echoreflectivity. Similar results have been found by Mimbs and coauthors[26] with the analysis of the echo-attenuation. In dogs, after the left anterior descending coronary artery ligation, they have demonstrated a good correlation between the infarct size (determined by the depletion of the creatine kinase) and the ultrasounds attenuation, indicating that the regional infarction is associated with changes in echoreflectivity, related to collagen accumulation[27].

In patients with left ventricular chronic disease (valvular, congenital and coronary artery disease) Shaw et al.[7] have compared the analysis of the pixel intensity of echo images with the collagen content. In this study a good correlation between the echo and the hystological pattern have been found.

In a group of hypertensive patients with mild to moderate left ventricular hypertrophy without left ventricular dysfunction Gigli et al.[28] have demonstrated that the inte-

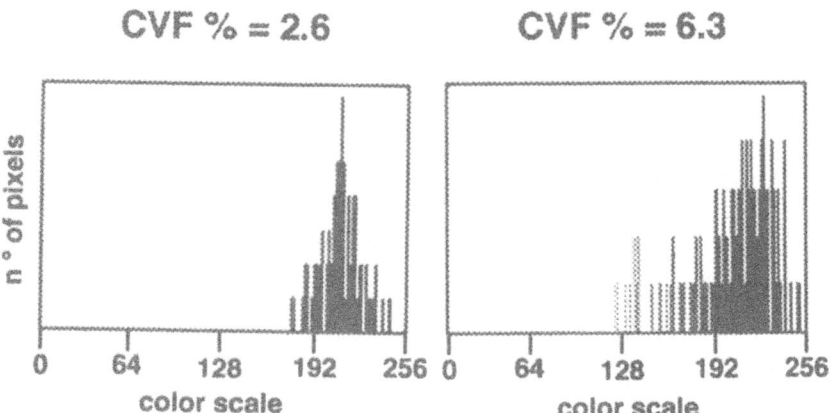

Figure 7. Color histograms derived respectively from a patient with a low (left panel) and a high (right panel) Collagen Volume Fraction (CVF). Normal CVF values are up to 2%.

grated backscatter is not altered, suggesting that collagen growth is not necessarily associated with the increase in left ventricular wall thickness. Similar findings have been observed in athletes with left ventricular hypertrophy[29]. Lucarini et al.[30] report no variations in integrated backscatter despite the regression of cardiac hypertrophy following antihypertensive treatment.

In order to assess the possibility of quantification of myocardial fibrous tissue by using gray scale analysis, we have recently studied a group of 9 hypertensive patients with left ventricular hypertrophy (LVMI > 125 g/m^2) and biopsy proven different degrees of myocardial fibrosis (collagen volume fraction %, CVF %, normal values > 2%). With the increase in CVF% we observed a progressive wider asymmetrical left shift of the myocardial color histogram (figure 7). The mean value of the color scale, that is directly related to the lightness of the image, was not relevant to collagen content, while a significant correlation (r=0.72) between the pixel color level frequency distribution and CVF% was found (figure 8). We advance the hypothesis that the increase in collagen network increases the casual constructive and destructive interactions of echoes whitin the myocardium. In a simplified model collagen fibers seem to act as diffuse reflectors inside the myocardium, returning echoes in all directions and thus producing a wider color spectrum.

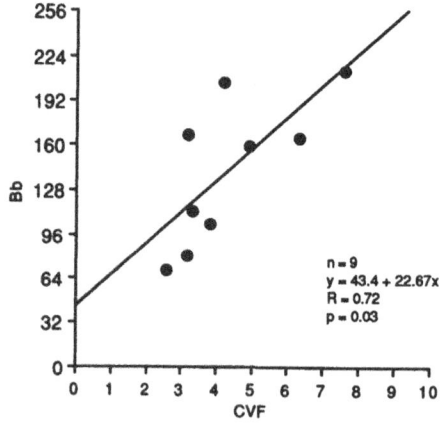

Figure 8. Correlation between Collagen Volume Fraction (CVF%) and Broad Band (Bb) about the color scale. Values are derived at end diastole; each dot represents one patient. The increase in collagen deposition produces an increase in septal echoreflectivity in hypertensive hypertrophic hearts.

Table 2. Factors involved in tissue echoreflectivity

ultrasound frequency and resolution power
focus depth
gray scale extension
echocardiographic window and view
changes due to cardiac cycle
signal attenuation due to tissue density
number and dimension of scatters
structural homogeneity of tissue components
collagen content
systolic thickening and contractility
coronary blood flow

5. CONCLUSIONS

Since myocardial fibrosis is increased in several heart diseases, the possibility of performing non-invasive myocardial characterization may be clinically, in particular in hypertensive patients, in whom reversal of left ventricular hypertrophy is considered a desirable goal of therapy.

There is little doubt that collagen deposition, due to its marked acoustic impedance (about 10,000 times higher than the impedance of surrounding tissues) has an important influence on the echo texture image from the myocardium[6]. Althought quantitative analysis of the ultrasound signals from myocardium has demonstrated an promising sensitivity for detection of collagen accumulation[31], the specificity of changes in ultrasonic reflectivity for the diagnosis of myocardial fibrosis is still uncertain, because the single scatters can not be solved at the transthoracic ultrasonic frequencies.

We cannot exclude that other possible contributing factors are involved in the genesis of an altered echoreflectivity. Diastolic dysfunction colud be one of the main contributors, through the altered mechanical performace[18], and the myocardial fiber disarray, observed in pathological forms of hypertrophic cardiomyopathy, might also play a role. The principal factors involved in tissue echoreflectivity are summarized in table 2.

Finally the diffusion of these techniques is hampered by the difficulties in setting up a system for ultrasonic tissue characterization. More recently, the addition of image processing capabilities to standard personal computers and the availability of analysis software has provided a low cost solution to improve image analysis and tissue characterization studies[23,24].

REFERENCES

1. Bhandari AK, Nanda NC. Myocardial texture characterization by two-dimensional echocardiography. Am J Cardiol 1983; 51: 817–825.
2. Miller JG, Perez JE and Sobel BE. Ultrasonic characterization of myocardium. Progress in Cardiovascular Diseases 1985; 27 (2): 85–110.
3. Price RR, Jones TB, Goddard J, Everette James A. Basic concepts of ultrasonic tissue characterization. Radiologic Clinics of North America 1980; vol 18 n°1: 21–30.
4. Pearlman ES, Weber KT, Janicki JS, Pietra GG and Fishman AP. Muscle fiber orientation and connective tissue content in the hypertrophied human heart. Lab Invest 1982; vol 46 n°2: 158–164.
5. Huysman JAN, et al. Changes in nonmyocyte tissue composition associated with pressure overload of hypetrophic human hearts. Pathol Res Pract 1989; 184: 577–581.

6. Kossoff G, Gossett WJ, Carpenter DA, Jellins J, Dadd MJ. Principles and classification of soft tissues by grey scale echography. Ultrasound Med Biol 1976; n°2: 89–105.
7. Shaw TRD, Logan-Sinclair RB, Surin C, et al. Relation between regional echo intensity and myocardial connettive tissue in chronic left ventricular disease. Br Heart J 1984; 51: 46–53.
8. Marini C, Ghelardini G, Picano E, et al. Effects of coronary blood flow on myocardial gray level amplitude in two dimensional echocardiography: an experimental study. Cardiovasc Res 1993; 27: 279–283.
9. Sagar KB, Pelc LR, Rhyne TL, Howard J and Warltier DC. Estimation of myocardial infarct size with ultrasonic tissue characterization. Circulation 1991; 83: 1419–1428.
10. Chandrasekaran K, Aylward PE, Fleagle SR, et al. Feasibility of identifying amyloid and hypertrophic cardiomyopathy with the use of computerized quantitative texture analysis of clinical echocardiographic data. J-Am-Coll-Cardiol. 1989 Mar 15; 13 (4): 832–40.
11. Rayleigh JWS. The theory of sounds. Dover Publications ed, New York 1945.
12. Roelandt J, van Dorp WG, Bom N, Laird JD, Hugenholtz PG. Resolution problems in echocardiology: a source of interpretation errors. Am J cardiol 1976; 37: 256–262.
13. Skorton DJ, Collins SM, Woskoff SD, Bean JA and Melton HE Jr. Range and azimuth-dependent variability of image texture in two-dimensional echocardiograms. Circulation 1983; 68 n°4:834–840.
14. Aygen M, Popp RL. Influence of orientation of myocardial fibers on echocardiographic images. Am J Cardiol 1987; 45: 248–263.
15. Ultrasonic Tissue Characterization. NBS Special Publication, U.S. Government Printing Office ed. Washington 1976; n° 453.
16. Sommer GF, Joynt LF, Carroll BA and Macovski A. Ultrasonic characterization of abdominal tissues via digital analysis of backscattered waveforms. Radiology 1981; 141: 811–817.
17. Rose JL and Goldberg BB. Frequency analysis. In Basic Phisics in Diagnostic Ultrasound, John Wiley and Sons ed, New York 1970; Chapter 7: 98–105.
18. Olshansky B., Collins S.M., Skorton D.J., Prasad N.V. Variation of left ventricular myocardial gray level on two-dimensional echocardiograms as a result of cardiac contraction. Circulation 1984; vol 70 n°6: 972–977.
19. Sagar KB, Pelc LE, Rhyne TL, Wann LS and Waltier DC. Influence of heart rate, preload, afterload and inotropic state on myocardial ultrasonic backscatter. Circulation 1988; vol 77 n°2: 478–483.
20. Ciulla M, Paliotti R, Magrini F. Effects of septal thickening during cardiac cycle on myocardial echoreflectivity in normal subjects: analysis in 256 gray scale images. High Blood Press 1994; vol 3 (suppl 1): 11.
21. Perez JE, Miller JG, Barzilai B, et al. Progress in quantitative ultrasonic characterization of myocardium: from the laboratory to the bedside. J Am Soc Echo 1988; vol 1 n°4: 294–305.
22. Ciulla M, Paliotti R, Hess DB, Tjahja E, Campbell SE, Magrini F and Weber KT. Echocardiographic patterns of myocardial fibrosis in hypertensive patients: endomyocarial biopsy versus ultrasonic tissue characterization. J Am Soc Echo 1997 in press.
23. Morris R. Image processing on the Macintosh. IEEE Computer 1990; 103–106.
24. Lennard P. Image analysis for all. Nature 1990; vol 347: 103–104.
25. Picano E, Pelosi G, Marzilli M, et al. In vivo quantitative ultrasonic evaluation of myocardial fibrosis in humans. Circulation 1990; 81: 58–64.
26. Mimbs JW, Yuhas DE, Miller JG, Weiss AN, Sobel BE. Detection of myocardial infarction in vitro based on altered attenuation of ultrasound. Circ Res 1977; 41: 192–198.
27. Mimbs JW, O'Donnell M, Bauwens D, Miller JG, Sobel BE. The dependence of ultrasonic attenuation and backscatter on collagen content in dog and rabbit hearts. Circ Res 1980; 47: 48–58.
28. Gigli G, Lattanzi F, Lucarini AR, et al. Normal utrasonic myocardial reflectivity in hypertensive patients. A tissue characterization study. Hypertension 1993; 21: 329–334.
29. Lattanzi F, Di Bello V, Picano E, Caputo MT, Talarico L, Di Muro C, Landini L, Santoro G, Giusti C, Distante A. Normal ultrasonic myocardial reflectivity in athletes with increased left ventricular mass. A tissue characterization study. Circulation 1992; 85: 1828–1834.
30. Lucarini AR, Gigli G, Lattanzi F, Picano E, Mazzarisi A, Iannetti M and Landini L. Regression of hypertensive myocardial hypertrophy does not affect ultrasonic myocardial reflectivity: a tissue characterization study. J Hypert 1994; 12: 73–79.
31. Hoyt RM, Skorton DJ, Collins SM, Melton HE. Ultrasonic backscatter and collagen in normal ventricular myocardium. Circ 1984; 69 (4): 775–782.

6

LOCAL ANGIOTENSIN II AND MYOCARDIAL FIBROSIS

Yao Sun*

Department of Internal Medicine
University of Missouri Health Sciences Center
Columbia, Missouri

1. INTRODUCTION

A wound healing response that eventuates in fibrous tissue formation appears at the site of myocardial infarction (MI). Fibrosis can also appear remote to the MI where it can cause an extensive structural remodeling of viable myocardium. Fibrosis, an abnormal increase in tissue collagen concentration, can adversely affect organ function.

Cells responsible for fibrous tissue formation at sites of repair consist principally of phenotypically transformed fibroblast-like cells having distinctive morphologic features and phenotypic characteristics termed *myofibroblasts* (myoFb), because they express alpha-smooth muscle actin microfilaments and are contractile (1). These cells are abundant at sites of tissue repair (1, 2). Interstitial fibroblasts are responsible for normal collagen turnover and are considered a source of myoFb. Signals responsible for this transformation in cell phenotype are under investigation. Recent *in vivo* and *in vitro* studies indicate that fibroblast-like cells are metabolically active — activity that extends beyond their synthesis and degradation of collagen. This includes their ability to generate substances such as AngII (3). It therefore is no longer tenable to consider metabolic activity of fibroblast-like cells as confined solely to the secretion of matrix components. The healing response is mediated by substances produced within infarcted tissue. The purpose of this manuscript will be to address the elaboration of AngII by myoFb in the infarcted heart and its contribution to fibrous tissue formation.

2. CARDIAC REPAIR POSTINFARCTION

Myocardial infarction in rats was created by left coronary artery ligation. Fibrosis of infarcted rat heart included: a) extensive myocardial infarction (MI) of the left ventricular

* Correspondence and reprints to: Yao Sun, M.D., Ph.D., University of Missouri-Columbia, Division of Cardiology, MA432 Medical Science Building, Columbia, Missouri 65212, USA. Tel: (314) 882-8580, Fax: (314) 884-4691

Hypertension and the Heart, edited by Zanchetti et al.
Plenum Press, New York, 1997

free wall; b) noninfarcted sites remote to MI; c) the visceral pericardium after opening of the parietal pericardium and manual handling of the heart; and d) placement of a foreign body (silk suture) into the myocardium around the left coronary artery (4). In the infarcted heart, type I collagen gene expression was determined by *in situ* hybridization; its fibrillar collagen composition by the collagen-specific stain picrosirius red; and its cellular elements using hematoxylin and eosin and/or specific immunohistochemistry for detection of cell phenotype (*vide infra*).

2.1 Collagen Gene Expression

By quantitative *in situ* hybridization, type I collagen gene expression is normally low in the myocardium of both ventricles. It is markedly increased at the site of infarction on day 3, remains elevated at week 1, 2, 4 and persists for as long as 3 months (5). Transcript for type I collagen is also increased at sites of pericardial fibrosis and endocardial fibrosis of intraventricular septum . Markedly increased type I collagen expression is further seen in noninfarcted myocardium of the septum and right ventricles at week 1, but not day 3, and remains high as long as week 4.

2.2 Collagen Accumulation

Type I collagen makes up about 80% of total collagen found in scar tissue and is therefore the most important collagen in repairing tissue. Microscopic evidence of early fibrillar collagen formation is seen at the site of MI at week 1. A fibrillar assembly of collagen that borders on necrotic tissue to represent early scar formation is seen at week 2. Continued collagen accumulation is evident at week 4 (Figure 1, panel A) and 8 (4). Necrotic cells have been completely replaced by fibrous tissue on week 4 and it is at this point in time that thinning of the infarct scar begins becoming more advanced at wk 8. Detailed aspects of scar remodeling has been reported by others (6, 7).

Increased fibrous tissue, evidenced by hydroxyproline assay and histochemistry, is observed by week 2 at remote sites in hearts with extensive MI. This likewise has been observed in the human myocardium (8). At these remote sites involving the right ventricular free wall and septum microscopic scars replace myocytes lost. Increased interstitial collagen formation is observed at these sites in the absence of myocyte necrosis. A perivascular fibrosis of intramyocardial coronary arteries is also seen at these sites (4). An endocardial fibrosis of the left ventricular aspect of the interventricular septum represents another aspect of the structural remodeling of the heart by fibrous tissue that appears remote to MI (4). In rats with or without MI, fibrosis of the visceral pericardium (Figure 1, panel B) and myocardium surrounding the silk ligature is evident at postoperative wk 2. Markedly increased type I collagen mRNA is colocalized with collagen accumulation in both infarcted and noninfarcted myocardium.

3. CELLS PRODUCING COLLAGEN AT SITES OF INJURY IN THE INFARCTED HEART

Cells responsible for type I collagen gene expression at the site of MI were identified by *in situ* hybridization (5) and found to be fibroblast-like cells, not cardiac myocytes, endothelial cells or vascular smooth muscle cells. These fibroblast-like cells, together with macrophages, surround necrotic myocytes. These cells were identified as myoFb by immu-

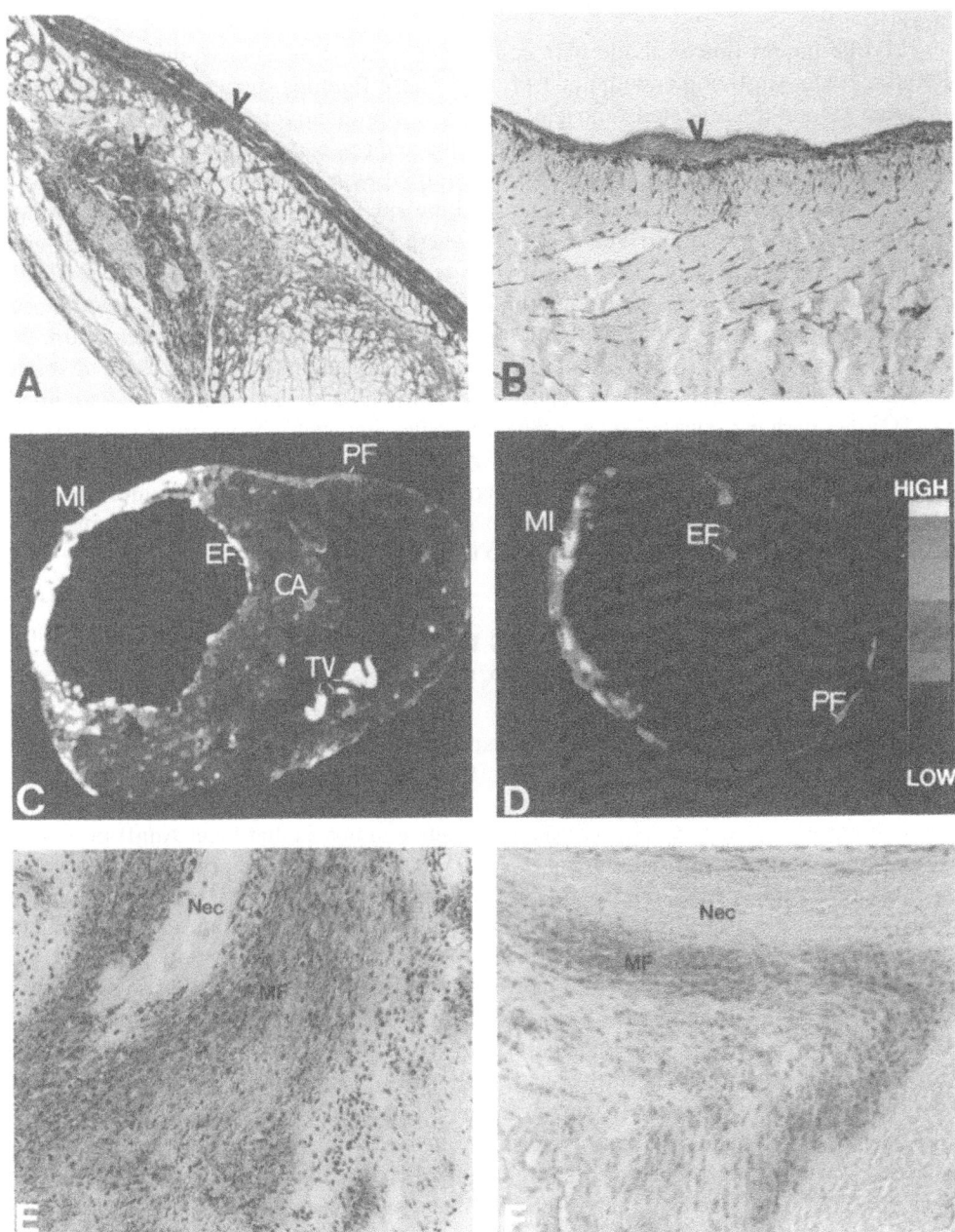

Figure 1. In the infarcted rat heart, fibrosis is evident at the site of MI (panel A, arrowhead, PSR, X120) and pericardium (panel B, arrowhead, PSR, X120). Autoradiographic ACE binding density (panel C) is markedly increased at sites of MI, endocardial and pericardial fibrosis compared to noninfarcted myocardium. Tricuspid valves (TV) normally contain high binding density of ACE (panel C). Cells expressing ACE at the site of MI are fibroblast-like cells surrounding necrotic tissue (Nec) (panel F). These ACE containing fibroblast-like cells also express α-smooth muscle actin and therefore, are myoFb (panel E, MF). Marked increase in autoradiographic AngII receptor binding density is colocalized with high ACE and fibrosis (panel D).

nohistochemistry (3). At the site of MI, myoFb first appear on day 3 postMI, become abundant and extensive thereafter (Figure 1, panel E). Unlike skin, where myoFb appear and then disappear by day 28 following injury (9), myoFb remain at the site of infarction for years (10).

MyoFb impart fibrous tissue with contractile activity. Substances that promote contraction include AngII and endothelin 1 (1, 11). These findings suggest diastolic dysfunction, often seen in the infarcted ventricle, could be a fibrocontractive disorder.

In situ hybridization localized fibroblast-like cells as expressing type I and III collagen mRNA at remote sites (5). MyoFb were identified by α-smooth muscle labeling in the fibrosed visceral pericardium, endocardium and the site of foreign-body fibrosis surrounding silk suture. In the study of Sun et al. (3), where microscopic scars replaced lost myocytes in the noninfarcted right ventricle, myoFb were also observed. Cleutjens et al. (5) did not find such scars remote to the MI and in this case interstitial fibroblasts (α-smooth muscle actin negative) were involved with interstitial fibrosis of noninfarcted myocardium. Differences in experimental preparation of the infarct model may explain these disparate findings. Factors responsible for the appearance of myoFb at or remote to MI remain uncertain. TGF-β_1, perhaps released by necrotic myocytes or macrophages involved in repair, could be implicated. Added to a wound healing chamber implanted subcutaneously, TGF-β_1 leads to the appearance of myoFb in subsequent granulation tissue that surrounds the chamber; exogenous administration of TGF-β_1 to cultured, serum-deprived skin fibroblasts is associated with their transformation to myoFb (12).

4. ANGIOTENSIN CONVERTING ENZYME (ACE) AND ANGII RECEPTORS IN THE INFARCTED HEART

In addition to its well described circulating endocrine properties, there is now accumulating evidence that locally generated AngII has important autocrine and paracrine functions in a variety of organs (13, 14). Locally generated AngII has been found to stimulate growth of cultured cells (15, 16). Increasing evidence indicates that local AngII production plays an important role in tissue repair (17, 18). ACE, a membrane bound ectoenzyme, is responsible for AngII generation from AngI. The multiple physiological effects of AngII are initiated by binding to specific receptors located on the plasma membrane. The existence of at least two subtypes of AngII receptors (AT$_1$ and AT$_2$) has been demonstrated.

In vitro quantitative autoradiography demonstrates the presence of ACE binding (^{125}I-351A) throughout the myocardium of each ventricle and atria in the normal rat heart. Binding density, however, is low at these sites. High-density ACE binding, on the other hand, is present in heart valve leaflets and adventitia of intramural coronary arteries (Figure 1, panel C) (19), where collagen turnover is expected to be high suggesting AngII, generated within connective tissue, is normally involved in fibrogenesis via AngII receptor-ligand binding. AngII receptor binding is normally low in myocardium of both left and right ventricles (20). Keeley et al. (21) found that 5 wks of enalapril administration (nonpressor dose) in 4 wk old rats retarded collagen formation in the right and left ventricles, aorta and superior mesenteric artery. Heart valves were not examined.

Three days after MI, ACE and AngII receptor binding density in the infarcted left ventricle was unchanged compared to normal myocardium. One week postMI, both ACE and AngII receptor binding density was markedly increased at the site of MI (4, 22). Such high ACE and AngII receptor binding in the infarcted ventricle was also seen on week 2, 4 (Figure 1, panels C and D) and 8.

One week postMI, marked increase in ACE and AngII receptor binding was seen at sites of fibrosis remote to infarction, including pericardial fibrosis (Figure 1, panels C and D), endocardial fibrosis (Figure 1, panels C and D), myocardial foreign body fibrosis, perivascular fibrosis and microscopic scars (4, 22). ACE and AngII receptor binding remained high at these sites of repair for at least 8 weeks. Each fibrous tissue site was, therefore, coincident with high-density ACE and AngII receptor binding. Displacement studies using either an AT_1 receptor antagonist (losartan) or AT_2 receptor antagonist (PD123177) demonstrated dominant AT_1 receptor binding at these sites (22). Furthermore, regulation of ACE expression at sites of repair was shown to be independent of circulating AngII or ALDO (23).

5. CELLS EXPRESSING ACE AND ANGII RECEPTORS IN THE INFARCTED HEART

Monoclonal antibody to ACE have been used to identify cells expressing this ecto-enzyme at the site of MI. Positively labeled cells include endothelial cells, found in blood vessels that appear in granulation tissue as part of neovascularization, macrophages, and myoFb (Figure 1, panel F) (3, 4). At remote fibrotic sites, myoFb are the primary cells expressing ACE (3). Each site is likewise coincident with high-density autoradiographic AngII receptor binding, predominantly of the AT_1 subtype. Predominant cells expressing AT_1 receptors at these sites were subsequently identified by emulsion autoradiography and immunolabeling as myoFb (24). Smooth muscle cells of blood vessels express low AT_1 receptors (24).

6. PHARMACOLOGICAL INTERVENTIONS

In vivo studies, using pharmacological agents that interfere with AngII generation (i.e., ACE inhibitors) or which bind to AT_1 receptors, support a role for locally generated AngII in regulating collagen turnover at sites of tissue repair in the heart and related structures.

Following experimental MI, elevations in circulating AngII and ALDO are not observed (23). Administration of an ACE inhibitor, either captopril or enalapril, for 6 wks reduced infarct size (percent of epicardial circumference of the left ventricle occupied by scar) and infarct area (planimetered scar area) (25). Similar findings have recently been reported for an AT_1 receptor antagonist (losartan) suggesting locally produced AngII contributes to fibrogenesis (26).

ACE inhibitors captopril or perindopril, initiated at the time of MI, prevents fibrosis at remote sites (27). A similar response was observed for losartan (26), implicating locally produced AngII in fibrogenesis at these sites. Autoradiographic ACE binding density at remote sites was attenuated by losartan, suggesting either the number of myoFb or their metabolic activity/cell was reduced (27).

7. SUMMARY

Tissue repair appears in the infarcted heart at both infarcted and noninfarcted myocardium. Experimental evidence gathered to date indicates that myoFb are the predominant cell responsible for collagen formation at sites of repair in the rat heart and related structures. These phenotypically transformed fibroblast-like cells are not normal residents of ventricular tissue. They appear on day 4 at sites of injury and remain abundant for weeks therefore. MyoFb express type I collagen mRNA and ACE and AT1 receptors. ACE inhibitors or AT_1 receptor antagonists attenuate collagen accumulation in both infarcted and noninfarcted myocardium. These findings suggest locally generated AngII may have an autocrine function in regulating myoFb collagen turnover.

REFERENCES

1. Gabbiani G., Hirschel B. J., Ryan G. B., Statkov P. R., and Majno G. Granulation tissue as a contractile organ. A study of structure and function. *J. Exp. Med.* 1972: 135: 719–734.
2. Sun Y. and Weber K. T. Angiotensin-converting enzyme and wound healing in diverse tissues of the rat. *J. Lab. Clin. Med.* 1996: 127: 94–101.
3. Sun Y. and Weber K. T. Angiotensin converting enzyme and myofibroblasts during tissue repair in the rat heart. *J. Mol. Cell. Cardiol.* 1996: 28: 851–858.
4. Sun Y., Cleutjens J. P. M., Diaz-Arias A. A., and Weber K. T. Cardiac angiotensin converting enzyme and myocardial fibrosis in the rat. *Cardiovasc. Res.* 1994: 28: 1423–143.
5. Cleutjens J. P. M., Verluyten M. J. A., Smits J. F. M., and Daemen M. J. A. P. Collagen remodeling after myocardial infarction in the rat heart. *Am. J. Pathol.* 1995: 147: 325–338.
6. Jugdutt B. I. and Amy R. W. M. Healing after myocardial infarction in the dog: changes in infarct hydroxyproline and topography. *J. Am. Coll. Cardiol.* 1986: 7: 91–102.
7. Whittaker P., Boughner D. R. and Kloner R. A. Analysis of healing after myocardial infarction using polarized light microscopy. *Am. J. Phthol.* 1989: 134, 879–893.
8. Volders P.G.A., Willems I.E.M.G., Cleutjens J.P.M., Arends J.-W., Havenith M.G., and Daemen M.J.A.P. Interstitial collagen is increased in the non-infarcted human myocardium after myocardial infarction. *J. Mol. Cell. Cardiol.* 1993: 25: 1317–1323.
9. Darby I., Skalli O., and Gabbiani G. α-Smooth muscle actin is transiently expressed by α-smooth muscle actin-positive cells in healing human myocardial scars. *Am. J. Pathol.* 1994: 145: 868–875.
10. Willems I. E. M. G., Havenith M. G., De Mey J. G. R., and Daemen M. J. A. P. The myofibroblasts during experimental wound healing. *Lab. Invest.* 1990: 63: 21–29.
11. Appleton I., Tomlinson A., Chander C. L., and Willoughby D. A. Effect of endothelin-1 on croton oil-induced granulation tissue in the rat. A pharmacologic and immunohistochemical study. *Lab. Invest.* 1992: 67: 703–710.
12. Desmouliere A., Geinoz A., Gabbiani F. and Gabbiani G. Transforming growth factor-β1 induces α-smooth muscle actin expression in granulation tissue myofibroblasts and in quiscent and growing cultured fibroblasts. *J. Cell Biol.* 1993: 122, 103–111.
13. Johnston C. I. Biochemistry and pharmacology of the renin-angiotensin system. *Drugs* 1990: 39(suppl 1), 21–31.
14. Sakaguchi K., Chai S. Y., Jackson B., Johnston C. I., Mendelsohn F. A. Inhibition of tissue angiotensin converting enzyme. Quantitation by autoradiography. *Hypertension* 1988: 11, 230–238
15. Scheling P., Fischer H., Ganten D., Angiotensin and cell growth: a link to cardiovascular hypertrophy? *Hypertension* 1991: 9, 3–15.
16. Baker K. M., Aceto J. F., Angiotensin II stimulation of protein synthesis and cell growth in chick heart cells. *Am. J. Physiol.* 1990: 259, H610–H618.
17. Weber K.T., Sun Y., Katwa L.C. Connective tissue: a metabolic entity? *J. Mol. Cell. Cardiol.* 1995: 27, 107–120.
18. Baker K. M. Booz G. W. Dostal D. E. Cardiac actions of angiotensin II: role of an intracardiac renin-angiotensin system. *Annu. Rev. Physio.* 1992: 54, 227–241.
19. Yamada H., Fabris B., Allen A. M., Jackson B., Johnston C. I., and Mendelsohn F. A. O. Localization of angiotensin converting enzyme in rat heart. *Circ. Res.* 1991: 68: 141–149.
20. Sun Y and Weber KT. Angiotensin II and aldosterone receptor binding in rat heart and kidney: response to chronic angiotensin II or aldosterone administration. *J. Lab. Clin. Med.* 1993:122.404–411.
21. Keeley F. W., Elmoselhi A., and Leenen F. H. H. Enalapril suppresses normal accumulation of elastin and collagen in cardiovascular tissues of growing rats. *Am. J. Physiol.* 1992: 262: H1013–H1021.
22. Sun Y. and Weber K. T. Angiotensin II receptor binding following myocardial infarction in the rat. *Cardiovasc. Res.* 1994: 28: 1623–1628.

23. Hodsman G. P., Kohzuki M., Howes L. G., Sumithran E., Tsunoda K., and Johnston C. I. Neurohumoral responses to chronic myocardial infarction in rats. *Circulation* 1988: 78: 376–381.

24. Sun Y. and Weber K. T. Cells expressing angiotensin II receptors in fibrous tissue of rat heart. *Cardiovasc. Res.* 1996: 31: 518–525.

25. Jugdutt B. I., Humen D. P., Khan M. I., and Schwarz-Michorowski B. L. Effect of left ventricular unloading with captopril on remodeling and function during healing of anterior transmural myocardial infarction in the dog. *Can. J. Cardiol.* 1992: 8: 151–163.

26. de Carvalho Frimm C., Sun Y., and Weber K. T Angiotensin II receptor blockade and myocardial fibrosis following infarction in the rat heart. . *J. Lab. Clin. Med.* in press.

27. Michel J.-B., Lattion A.-L., Salzmann J.-L., Cerol M. L., Philippe M., Camilleri J.-P., et al. Hormonal and cardiac effects of converting enzyme inhibition in rat myocardial infarction. *Circ. Res.* 1988: 62: 641–650.

7

LEFT VENTRICULAR ANATOMY AND FUNCTION IN PRIMARY ALDOSTERONISM AND RENOVASCULAR HYPERTENSION

Achille C. Pessina, Alfredo Sacchetto, and Gian Paolo Rossi[*]

Department of Clinical & Experimental Medicine
University of Padua Medical School and Azienda Ospedaliera di Padova

SUMMARY

Left ventricular hypertrophy (LVH) is a common finding in hypertension and represents a detrimental outcome since it is associated with increased morbidity and mortality. For similar elevation of blood pressure the severity and type of LVH vary considerably in relation to several factors. Compelling evidence suggests that both the renin-angiotensin system (RAS) and the aldosterone excess play an important role in the pathogenesis of LVH, since experimentally angiotensin II has been found to cause myocardial cells hypertrophy and/or hyperplasia and excess aldosterone has been related to extracellular matrix and collagen deposition and therefore to myocardial fibrosis. Secondary forms of hypertension offer models for investigating the relative role of the RAS and aldosterone on the heart in humans. Being rare in the population of hypertensive patients, they furnish an example of the so called Bateson's approach to the understanding of diseases "Treasure your exceptions." In this paper, we review the data concerning the LV changes in primary aldosteronism and renovascular hypertension and discuss the insight that they have provided into the pathogenesis of LVH.

INTRODUCTION

Left ventricular hypertrophy (LVH) is a common finding in hypertensives, even in patients with mild hypertension without EKG changes[1], and represents a detrimental consequence of hypertension since it is associated with increased morbidity and mortality[2,3]. Furthermore, a growing amount of evidence suggests that regression of LVH is associated with a more favourable outcome as compared to either lack of regression or progression[4].

---

* Correspondence: Gian Paolo Rossi, M.D., FACC, Dipartimento di Medicina Clinica e Sperimentale, Policlinico Universitario, via Giustiniani, 2, 35126 Padova. Tel.: 049-821-2301, Fax: 049-875-4179 or 880-2252

Hypertension and the Heart, edited by Zanchetti et al.
Plenum Press, New York, 1997

It has been appreciated since long that for similar elevation of blood pressure (BP) the severity and type of LVH vary considerably in relation to genetic, demographic and bio-humoral factors[5,6]. Accordingly, the concept of a multifactorial aetiology of LVH is now widely accepted. Compelling evidence suggests that both the renin-angiotensin system (RAS) and the aldosterone excess play an important role in the pathogenesis of LVH. In fact, experimentally angiotensin II was found to cause myocardial cells hypertrophy and/or hyperplasia[5-7] and excess aldosterone has been related to extracellular matrix and collagen deposition and therefore to myocardial fibrosis[8-15]. Primary aldosteronism (PA) and renovascular hypertension (RVH) are rare causes of hypertension but, being charac-terised by hyperaldosteronism and contrasting levels of plasma renin activity, offer two models for investigating the relative role of the RAS and aldosterone on the heart in humans. In other terms, they furnish an example of the so called Bateson's approach "*Treasure your exceptions*" to the understanding of diseases. In this paper, we review the data concerning the LV changes in these two forms of secondary hypertension and discuss the insight that they have provided into the pathogenesis of LVH.

PRIMARY ALDOSTERONISM (PA)

In 1973, in a seminal paper Tarazi et al. reported that cardiac index was increased in patients with PA as compared to essential hypertensives (EH), a finding which could not be accounted for by an increased plasma volume[16]. The hypothesis of an enhanced contractility due to either a direct inotropic effect of aldosterone or to hypokalemia was therefore put for-ward, but could not be ascertained due to the lack of direct indexes of myocardial contractil-ity. In addition, no information on changes in LV wall thickness and mass was attainable. To investigate these issues we recently compared the Doppler echocardiography findings of 34 consecutive patients with confirmed PA with 34 EH, who were individually matched for demography, casual BP values, and known duration of hypertension[17]. The two groups dif-fered significantly for plasma aldosterone, which was higher (1,107±774 pmol/L vs 206±99, p<0.0001), and for serum potassium, supine baseline and captopril-stimulated plasma renin activity, which were lower in PA than in EH patients. The PA patients were found to have significantly thicker interventricular septum and LV posterior wall as compared to EH patients, whereas the end-systolic and end-diastolic LV diameter were similar. Stepwise multiple regression analysis showed that both the interventricular septum and the posterior wall thickness were directly related with plasma aldosterone levels and not with BP. Signifi-cantly more PA than EH patients had either LVH or LV concentric remodelling (Fig. 1) and therefore LVMI resulted to be significantly higher in the PA, as compared to the EH group.

LV ejection fraction (67±2% vs 62±1, p=0.22) and cardiac output (6.45±0.31 vs 5.53±20.21 L·min^{-1}, p=0.017) were also higher in PA than in matched EH patients[17], in keeping with the aforementioned Tarazi's report[17]. In order to establish whether an enhanced contractility might contribute to these enhanced load-dependent indexes of LV function, we determined the systolic midwall fractional shortening in our patients. This is an index of LV chamber dynamics that has been shown to more accurately reflect the LV myocardial performance, as compared to the endocardial fractional shortening[18,19]. We also assessed the systolic midwall fractional shortening/end-systolic meridional wall stress relationship, which was shown to identify a subgroup of hypertensive subjects with reduced LV function who are at increased cardiovascular risk[20]. No significant difference of this relationship between PA and EH patients was evident, suggesting that no change in the inotropic state of the LV occurred in our PA patients.

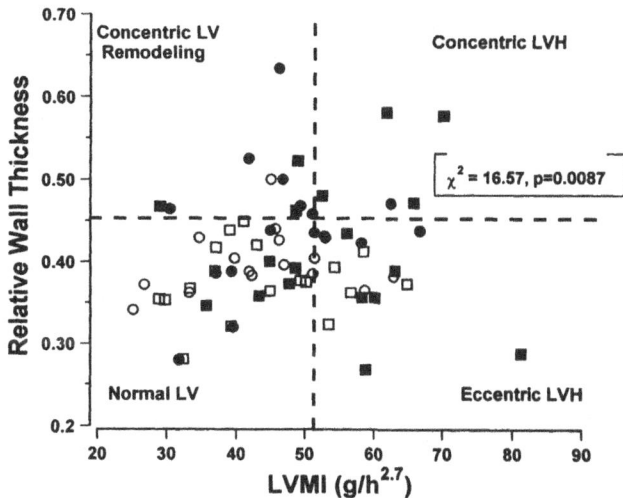

Figure 1. Individual values of LVMI and RWT in patients with primary aldosteronism (closed symbols) and matched EH (open symbols) patients (men = squares, women = circles). Vertical lines indicate the 97.5th percentile of the normal distribution $(51 g/m^2)^{17}$ in adult men and women. Horizontal line divides those with concentric LVH, or LV concentric remodeling, from those with eccentric LVH, or normal LV, respectively. Patients with primary aldosteronism had a significantly higher proportion of LVH and LV concentric remodeling by χ^2 test.

Since, as already mentioned, excess aldosterone was related to myocardial fibrosis, we sought for the changes of diastolic function. We measured the ratio of early and late diastolic transmitral flow velocity integral (E_i/A_i) in our patients. We found that it was significantly lower (0.91 ± 0.05 vs 1.25 ± 0.08, p<0.001) in the PA, as compared to EH group, and the atrial contribution to left ventricular filling (ACLVF) was significantly increased ($54.3\pm1.5\%$ vs 45.5 ± 1.3, p<0.001). In addition, these changes of LV filling were at least in part accounted for by a prolongation of the PQ interval in PA patients. Finally the E_i/A_i and ACLVF were inversely and directly related, respectively, with age and plasma aldosterone. Collectively these findings suggested that the LV of PA patients is more dependent upon the atrial kick for its filling.

FINDINGS IN CONN'S ADENOMA

The excess of aldosterone and the suppression of renin are usually even more marked in patients with Conn's adenoma, than in those with idiopathic hyperaldosteronism. We therefore carried out similar analyses in 26 PA patients with surgically confirmed Conn's adenoma, who were individually matched with EH patients in terms of demography and casual BP values. Although the two groups had superimposable average 24-hr BP values as well as average daytime and night-time BP and variability (as assessed from SD from the mean)[21], in patients with Conn's adenoma we found even more marked differences in terms of interventricular septum and LV free wall thickness, LVMI (118 ± 5 g/m^2 vs 100 ± 4, p=0.009), and changes of transmitral Doppler flow velocity indexes, as compared to EH. The integral of the early diastolic filling wave (E_i) (p=0.011), and the ratio E_i/A_i (A wave integral) (0.99 ± 0.08 vs 1.24 ± 0.10, p=0.038) were lower, and the atrial contribution to LV filling higher ($52\pm2\%$ vs 46 ± 2, p=0.038) in APA than in EH patients. Based on these findings, we concluded that excess aldosterone with suppression of the RAS is associated to an increase of LVMI and an

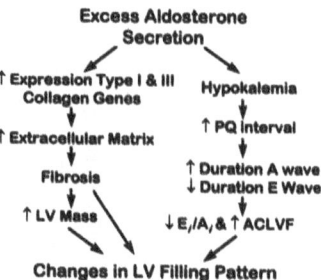

Figure 2. Schematic representation of the mechanisms associated with the changes in LV filling pattern determined with transmittal Doppler flow velocity in primary aldosteronism patients. E_i = E (early diastolic wave) integral; A_i = (late diastolic wave) integral; ACLV = Atrial contribution to left ventricular filling.

excess of LVH. This is in keeping with the results of Denolle et al[22], who also observed an increased LVMI in Conn's adenoma patients compared to both renovascular hypertensives and pheochromocytoma patients. However, we also observed an excess of LV concentric remodelling in patients with Conn's adenoma, as compared to EH patients with similar BP values. At variance with these results, Shigematsu et al[23] recently reported a very high prevalence of eccentric LVH in 23 PA compared to 116 EH patients (57% vs 22%, χ^2=11.1, p< 0.01). Based on the finding that most of their PA subjects with eccentric LVH had negligible evdence of target organ damage, they also suggested that LVH may precede the onset of other target organs damage, namely hypertensive retinopathy and renal involvement, in PA patients. This contention is consistent with our findings of no difference in the extent and severity of carotid artery lesions between PA and EH, as assessed with a high resolution ultrasound technique[24]. It also agrees with our observation of no difference in serum creatinine and blood urea nitrogen in a large series of PA[25], but not with that of Halimi and Mimran[26] that urinary β_2-microglobulin and albumin excretion rate is increased in untreated PA as compared to EH[26].

As regards diastolic function, the changes of LV filling in PA patients with Conn's adenoma, which we described[17,21] might be due in part to the prolongation of AV conduction time, due to hypertrophy, hypokalemia, and the effect of excess aldosterone, and in part to myocardial fibrosis. A schematic illustration of this hypothesis is depicted in Fig. 2.

EFFECTS OF ADRENALECTOMY

Twenty-five PA patients were studied again echocardiographically one year after removal of a Conn's adenoma or the initial evaluation while on medical therapy. A highly significant decrease of LV wall thickness and mass was observed in the surgically-treated patients, and to a much lesser extent in those pharmacologically treated[17,21]. Treatment was based on a multiple drug regimen and included aldosterone antagonists which stimulate the RAS. In the former patients the surgical excision of the tumour determined a regression to normal also of LV filling abnormalities, which did not occur in the latter patients despite a similar degree of control of BP. This regression of LVH is in agreement with the findings of Denolle et al.[22] Although caution is advised before drawing conclusions since the patients were not randomized to either surgical or medical treatment, these findings strengthen the contention that excess aldosterone may play an etiologic role in the LV morphological and functional changes that were observed.

RENOVASCULAR HYPERTENSION (RVH)

Although renin as been proposed as a risk factor for heart attack more than two decades ago[27,28], limited data concerning cardiac structure and function in RVH are available.

According to a study, patients with bilateral renal artery stenosis would be particularly susceptible to develop recurrent pulmonary oedema[29], a finding which was attributed to volume overload. In another study, patients with RVH were found to have a decreased LV systolic function, as assessed by LV fractional shortening, as compared to age- and sex-matched EH subjects[30]. The latter was subnormal (less than 26%) in 19% of 42 RVH vs. 0% of 42 matched EH (p<0.005). This depressed systolic function appeared to result from a greater LV dilatation and septal, but not LV posterior wall hypertrophy. These changes failed to offset the pressure overload, thereby accounting for an abnormally high end systolic stress. Of interest, subjects with bilateral renovascular stenosis had a higher cardiac output (3.9 ± 1.1 l/min/m^2) than those with unilateral stenosis (3.2 ± 1.1 l/min/m^2 p<0.05), a finding which was attributed to volume overload in the former. Patients with RVH and PA were compared from the echocardiographic standpoint in two studies. In a Japanese study 19 PA patients were compared with 19 demographically similar RVH patients with unilateral renal artery stenosis[31]. Although no difference of LV wall thickness, relative wall thickness and LVMI between groups was observed, LV end diastolic dimension was increased in PA patients. At variance, in a French study[22] LVMI tended to be higher and LV fractional shortening lower in 40 RVH as compared to 21 PA patients. This is in keeping with the aforementioned study by Vensel et al.[30]

CONCLUSIONS AND PERSPECTIVES

A definite proof of the contribution of the renin-angiotensin aldosterone system to the pathogenesis of LVH and myocardial fibrosis in humans is still lacking, as ethical reasons have prevented the attainment of conclusive histological evidence thus far. However, compelling experimental evidence as well as several clinical data are consistent with this contention. It is conceivable that upcoming new technologies for assessing the relative contribution of cardiac myocytes and fibrosis to LVH, such as MR imaging, ultrasonic backscatter analysis[32,33] and computer assisted videodensitometry, might provide in the near future a better insight into the role of the RAS and aldosterone in the pathogenesis of LVH as well as into the functional correlates of the different types of LVH in hypertensive patients. Investigation of secondary forms of hypertension, such as PA and RVH, where the mechanisms increasing blood pressure are better understood, will help to clarify the pathogenic mechanisms of one of the most common forms of heart disease.

REFERENCES

1. Liebson PR, Grandits G, Prineas R, Dianzumba S, Flack JM, Cutler JA, Grimm R, Stamler J: Echocardiographic correlates of left ventricular structure among 844 mildly hypertensive men and women in the Treatment of Mild Hypertension Study (TOMHS). *Circulation* 1993; 87:476–486.
2. Levy D, Garrison RJ, Savage DD, Kannel WB, Castelli WP: Prognostic implications of echocardiographically determined left ventricular mass in the Framingham Heart Study. *N Engl J Med* 1990; 322:1561–1566.
3. Koren MJ, Devereux RB, Casale PN, Savage DD, Laragh JH: Relation of left ventricular mass and geometry to morbidity and mortality in uncomplicated essential hypertension. *Ann Intern Med* 1991; 114:345–352.
4. White WB, Dey HM, Schulman P: Assessment of the daily blood pressure load as a determinant of cardiac function in patients with mild-to-moderate hypertension. *Am Heart J* 1989; 118:782–795.
5. Morgan HE, Baker KM: Cardiac hypertrophy. Mechanical, neural, and endocrine dependence. *Circulation* 1991; 83:13–25.
6. Iwai N, Ohmichi N, Nakamura Y, Kinoshita M: DD genotype of the angiotensin-converting enzyme gene is a risk factor for left ventricular hypertrophy. *Circulation* 1994; 90:2622–2628.

7. Geisterfer AA, Peach MJ, Owens GK: Angiotensin II induces hypertrophy, not hyperplasia, of cultured rat aortic smooth muscle cells. *Circ Res* 1988; 62:749–756.

8. Weber KT: Cardiac interstitium in health and disease: the fibrillar collagen network. *J Am Coll Cardiol* 1989; 13:1637–1652.

9. Weber KT, Sun Y, Campbell SE, Slight SH, Ganjam VK, Griffing GT, Swinfard RW, Diaz-Arias AA: Chronic mineralocorticoid excess and cardiovascular remodeling. *Steroids* 1995; 60:125–132.

10. Jalil JE, Doering CW, Janicki JS, Pick R, Clark WA, Abrahams C, Weber KT: Structural vs. contractile protein remodeling and myocardial stiffness in hypertrophied rat left ventricle. *J Mol Cell Cardiol* 1988; 20: 1179–1187.

11. Weber KT, Brilla CG, Campbell SE: Regulatory mechanisms of myocardial hypertrophy and fibrosis: results of in vivo studies. *Cardiology* 1992; 81:266–273.

12. Weber KT, Janicki JS, Pick R, Abrahams C, Shroff SG, Bashey RI, Chen, RM. Collagen in the hypertrophied, pressure-overloaded myocardium. *Circulation* 1987; 75:I40–7.

13. Weber KT, Brilla CG, Janicki JS, Reddy HK, Campbell SE: Myocardial fibrosis: role of ventricular systolic pressure, arterial hypertension, and circulating hormones. *Basic Res Cardiol* 1991; 86 Suppl 3:25–31.

14. Brilla CG, Zhou G, Matsubara L, Weber KT: Collagen metabolism in cultured adult rat cardiac fibroblasts: response to angiotensin II and aldosterone. *J Mol Cell Cardiol* 1994; 26:809–820.

15. Young M, Fullerton M, Dilley R, Funder J: Mineralocorticoids, hypertension, and cardiac fibrosis. *J Clin Invest* 1994; 93:2578–2583.

16. Tarazi RC, Ibrahim M, Bravo EL, Dustan HP: Hemodynamic characteristics of primary aldosteronism. *N Engl J Med* 1973; 289:1330–1335.

17. Rossi GP, Sacchetto A, Visentin P, Canali C, Graniero GR, Palatini P, Pessina AC: Changes in left ventricular anatomy and function in hypertension and primary aldosteronism. *Hypertension* 1996; 27:1039–1045.

18. Shimizu G, Hirota Y, Kita Y, Kawamura K, Saito T, Gaasch WH: Left Ventricular wall mechanics in systemic arterial hypertension: myocardial function is depressed in pressure-overload hypertrophy. *Circulation* 1991; 83:1676–1684.

19. de Simone G, Devereux RB, Roman MJ, Ganau A, Saba PS, Alderman MH, Laragh JH: Assessment of Left ventricular function by the Midwall Fractional Shortening/End-Systolic Stress relation in human hypertension. *J Am Coll Cardiol* 1994; 23:1444–1451.

20. de Simone G, Devereux RB, Koren MJ, Mensah GA, Casale PN, Laragh JH: Midwall Left Ventricular mechanics. An independent predictor of cardiovascular risk in essential hypertension. *Circulation* 1996; 93: 259–265.

21. Rossi GP, Sacchetto A, Pavan E, Palatini P, Graniero GR, Canali C, Pessina AC: Remodeling of the left ventricle in primary aldosteronism due to Conn's adenoma. *Circulation* 1997; 95: 1471–1478.

22. Denolle T, Chatellier G, Julien J, Battaglia C, Luo P, Plouin PF: Left ventricular mass and geometry before and after etiologic treatment in renovascular hypertension, aldosterone-producing adenoma, and pheochromocytoma. *Am J Hypertens* 1993; 6:907–913.

23. Shigematsu Y, Hamada M, Okayama H, Hara Y, Hayashi Y, Kodama K, Kohara K, Hiwada K: Left ventricular hypertrophy precedes other target-organ damage in primary aldosteronism. *Hypertension* 1997; 29:723–727.

24. Rossi G, Rossi A, Zanin L, Calabro A, Crepaldi G, Pessina AC: Prevalence of extracranial carotid artery lesions at duplex in primary aldosteronism. *Am J Hypertens* 1993; 6:8–14.

25. Rossi GP, Rossi E, Pavan E, Rosati N, Zecchel R, Sacchetto A, Perazzolo F, Semplicini A, Pessina AC: Identification of Conn's adenoma (CA) with a multivariate discriminant analysis (MDA). *Am J Hypertens* 1997; in press: (Abstract).

26. Halimi JM, Mimran A: Albuminuria in untreated patients with primary aldosteronism or essential hypertension. *J Hypertens* 1995; 13:1801–1802.

27. Alderman MH, Madhavan S, Ooi WL, Cohen H, Sealey JE, Laragh JH: Association of the renin-sodium profile with the risk of myocardial infarction in patients with hypertension. *N Engl J Med* 1991; 324:1098–1104.

28. Brunner HR, Laragh JH, Baer L, Newton MA, Goodwin FT, Krakoff LR, Bard RH, Buhler FR: Essential hypertension:renin and aldosterone, heart attack and stroke. *N Engl J Med* 1972; 286:441–449.

29. Pickering TG, Herman L, Devereux RB, Sotelo JE, James GD, Sos TA, Silane MF, Laragh JH: Recurrent pulmonary oedema in hypertension due to bilateral renal artery stenosis: treatment by angioplasty or surgical revascularisation. *Lancet* 1988; 2:551–552.

30. Vensel LA, Devereux RB, Pickering TG, Herrold EM, Borer JS, Laragh, JH. Cardiac structure and function in renovascular hypertension produced by unilateral and bilateral renal artery stenosis. *Am J Cardiol* 1986; 58:575–582.

31. Suzuki T, Abe H, Nagata S, Saitoh F, Iwata S, Ashizawa A, Kuramochi, M, Omae T: Left ventricular structural characteristics in unilateral renovascular hypertension and primary aldosteronism. *Am J Cardiol* 1988; 62:1224–1227.

32. Wong AK, Verdonk ED, Hoffmeister BK, Miller JG, Wickline SA: Detection of unique transmural architecture of human idiopathic cardiomyopathy by ultrasonic tissue characterization. *Circulation* 1992; 86: 1108–1115.

33. Lucarini AR, Gigli G, Lattanzi F, Picano E, Mazzarisi A, Iannetti M, Landini L: Regression of hypertensive myocardial hypertrophy does not affect ultrasonic myocardial reflectivity: a tissue characterization study. *J Hypertens.* 1994; 12:73–79.

8

HYPERTENSION DIFFERENTIALLY AFFECTS THE EXPRESSION OF THE GAP JUNCTION PROTEIN CONNEXIN43 IN CARDIAC MYOCYTES AND AORTIC SMOOTH MUSCLE CELLS

Jacques-Antoine Haefliger,[1][*] Einar Castillo,[1] Gérard Waeber,[1] Jean-François Aubert,[2] Pascal Nicod,[1] Bernard Waeber,[2] and Paolo Meda[3]

[1]Department of Internal Medicine B
[2]Division of Hypertension
University Hospital
CHUV-1011 Lausanne
[3]Department of Morphology
University of Geneva
CMU,1211 Genève 4
Switzerland

ABSTRACT

Electrical and mechanical coupling of myocytes in heart and of smooth muscle cells in the aortic wall is thought to be mediated by intercellular channels aggregated at gap junctions. Connexin43 (Cx43) is one of the predominant membrane proteins forming junctional channels in the cardiovascular system. This study was undertaken to assess its expression during experimental hypertension. Rats were made hypertensive by clipping one renal artery (two-kidney, one-clip renal hypertension) or by administering deoxycorticosterone and salt (DOCA-salt hypertension). After four weeks, rats from both models showed a similar increase in intra-arterial mean blood pressure, as well as in the thickness of both aorta and heart walls. Northern blot analysis showed that, compared to controls, hypertensive rats expressed twice more Cx43 in aorta, but not in heart. These results suggest that localized mechanical forces induced by hypertension are major tissue-specific regulators of Cx43 expression.

* Corresponding author: J.-A. Haefliger, PhD, Department of Internal Medicine B, Laboratory of Molecular Biology 19-135, Centre Hospitalier Universitaire Vaudois, CHUV-1011 Lausanne, Switzerland. Tel: (41) 21 340.09.27, Fax: (41) 21 314.06.30, E-mail: jhaeflig@chuv.hospvd.ch

Hypertension and the Heart, edited by Zanchetti et al.
Plenum Press, New York, 1997

1. INTRODUCTION

1.1. Connexins and Gap Junction Channels

Virtually all cells of multicellular systems are connected by gap junctions[1,2]. These structures are seen at sites where the plasma membranes of two adjacent cells become closely apposed, reducing the intercellular space, which is usually about 200 nm wide, to a narrow gap of 2 nm (Figures 1 and 2). In these regions, the two interacting membranes feature specialized microdomains characterized by the concentration of uniformely large protein assemblies named connexins (Figures 1 and 2).

These structures provide the wall of intercellular channels, that allow for the passage of ions as well as for the exchange of metabolites and second messengers up to 1kDa[3,4] from one cell to another. Such a direct cell-to-cell exchange of molecules can be visualized using exogenous tracers, such as Lucifer Yellow. After microinjection into individual cells, the intercellular diffusion of this tracer, which cannot cross the cell membrane, can be directly observed under a fluorescence microscope (Figure 2)[5]. Gap junction channels are formed by the hexameric assembly of membrane-spanning proteins (Figures 1 and 2), known as connexins, which in mammals belong to a family of 13 members[2]. Four of these proteins, referred to as Cx43, Cx45, Cx40 and Cx37 have been identified in the cardiovascular system[6,7]. As yet, little is known about their role and their possible changes in cardiovascular diseases.

1.2. Connexins of Muscle Cells of Heart and Aorta

Gap junctions ensure the electrical and mechanical coupling of different types of muscle cells[8,9]. Such a role is critical in the heart, since proper propulsion of blood in the circulatory system obligatory depends on the coordinated contraction of both atrial and ventricular cardiomyocytes. This contraction, in turn, is mediated by the rapid propagation of action potentials to multiple cells that should depolarize in coordination. These events are dependent on gap junctional communication, whereby adjacent cardiomyocytes exchange current-carrying ions. By diffusing from one cell to the next, these ions synchronize the electrical and mechanical activity of neighbor cells[10].

Coordination of smooth muscle cells of the vascular wall is also critical to the local modulation of vasomotor tone, thus contributing to the proper function of large vessels. The aorta, which is a sparsely innervated and electrically quiescent vascular tissue, is likely to be particulary dependent on gap junctional communication for coordinating the responses of smooth muscle cells to diverse neural and endothelial signals[11–17]. Thus, conditions perturbing the function of the aortic wall, as observed during chronic hypertension, are expected to be associated to alterations of connexins, gap junctions or coupling.

1.3. Models of Hypertension

To test this hypothesis, we have assessed whether the expression of Cx43, the physiologically predominant connexin of myocardial cells[10] and aortic smooth muscle cells[16,18], is altered during chronic hypertension. To this end, we have investigated two rat models characterized by a similar degree of hypertension and hypertrophy of both aorta and heart, but differing markedly by the mechanism causing these changes. In the two kidney, one-clip model (2K,1C), hypertension was produced by clipping one renal artery, leading to stimulation of renin secretion and to an angiotensin II-dependent elevation of blood pres-

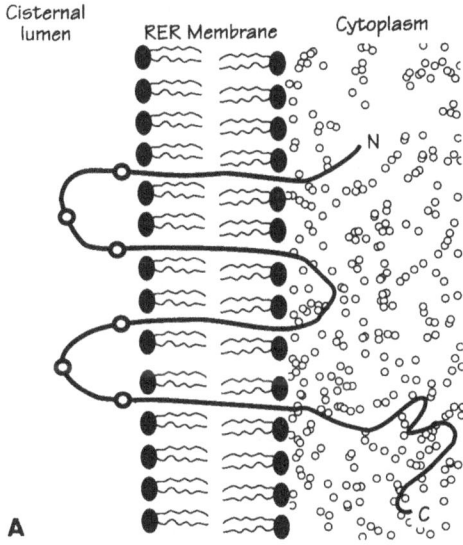

A

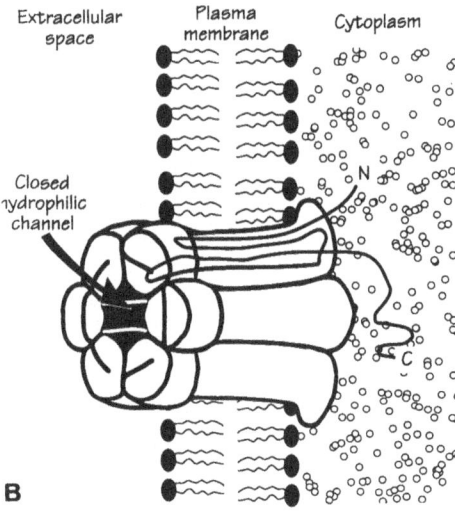

B

Figure 1. Topography of a connexin channel. **A)** During biosynthesis, connexin proteins are inserted in the membrane of rough endoplasmic reticulum (RER), which they cross four times. This arrangement provides for two loops in the cisternal lumen, and for the location of both C- and N-termini in the cytoplasm. All connexins feature three cysteine residues (open circles) in the two intracisternal loops. The C-terminus varies in sequence and length in different connexins. **B)** During their intracellular transport, connexins arrange as hexamers to form a tubular structure (called connexin) around a hydrophilic space of 2 nm diameter that extends across the entire length of the membrane. **C)** At gap junctions, connexins of one cell dock with those made by an adjacent cell. The alignment of two apposed connexins forms the wall of a channel, which directly links the cytoplasms of two neighbour cells. Modified from *Méd. Hyg.*, 1997, Vol. 55, pp. 270–274,[5] by copyright permission of the editor.

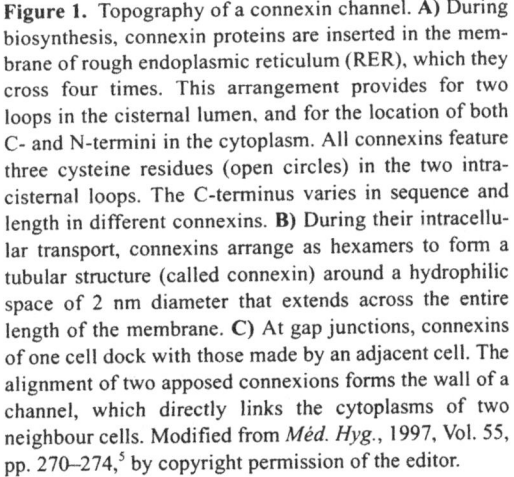

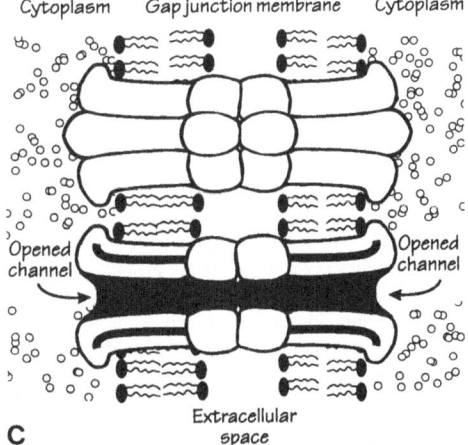

C

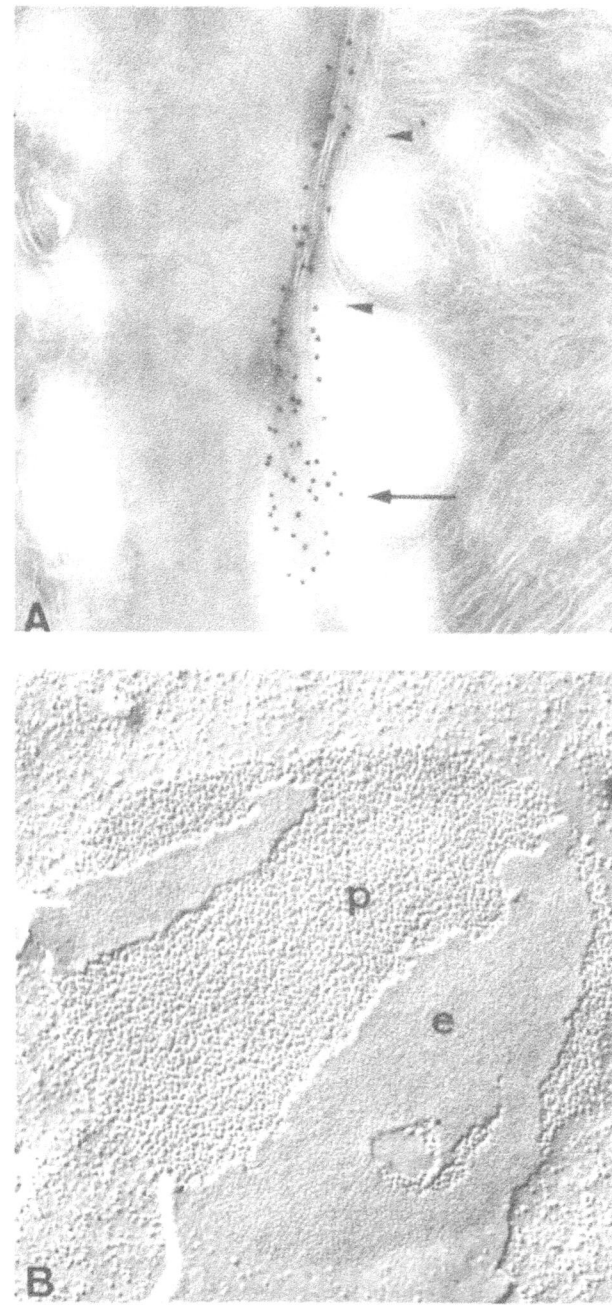

Figure 2. Connexins, gap junctions, and junctional coupling. **A)** Immunostaining with antibodies and protein A-gold particles reveals the plaque arrangement of connexins in regions where two plasma membranes are closely apposed, reducing the intercellular space to a gap of 2 nm (arrowheads). **B)** By freeze-fracture electron microscopy, gap junctions are identified as intramembrane aggregates of proteic particles, each representing a connexin, on the protoplasmic face (P) of the membrane. The imprints of connexins which are observed on the exoplasmic face (E) of the membrane indicate that gap junction channels entirely cross the plasma membranes of two adjacent cells.

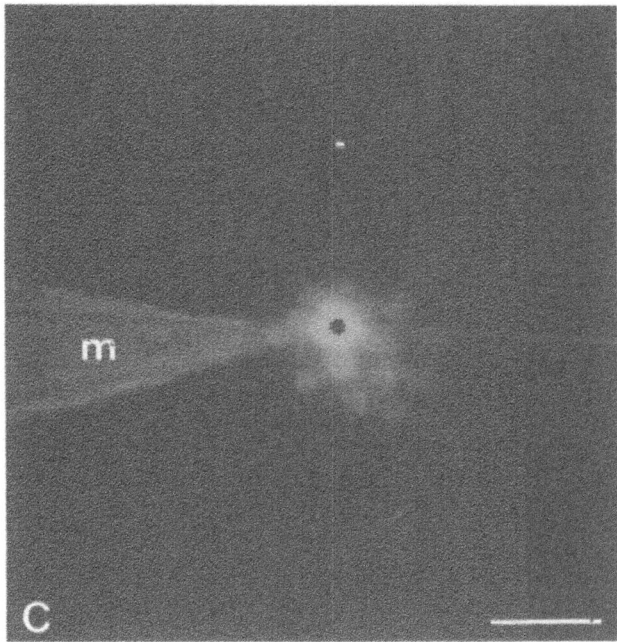

Figure 2. *(Continued.)* **C)** Microinjection of one cell with Lucifer Yellow, is immediately followed by the passage of this vital tracer in neighbouring cells connected by gap junction channels. This event is referred to as intercellular or junctional coupling. The microelectrode used to inject the dye is labelled by m. Bar represents 190 nm in A and B, and 22 μm in C. Reproduced from *Méd. Hyg.*, 1997, Vol. 55, pp. 270–274,[5] by copyright permission of the editor.

sure[19,20]. In the mineralocorticoid-salt induced model (DOCA-salt), hypertension results from sodium retention while renin secretion is suppressed[21-23].

2. RESULTS

2.1. Characteristics of Rats

The characteristics of the different groups of rats studied are shown in Table 1. There was no significant difference in body weight between 2K,1C and sham-operated rats. In contrast, body weight of DOCA-salt hypertensive rats was significantly lower than that of the corresponding controls. Mean intra-arterial blood pressure of both 2K,1C and DOCA-salt animals was similarly elevated compared to that of corresponding normotensive controls. There was no significant difference in heart rate between the four groups of animals (not shown).

2.2. Effects of Hypertension on the Aorta

As shown in Table 1 and Figure 3, the thickness of the aortic wall (intima plus media layers) was significantly larger in hypertensive than in normotensive animals, resulting in a 30% increase of the vessel cross-sectional area, in spite of a constant lumen radius. These changes resulted from an enlargment of smooth muscle cells, whose numeri-

Table 1. Characteristics of normotensive and hypertensive rats

Groups	Number of rats	Body weight (g)	Mean blood pressure (mm Hg)	Lumen radius (μm)	Media-intima thickness (μm)	Cross sectional area (10^4 μm^2)	Smooth muscle cells Numerical density (μm^{-2})	Profile area (μm^2)
2K,1C	9	295 ± 9	203.4 ± 7.9***	632 ± 7	78.6 ± 2.8***	33.2 ± 1.2***	4.4 ± 0.1*** n=96	70.1 ± 1.8*** m=399
Sham	9	294 ± 6	128.4 ± 1.5	636 ± 10	55.6 ± 1.6	23.2 ± 0.7	4.9 ± 0.1 n=88	61.4 ± 1.3 m=320
DOCA-salt	6	248 ± 7***	192.3 ± 8.5***	626 ± 14	81.7 ± 1.8***	34.1 ± 0.5**	3.8 ± 0.1*** n=24	68.5 ± 1.8*** m=240
Controls	6	296 ± 9	134.3 ± 3.3	649 ± 21	56.3 ± 2.4	23.9 ± 1.2	4.3 ± 0.1 n=24	60.6 ± 1.6 m=240

2K,1C: two-kidney, one-clip hypertension model; DOCA-salt: deoxycorticosterone-salt hypertension model
Numerical density = number of cells/1000 μm^2; (n = number of aortic fields measured)
Profile area = average size of smooth muscle cells; (m = number of smooth muscle cells measured)
**p.01 vs control
***p.001 vs sham or control
Reproduced from *Circulation*, 1997, Vol. 95, pp. 1007–1014,[24] by copyright permission of the American Heart Association.

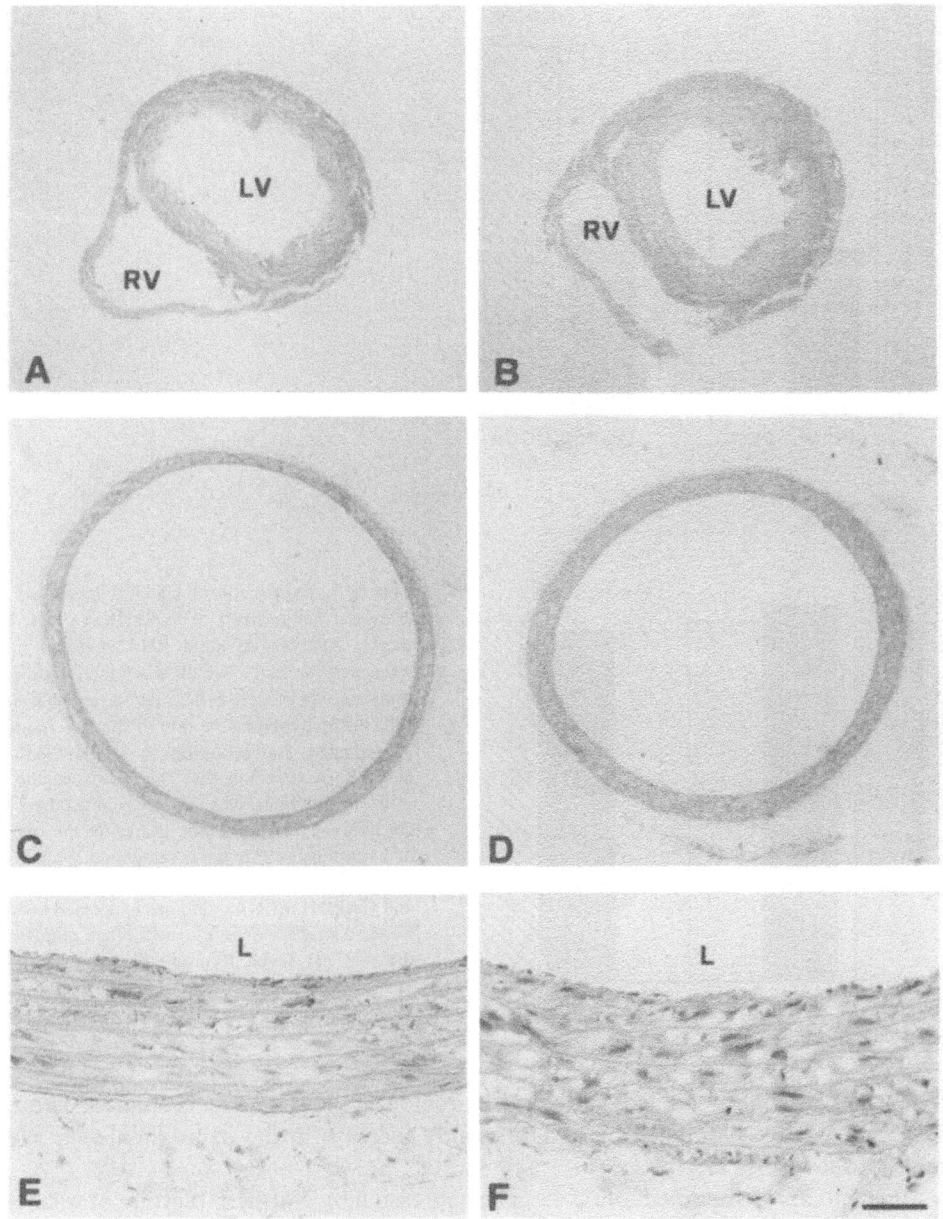

Figure 3. Thickening of ventricular and aortic walls in hypertensive rats. After four weeks of hypertension, left ventricular wall (LV) was thicker in 2K,1C (B) and DOCA-salt treated hypertensive rats than in normotensive controls (A), whereas no difference was observed in the right ventricule (RV). Also, the aorta of 2K,1C (D), and DOCA-salt treated rats showed a significantly thicker wall than that of normotensive controls (C), in spite of a similar internal diameter. At higher magnification, the thickened arterial wall of hypertensive rats (F) contained smooth muscle cells that were hypertrophic compared to those of corresponding controls (E). L indicates the lumen of the vessel. The bar represents 2 mm in A and B, 320 μm in D and C and 43 μm in F and E. Modified from *Circulation*, 1997, Vol. 95, pp. 1007–1014,[24] by copyright permission of the American Heart Association.

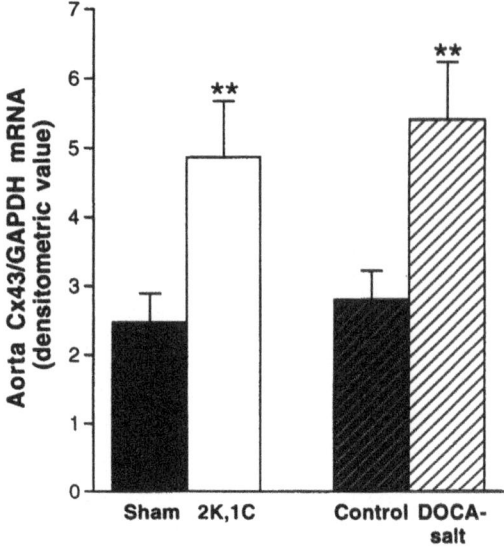

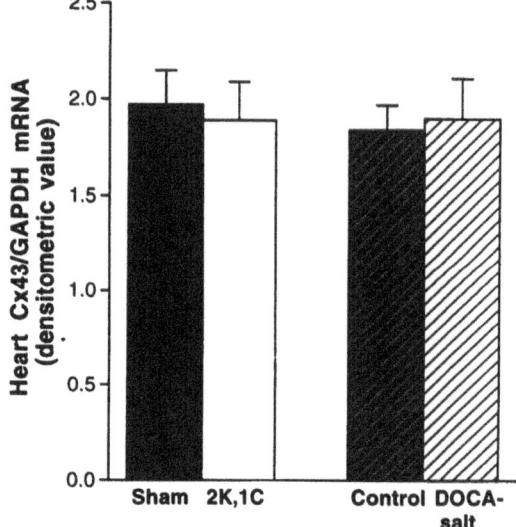

Figure 4. Expression of Cx43 is increased in the aorta but not in heart of hypertensive rats. **Upper panel:** Analysis of aorta RNA revealed that the transcript for Cx43, which was mostly contributed to by smooth muscle cells, was increased about two fold in the hypertensive rats of the two models we investigated. **Lower panel:** A similar analysis of heart RNA revealed that the levels of the Cx43 transcript, which was mostly contributed to by cardiomyocytes, were not altered in the two types of hypertensive rats we investigated. Values represent ratios of densitometric measurements of Cx43 and GAPDH mRNAs, and are expressed as mean ± SEM. Asterisks denote a difference significant at the p < .01 level. Reproduced from *Circulation*, 1997, Vol. 95, pp. 1007–1014,[24] by copyright permission of the American Heart Association.

cal density was slightly reduced in the media region of the two models studied. These cellular changes were paralleled by a significantly increase in the expression of α-skeletal actin (not shown).

Quantitative assessment of Cx43 gene expression by Northern blotting of total RNA, showed significantly higher values in the aorta of hypertensive than of normotensive rats (Figure 4). These changes were paralleled by a modest but sizeable increase in the amount of Cx43 protein that could be immunolabelled on cryosections of aorta[24].

2.3. Effects of Hypertension on the Heart

Hypertensive rats showed a 30% increase in heart index compared to normotensive counterparts (not shown). In agreement with this change, Northern blot analysis showed a two fold increase in the expression of α-skeletal actin mRNA in the two groups of hypertensive rats (not shown) and histology revealed a thickening of the left ventricular wall (Figure 3)

Quantitative assessment by Northern blot analysis, showed that Cx43 expression was similar in the hypertrophied hearts of hypertensive rats and in those of normotensive controls (Figure 4). This finding correlated with the absence of significant differences in the amount of Cx43 which could be immunolabelled in heart muscle (not shown).

3. DISCUSSION

We have examined the effects of chronic experimental hypertension on the expression of Cx43, the major native connexin of the cardiovascular system[25,26]. We have found that hypertension is associated with increased levels of Cx43 within the wall of the aorta, in two different rat models that are characterized by comparable changes in blood pressure but that differ in the mechanism leading to these changes.

In the 2K,1C model, the development of hypertension results from the constriction of one renal artery and the ensuing activation of the renin-angiotensin system[20], as reflected by enhanced renin mRNA levels in the hypoperfused kidney and by elevated plasma renin activity[27]. The further proteolytic cleavage of angiotensinogen by renin and the processing of angiotensin I by the angiotensin converting enzyme leads to the generation of the biologically active angiotensin II (AngII). AngII is a most potent vasoconstrictor peptide which also plays a role in the development of vascular and cardiac hypertrophy[28,29]. Therefore, cellular changes observed in 2K,1C rats could be due to both the increased blood pressure and the increased levels of AngII. To discriminate between these possibilities, we have studied the DOCA-salt model, which is characterized by the functional suppression of the renin-angiotensin system. In this model, hypertension is induced by administration of a salt-retaining mineralocorticoid in association with a high sodium intake[21].

After one month, the increase in blood pressure achieved in the two models was comparable, and the two groups of hypertensive animals also exhibited a similar degree of thickening of the aorta wall, which was mostly accounted for by the hypertrophy of smooth muscle cells and the accumulation of extracellular materials. All hypertensive rats also featured a comparable two fold increase in the level of Cx43 expressed by the smooth muscle cells of the aortic media. This change could not be related to the circulating levels of AngII which differed considerably in the 2K,1C and the DOCA-salt hypertensive rats and, hence, is likely to be associated with the elevation of blood pressure.

The molecular mechanism leading to the pressure-induced increase in the expression of the Cx43 gene remains to be elucidated. The presence of multiple promoters in the 5' untranslated region of this gene[30,31] raises the possibility that the tissue-specific regulation of the increase we observed is controlled by distinct transcription factors[32-35]. Of particular interest is this context is the recent finding that transcription of Cx43 gene may be promoted by an increase in the expression of c-fos[36], since the mRNA coding for this transcription factor accumulates in smooth muscle cells of rat aortas following exposure to angiotensin II[37,38], that contributes to hypertension in the 2K,1C model.

The reasons why Cx43 increases during hypertension also remain to be elucidated. In view of several electrophysiological studies which have suggested that gap junction proteins may coordinate the mechanical contraction of smooth muscle cells[12,13,39], it is possible that Cx43 is implicated in modulating the vasomotor tone of the aortic wall. Certainly, Cx43 channels can provide an intercellular pathway for the syncitial functioning of smooth muscle cells, that could be recruited for synchronous contraction through propagation of gap junction-permeant second messengers[16].

Under the conditions we studied, hypertensive animals also featured a significant cardiac hypertrophy[24], but failed to show significant differences in the level of expression of Cx43 between myocardial cells. This finding suggests that Cx43 is not involved in the myocardial adaptation that accompanies a hypertension-induced increase in heart load. Obviously, this conclusion does not rule out the possibility of changes in other connexins (Cx45, Cx40, Cx37) which colocalize with Cx43 at myocardial[7,40] and endothelial cell gap junctions[18]. Indeed, the recent inactivation of the Cx43 gene in transgenic mice[41] suggests that, at least under certain conditions, Cx43 may be functionally replaced by another connexin. Thus, lack of Cx43 was compatible with survival of mouse embryos to term. However, homozygous knock-out embryos died at birth, as a result of the blockage of the right ventricular outflow tract[41]. This finding emphasises the possibility that Cx40, and perhaps also Cx45 and Cx37, have the potential to functionally compensate for Cx43[42].

In summary, we have found that the expression of Cx43 is differentially regulated in the hypertrophic muscle cells of heart and aorta, and that this differential regulation takes place in rats made similarly hypertensive by different mechanisms. Further studies are however needed to understand how the changes in Cx43 expression participate to the adaptative response of the aorta to high blood pressure.

ACKNOWLEDGMENTS

J.-A.H. is supported by a career award from the Max Cloëtta Foundation. This work was supported by grants from the Swiss National Science Foundation (31-46770.96 to J.-A.H., 32-31915.91 and 32-29317.91 to G.W., 32-0338.05 to B.W., 32-43086.95 to P.M.) and the European Union BMH4-CT96-1427 (to P.M.).

REFERENCES

1. Meda P: Molecular biology of gap junction proteins. Mol Biol of diabetes, Part I 1994;14:333–356.
2. Bennett MVL, Barrio LC, Bargiello TA, Spray DC, Hertzberg E, Saez JC: Gap junctions: new tools, new answers, new questions. Neuron 1991;6:305–320.
3. Beyer EC, Goodenough DA, Paul DL: The connexins, a family of related gap junction proteins, in Herzberg EL, Johnson RG (eds): Gap Junction. New-York, Alan R. Liss, 1988, pp 167–175.
4. Loewenstein WR: Junctional intercellular communication. The cell-to-cell membrane channel. Physiological Reviews 1981;61:829–913.
5. Haefliger J-A, Waeber G, Meda P: Communication intercellulaire par les canaux jonctionnels "GAP": Rôle en endocrinologie. Méd Hyg 1997;55:270–274.
6. Haefliger J-A, Bruzzone R, Jenkins NA, Gilbert DJ, Copeland NG, Paul DL: Four novel members of the connexin family of gap junction proteins: molecular cloning, expression and chromosome mapping. J Biol Chem 1992;267:2057–2064.
7. Kanter HL, Laing JG, Beyer EC, Green KG, Saffitz JE: Multiple connexins colocalize in canine ventricular myocyte gap junctions. Circ Res 1993;73:344–350.
8. Spray DC, Burt JM: Structure-activity relations of cardiac gap-junction channel. Am J of Physiol 1990; 258:C195–C205.
9. Christ GJ: Modulation of a_1-adrenergic contractility in isolated vascular tissue by heptanol: A functional demonstration of the potential importance of intercellular communication to vascular response generation. Life Sciences 1995;56:709–721.
10. Severs NJ: Pathophysiology of gap junctions in heart disease. Journal of Cardiovascular Electrophysiology 1994;5:462–475.
11. Segal SS: Cell-to-Cell communication coordinates blood flow control. Hypertension 1994;23:1113–1120.

12. Segal SS, Duling BR: Flow control among microvessels coordinated by intercellular conduction. Science 1986;234:868–870.

13. Larson DM, Haudenschild CC, Beyer EC: Gap junction messenger RNA expression by vascular wall cells. Circ Res 1990;66:1074–1080.

14. Moore LK, Beyer EC, Burt JM: Characterisation of gap junction channels in A7r5 vascular smooth muscle cells. American J physiol 1991;260:C975–C981.

15. Christ GJ, Moreno AP, Parker ME, Gondre CM, Valcic M, Melman A, Spray DC: Intercellular communication through gap junctions: A potential role in pharmacomechanical coupling and syncytial tissue contraction in vascular smooth muscle isolated from the human corpus cavernosum. Life Science 1991;49:PL-195–PL-200.

16. Christ GJ, Brink PR, Zhao W, Moss J, Gondré CM, Roy C, Spray DC: Gap junctions modulate tissue contractility and alpha adrenergic agonist efficacy in isolated rat aorta. The journal of pharmacology and experimental therapeutics 1993;266:1054–1065.

17. Christ GJ, Spray DC, El-Sabban M, Moore LK, Brink PR: Gap junction in vascular tissues. Evaluating the role of the intercellular communication in the modulation of vasomotor tone. Circ Res 1996;79:631–646.

18. Bruzzone R, Haefliger J-A, Gimlich RL, Paul DL: Connexin40, a component of gap junctions in vascular endothelium, is restricted in its ability to interact with other connexins. Mol Biol of the Cell 1993;4:7–20.

19. Goldblatt H, Lynch J, Hanzal RF, Summerville WW: Studies on experimental hypertension: production of persistent elevation of systolic blood pression by means of renal ischemia. J Exp Med 1934;59:347–379.

20. Leenen FHH, De Jong W, De Wied D: Renal venous and peripheral plasma renin activity in renal hypertension. Am J Physiol 1973;225:1513–1518.

21. Gavras H, Brunner HR, Larah JH, Vaughn ED, Koss M, Cote LJ, Gavras I: Malignant hypertension resulting from deoxycorticosterone acetate and salt excess. Circ Res 1975;36:300–309.

22. Schiffrin EL, St-Louis J: Decreased density of vascular receptors for atrial natriuretic peptide in DOCA-salt hypertensive rats. Hypertension 1987;9:504–512.

23. Liu DT, Birchall I, Hewitson T, Kincaid-Smith P, Whitworth JA: Effect of dietary calcium on the development of hypertension and hypertensive vascular lesions in DOCA-salt and two-kidney, one clip hypertensive rats. Journal of Hypertension 1994;12:145–153.

24. Haefliger J-A, Castillo E, Waeber G, Bergonzelli GE, Aubert J-F, Sutter E, Nicod P, Waeber B, Meda P: Hypertension increases connexin43 In a tissue specific manner. Circulation 1997;95:1007–1014.

25. Beyer EC, Paul DL, Goodenough DA: Connexin 43: A protein from rat heart homologous to a gap junction protein from liver. J Cell Biol 1987;105:2621–2629.

26. Beyer EC, Kistler J, Paul DL, Goodenough DA: Antisera directed against connexin43 peptides react with a 43-KD protein localized to gap junctions in myocardium and other tissues. J Cell Biol 1989;108:595–605.

27. Haefliger J-A, Bergonzelli G, Waeber G, Aubert J-F, Nussberger J, Gavras H, Nicod P, Waeber B: Renin and angiotensin II receptor gene expression in kidneys of renal hypertensive rats. Hypertension 1995;26:733–737.

28. Levy BI, Michel J-B, Salzmann J-L, Azizi M, Poitevin P, Safar M, Camilleri J-P: Effects of chronic inhibition of converting enzyme on mechanical and structural properties of arteries in rat renovascular hypertension. Circulation Research 1988;63:227–239.

29. Morishita R, Higaki J, Miyazaki M, Ogihara T: Possible Role of the Vascular Renin-Angiotensin System in Hypertension and Vascular Hypertrophy. Hypertension 1992;19:II-62–II-67.

30. Yu W, Dahl G, Werner R: The connexin43 gene is responsive to oestrogen. Proc R Soc Lond B Biol Sci 1994;255:125–132.

31. Chen Z-Q, Lefebvre DL, Bai X-H, Reaume A, Rossant J, Lye SJ: Identification of two regulatory elements within the promoter region of the mouse Cx-43 gene. J Biol Chem 1995;270:3863–3868.

32. Risek B, Guthrie S, Kumar N, Gilula NB: Modulation of gap junction transcript and protein expression during pregnancy in the rat. J Cell Biol 1990;110:269–282.

33. Chow L, Lye SJ: Expression of the gap junction protein, Connexin-43 is increased of the human myometrium towards term and with the onset of labour. Am J Obstet Gynecol 1994;170:788–795.

34. Petrocelli T, Lye SJ: Regulation of transcripts encoding the myometrial gap junction protein, connexin-43, by estrogen and progesterone. Endocrinology 1993;133:284–290.

35. Piersanti M, Lye SJ: Increase in messenger ribonucleic acid encoding the myometrial gap junction protein, connexin-43, requires protein synthesis and is associated with increased expression of the activator protein-1, c-fos. Endocrinology 1995;136:3571–3578.

36. Lefebvre DL, Piersanti M, Bai X-H, Chen Z-Q, Lye SJ: Myometrial transcriptional regulation of the gap junction gene, connexin-43. Reprod Fertil Devel 1996;7:603–611.

37. Taubman MB, Berk BC, Izumo S, Tsuda T, Alexander RW, Nadal-Ginard B: Angiotensin II induces c-fos mRNA in aortic smooth muscle. J Biol Chem 1989;264:526–530.

38. Naftilan AJ, Pratt RE, Eldridge CS, Lin HL, Dzau VJ: Angiotensin II induces c-fos expression in smooth muscle via transcriptional control. Hypertension 1989;13:706–711.
39. Wathers DC, Porter DG: Effect of uterine distension and estrogen treatment on gap junction formation in the myometrium of the rat. J Reprod and Fert 1982;65:497–505.
40. Bastide B, Neyses L, Ganten D, Paul M, Willecke K, Traub O: Gap Junction Protein Connexin40 is preferentially expressed in vascular endothelium and conductive bundles of rat and is increased under hypertensive conditions. Circ Res 1993;73:1138–1149.
41. Reaume AG, de Sousa PA, Kulkarni S, Langille BL, Zhu D, Davies TC, Juneja SC, Kidder GM, Rossant J: Cardiac malformation in neonatal mice lacking connexin43. Science 1995;267:1831–1834.
42. Gros DB, Jongsma HJ: Connexins in mammalian heart function. Bioessays 1996;18:719–730.

9

MODULATION OF CARDIAC HYPERTROPHY BY ESTROGENS

Theo Pelzer, Asiya Shamim, Simone Wölfges, Michael Schumann, and Ludwig Neyses*

Department of Medicine
University of Würzburg
Josef-Schneider-Str. 2
D-97080 Würzburg
Germany

1. SUMMARY

Gender-specific differences in heart disease have long been known but it has only been since the advent of molecular biology that it has become possible to investigate the molecular mechanisms.

Most biochemical work in the last 50 years has focused on the characterization of the steroid hormones involved in gender specificity. More recently, the cloning of the steroid receptors and characterization of the signaling pathways through these proteins has given new insights into the mechanisms underlying the mode of action of steroid hormones. It has also become clear that the steroid receptors can be classified into families (receptors for thyroid hormone, glucocorticoids, estrogens, androgens, retinoic acid, and so called orphan receptors of mostly unknown function). The structures of these receptors show very close resemblance and all are DNA-binding proteins acting as transcription factors. Some (if not all) act as repressors of transcription of some genes in the native state and are converted to activators (or perhaps repressors of other genes) upon binding of the cognate hormone.

Naturally, classical target tissues for estrogens and androgens have been studied first and only in very recent years has it been recognized that estrogens and androgens act on a much wider spectrum of tissues.

In the cardiovascular field, the beneficial effect of estrogen replacement therapy in postmenopausal women which reduces the incidence of cardiovascular disease by some 40% and the lower incidence of cardiovascular disease in premenopausal women have mostly been explained by the beneficial action of estrogens on the lipid profile (increase

* Corresponding author: Tel.: +49-931-201-2774, Fax.: +49-931-210-2291.

Hypertension and the Heart, edited by Zanchetti et al.
Plenum Press, New York, 1997

83

in HDL and decrease in LDL cholesterol). Recently, functional estrogen receptors have also been shown in vascular smooth muscle cells and in the endothelium.

Our own group has characterized the presence of estrogen receptors in the myocardium and in cardiac fibroblasts. We have also shown that these receptors are transcriptionally active because they are able to drive a minigene composed of a triple estrogen responsive DNA regulatory element (promoter) coupled to the firefly luciferase gene which serves as a reporter by way of its ability to drive a light-emitting reaction.

We are in the process of characterizing the target genes for estrogen in the myocardium. A specific series of immediate-early genes is induced by estradiol (the major pre-menopausal estrogen) and we have also characterized a number of tissue-specific genes whose expression is driven by estrogens in the myocardium.

The ultimate goal of these investigations is to explore the use of estrogens in the treatment of cardiac hypertrophy (and failure) by way of their properties to counteract (at least some of) the pathological switches in gene expression in these disease entities.

2. INTRODUCTION

The beneficial effect of estrogens on lipid metabolism (1) and the formation of atherosclerotic plaques in arterial vessels (2) has long been described, but the magnitude of these effects does not fully explain their protective action (3). Thus, additional and presently unknown mechanisms must be operative. In our current understanding, the effects of estrogens are either genomic (i.e. mediated by changes in gene expression) or non-genomic (i.e. independent of changes in gene expression) and will be discussed in this order. The genomic action of estrogens in the heart also affects directly the gene expression of cardiac myocytes; these effects are currently a major interest of our own laboratory.

In this context, gender specific differences in the incidence of cardiovascular disease were first recognized more than 50 years ago (4). Whereas the risk of heart disease in men increases constantly with age, pre-menopausal women have a significantly lower risk that increases rapidly to levels comparable with their male counterparts after menopause if they do not receive estrogens. In fact, the cardiovascular mortality in postmenopausal women receiving estrogen substitution is 30% to 50% less than in their untreated counterparts (5). Thus, estrogens are among the major determinants of cardiovascular disease. From this viewpoint it seems tempting to employ estrogens in the prevention and therapy of heart disease. However, at present the therapeutic application of estrogens in heart disease is limited by the fact that the underlying mechanisms are only partially understood.

We will here discuss general principles of estrogen action and some of the newer findings on the action of estrogens on the myocardium. Effects on the coronary vasculature (smooth muscle cells and endothelium) which have also been demonstrated recently (6) will not be discussed.

3. GENERAL PRINCIPLES OF ESTROGEN ACTION

Estrogens are members of the steroid hormone family, which also include adrenal steroids and vitamin D3. Biochemical studies in the 1970s and 1980s demonstrated that steroids reversibly bind to specific intracellular receptor proteins. Ligand binding induces a conformational change of the receptor. This facilitates binding of the hormone-receptor complex to highly conserved DNA sequences, termed hormone response elements (HRE), in the promoter region of specific target genes (7). In the case of the estrogen receptor (ER), hormone binding is followed by binding to a short cis-acting sequence (consensus: 5' AGGTCA 3'; ref. 8) termed "estrogen response element" (ERE). In a "classical" ERE two of these sequences are arranged as palindromes, separated by three random base pairs. ER bound to the ERE transactivates or transrepresses transcription of the target gene by interaction with the basic transcription machinery or with additional transcription factors (7–9). ER, like other steroid hormone receptors, contain different domains which confer different properties on the protein. The hormone binding domain (HBD, ref. 10) also contains a dimerization surface responsible for homo-dimerization of the ER. The mechanism by which the ER regulates expression of target genes has been studied in detail. In analogy to many other phosphorylation processes in signal transduction, the transcriptional activity of the ER is also regulated by phosphorylation. Chambon et al were able to show that the affinity of ER to the ERE is increased by tyrosine phosphorylation (11). In addition, the ER can also be phosphorylated by MAP-kinase, which increases binding to the ERE and thus transactivates gene expression (12). The transcriptional activation of target genes by the ER is thought to be mediated by direct or indirect physical interaction of ER with the basal transcription machinery (13). As discussed above, transcriptional activation of the ER is also dependent on the presence of specific DNA binding motifs in the regulatory region of the target gene. The DNA sequence requirements for ER binding to EREs have been determined in detail (8). Binding of the ER to "classical" (i.e. palindromic) EREs is the best established mechanism for ER mediated gene expression (classical sequence: AGGTCANNNTGACCT, where N may be any nucleotide). Recent data suggest that the ER may also bind promiscuously to direct repeats or even single copies of ERE half-sites (14). In addition, estrogen response elements may not be strictly mandatory for transcriptional regulation by the ER. The ovalbumin promoter contains an ERE half-site with striking similarity to an AP-1 site, which binds transcription factors of the jun-fos gene family and may also be transactivated by the estrogen receptor (15). Null-mutations for the estrogen receptor have been generated in the mouse system (16). Mice of both sexes are viable but infertile. Infertility in males was unexpected, but the testes of receptor deficient males are small and the morphology of seminiferous tubules is altered. Although the animals are not described to have a prominent cardiovascular phenotype, this does not argue against the relevance of estrogens in the heart, which may be relevant under circumstances not encountered in the transgenic animals (e.g. hypertension, atherosclerosis etc.). It just means that the estrogen receptor is not morphogenic during development or that its loss of function can be compensated for by other proteins. Hemodynamic studies and analysis of gene expression in knockout animals will be a prerequisite in dissecting genomic and non-genomic effects of estrogens in mice.

4. ESTROGEN ACTION ON THE MYOCARDIUM

Until recently, the myocardium was thought to lack estrogen receptors. Surprisingly, studies in our own lab have shown that cardiac myocytes express ER mRNA and protein as determined by Northern and Western analysis (17). Furthermore, addition of E2 to cultured neonatal cardiac myocytes resulted in nuclear translocation of the ER. These estrogen receptors are transcriptionally competent, since they induce transcription of a luciferase reporter gene that contains a trimer of EREs. Also the endogenous progesterone gene, which is well known to be E2 responsive in non-cardiac tissues, is up-regulated by the ER in cardiac myocytes. These data indicate that estrogens are able to regulate gene expression in the myocardium. Thus, transcriptional regulation of several genes relevant to the myocardium may occur via estrogen receptors.

In order to get a better understanding on the role of estrogens in cardiac hypertrophy we are currently investigating the effects of E2 on overall protein synthesis of the rat heart. Changes in myocardial gene expression during hypertrophy are thought to be mediated in part by proto-oncogenes. The proto-oncogenes c-fos, c-jun, egr-1 and c-myc are induced rapidly and transiently after exposure of cardiac myocytes to external hypertrophic stimuli (18). These transcription factors bind to defined DNA sequences located in the promoter/enhancer region of specific downstream target genes where they regulate transcriptional activity of the gene. Studies in non-cardiac tissues indicate, that the expression of several proto-oncogenes is regulated by estrogens (19, 20, 21). We have shown in a previous study that egr-1, which is transcriptionally regulated by E2 in non-cardiac tissues, is required for the transduction of hypertrophic stimuli in cardiac myocytes (22). Thus, transcriptional control of cardiac gene expression during hypertrophy could be regulated by interference of the ER with proto-oncogene expression. An alternative or additional point of convergence between ER and proto-oncogene mediated gene expression pathways may be the target promoter of downstream genes. This hypothesis is supported by reports on direct ER interactions with c-fos and c-jun as discussed before.

Evidence that E2 mediates the expression of structural genes in the myocardium comes from studies that show estrogen dependent expression of the myosin heavy chain genes (MHC) in the rat heart. Cardiac hypertrophy in spontaneously hypertensive rats (SHR) leads to a shift in the expression of isomyosins in the heart from the V1 (α/α) to the V3 (α/β) isoform. Myofibrillar ATPase activity and contractility of cardiac myocytes expressing the V3 isoform is significantly reduced. Morano et al were able to show that female SHR rats are able to maintain at least equal ratios of V1 versus V3 isomyosin, whereas in male SHR rats the V3 isoform is clearly predominant (23). Furthermore, substitution of ovarectomized female rats with physiological levels of 17β-estradiol prevented the decline of V1 isomyosin seen in unsubstituted animals (24). The exact mechanism by which estrogens and also testosterone (25) regulate MHC expression is at present not well understood. Besides changes in the expression of contractile proteins, cardiac hypertrophy leads to increases in overall protein synthesis and induces specific changes in myocardial gene expression. In a first approximation, these may be summarized as the hypertrophic gene program (review in 26).

Transcriptional control of cardiac gene expression by estrogens potentially includes a variety of additional genes important for cardiac function. These genes are either known to be regulated by estrogen in non-myocardial tissues or they contain EREs in their promoter region. None of these has actually been shown to be regulated by estrogens in the myocardium. At first, the estrogen receptor gene itself is upregulated in a feed back loop. Differences in gender dependent gene expression may thus be explained by the fact that males first have to up-regulate their estrogen receptors until maximal transcriptional activation of ER responsive target genes occurs. Cardiac hypertrophy is associated with an increase in life-threatening arrhythmias. Propagation of the electrical impulse in the heart is facilitated by highly specialized intercellular channels, which are formed by proteins of the connexin (CX) gene family (27, 28). The expression of the predominant connexin in the heart (CX43) may be regulated by estrogens, since the promoter of the rat CX43 gene contains several ERE half-sites (29). Furthermore, promoter constructs of CX43 are E2 responsive in non-myocyte cell lines (30). Previous studies also indicate altered connexin expression in the hypertrophied rat myocardium (31). Further genes which might be transcriptionally regulated by the ER in the myocardium are the calcium-dependent and calcium-independent isoforms of the nitric oxide synthase gene as well as the angiotensin-I converting enzyme (ACE). The activities of these enzymes are either known to be regulated by E2 in vascular cells or they contain EREs in their promoter regions (32, 33, 34).

5. NON-GENOMIC EFFECTS OF ESTROGENS IN THE MYOCARDIUM

Non-genomic effects of steroid hormones are independent of receptor mediated gene expression. This mechanism does not require de novo protein synthesis and is thus characterized by its rapid onset of action within minutes after application of the hormone. In contrast, the genomic action of E2 may require several hours for target gene expression before significant effects can be observed. At present our knowledge on non-genomic effects of estrogens in the myocardium itself is very limited. Jiang et al report on a calcium antagonistic effect of E2 in guinea-pig cardiac myocytes (35). However the concentrations of E2 in these experiments were in the micromolar range which exceeds the physiological level by three orders of magnitude. However E2 at physiological levels might for instance also regulate the electrophysiological properties of cardiac myocytes as it does in vascular smooth muscle cells. The techniques to answer these questions are at hand and initial studies may open an additional and promising field of research.

6. POTENTIAL CLINICAL APPLICATIONS

The previously somewhat vague function of estrogens in the heart can now be precisely defined using modern molecular methods. Estrogens are already established drugs in the prevention or treatment of osteoporosis and gynaecological disorders. But the therapeutic application of these compounds in heart disease is at present limited mainly for two reasons. First, the question if estrogens, even in combination with progesterones, increase the incidence of breast cancer has not been finally answered. Second, the application of female sex hormones in male patients causes a variety of side effects reaching from cosmetical problems and impotence to an increased risk of testicular cancer. Further research should thus be directed to the elucidation of the regulatory pathway of estrogen mediated gene expression in the heart. The identification of downstream and eventually heart specific target genes of estrogens and synthesis of novel estrogen-analogs should circumvent the unfavourable side effects of estrogens in men and women.

ACKNOWLEDGMENTS

The authors are grateful to S. Oberdorf-Maass for excellent technical assistance and to the members of the laboratory for conceptual discussions. We also thank Dr. Mike Mendelsohn and Dr. Richard Karas, Boston for conceptual input.

Part of this work has been made possible by a grant from the 'Deutsche Forschungsgemeinschaft' (German Research Association, TP B6, SFB 355).

REFERENCES

1. Bush TL, Barrett-Connor E, Cowan LD, Criqui MH, Wallace RB, Suchindran CM, Tyroler HA, Rifkind BM. Cardiovascular mortality and noncontraceptive use of estrogen in women: results from the Lipid Research Clinics Program follow-up study. Circulation 1987; 75:1102–1109.

2. Hong MK, Romm PA, Reagan K, Green CE, Rackley CE. Effects of estrogen replacement therapy on serum lipid values and angiographically defined coronary artery disease in postmenopausal women. Am J Cardiol 1992; 69:176–178.

3. Adams MR, Clarkson TB, Kaplan JR, Koritnik DR. Ovarian secretions and arteriosclerosis. In: Gutmann JN, DeCherney AH, Sarrel PM, eds. Ovarian secretions and cardiovascular and neurological function. New York: Raven Press 1990.

4. Glendy RE, Levine SA, White PD. Coronary disease in youth: comparison of 100 patients under 40 with 300 persons past 80. JAMA 1937; 109:1775–1781.

5. Stampfer MJ, Colditz GA, Willett WC, Manson JE, Rosner B, Speizer FE, Hennekens CH. Postmenopausal estrogen therapy and cardiovascular disease. N Engl J Med 1991; 325:756–762.

6. Karas RH, Patterson BL, Mendelsohn ME. Human vascular smooth muscle cells contain functional estrogen receptor. Circulation 89: 1943–1950, 1994.

7. Beato M, Herrlich P, Schütz G. Steroid hormone receptors: many actors in search for a plot. Cell 1995; 83: 851–857.

8. Klein-Hitpass L, Schorpp M, Wagner W, Ryffel GU. An estrogen responsive element derived from the 5' flanking region of the xenopus vitellogenin A12 gene functions in transfected human cells. Cell 1986; 46:1053–1061.

9. Walter P, Green S, Krust A, Bornert JM, Jeltsch JM, Staub A, Jensen E, Scrace G, Waterfield M, Chambon P. Cloning of the human estrogen receptor cDNA. Proc Natl Acad Sci USA 1985; 82:7889–7893.

10. Kumar V, Green S, Staub A, Chambon P. Localisation of the estradiol-binding and putative DNA-binding domains of the human estrogen receptor. EMBO J 1986; 5:2231–2236.

11. Migliaccio A, Di Domenico M, Green S, de Falco A, Kajtaniac EL, Blasi F, Chambon P, Auricchio F. Phosphorylation on tyrosine of in vitro synthezised human estrogen receptor activates its hormone binding. Mol Endocrinol 1989; 3:1061–1069.

12. Kato S, Endoh H, Masuhiro Y, Kitamoto T, Uchiyama S, Sasaki H, Masushige S, Gotoh Y, Nishida E, Kawashima H, Metzger D, Chambon P. Activation of the estrogen receptor through phosphorylation by mitogen-activated protein kinase. Science 1995; 270:1491–1494.

13. Jacq X, Brou C, Lutz Y, Davidson I, Chambon P, Tora L. Human TAFII30 is present in a distinct TFIID complex and is required for transcriptional activation by the estrogen receptor. Cell 1994; 79:107–117.

14. Kato S, Sasaki H, Suzawa M, Masushige S, Tora L, Chambon P, Gronemeyer H. Widely spaced, directly repeated PuGGTCA elements act as promiscuous enhancers for different classes of nuclear receptors. Mol Cell Biol 1995; 15:5858–5867.

15. Gaub MP, Bellard M, Scheuer I, Chambon P, Sassone-Corsi P. Activation of the ovalbumin gene by the estrogen receptor involves the fos-jun complex. Cell 1990; 63:1267–1276.

16. Lubahn DB, Moyer JS, Golding TS, Couse JF, Korach KS, Smithies O. Alteration of reproductive function but not prenatal sexual development after insertional disruption of the mouse estrogen receptor gene. Proc Natl Acad Sci USA 1993; 90:11162–11166.

17. Grohe C, Kahlert S, Löbbert K, Stimpel M, Karas RH, Vetter H, Neyses L. Cardiac myocytes and fibroblasts contain functional estrogen receptors. (submitted)

18. Neyses , Nouskas J, Luycken J, Fronhoffs S, Oberdorf S, Williams RS, Sukhatme VP, Vetter H. Induction of immediate-early genes by angiotensin-2 and endothelin-1 in adult rat cardiomyocytes. J Hypertens 1993; 11:927–934.

19. Dubik D, Dembinski TC, Shiu RPC. Stimulation of the c-myc oncogene expression associated with estrogen-induced proliferation of human breast cancer cells. Cancer Res 1987; 47:6517–6521.

20. Weisz A, Rosales R. Identification of an estrogen response element upstream of the human c-fos gene that binds the estrogen receptor and the AP-1 transcription factor. Nucleic Acids Res 1990; 18:5097–5106.

21. Cicatiello L, Sica V, Bresciani F, Weisz A. Identification of a specific pattern of "immediate-early" gene activation induced by estrogen during mitogenic stimulation of rat uterine cells. Receptor 1993; 3:17–30.

22. Neyses L, Nouskas J, Vetter H. Inhibition of endothelin-1 induced myocardial protein synthesis by an antisense oligonucleotide against the early growth response gene-1. Biochem Biophys Res Commun 1991; 181:22–27.

23. Morano I, Gagelmann M, Arner A, Ganten U, Rüegg JC. Myosin isoenzymes of vascular smooth and cardiac muscle in the spontaneously hypertensive and normotensive male and female rat: a comparative study. Circ Res 1986; 59:456–462.

24. Malhotra A, Buttrick P, Scheuer J. Effects of sex hormones on development of physiological and pathological cardiac hypertrophy in male and female rats. Am J Physiol 1990; 259:H866–H871.

25. Morano I, Gerstner J, Rüegg JC, Ganten U. Regulation of myosin heavy chain expression in the hearts of hypertensive rats by testosterone. Circ Res 1990; 66:1585–1590.

26. Neyses L, Pelzer T. The biological cascade leading to hypertrophy. Eur Heart J, 1995; 16 (Suppl. N):8–11.

27. Beyer EC, Paul DL, Goodenough DA. The connexin family of gap junction proteins. J Membrane Biol 1990; 116:187–194.

28. Willecke K, Hennemann H, Dahl E, Jungbluth S, Heynkes R. The diversity of connexin genes encoding gap junctional proteins. Eur J Cell Biol 1991; 56:1–7.

29. De Leon JR, Buttrick PM, Fishman GI. Functional analysis of the connexin-43 gene promoter in vivo and in vitro. J Mol Cell Cardiol 1994; 26:379–389.

30. Yu W, Dahl G, Werner R. The connexin-43 gene is responsive to estrogen. Proc R Soc Lond 1994; 255:125–132.

31. Bastide B, Neyses L, Ganten D, Paul M, Willecke K, Traub O. The gap junction protein connexin-40 is preferentially expressed in vascular endothelium as well as conductive bundles of rat myocardium and is increased under hypertensive conditions. Circ Res 1993: 73:1138–1149.

32. Weiner C, Lizasoain I, Baylis SA, Knowles RG, Charles IG, Moncada S. Induction of calcium-dependent nitric oxide synthases by sex hormones. Proc Natl Acad Sci 1994; 91:5212–5216.

33. Proudler AJ, Ahmed Al H, Crook D, Fogelman I, Rymer JM, Stevenson JC. Hormone replacement therapy and serum angiotensin-converting-enzyme activity in postmenopausal women. Lancet 1995; 346:89–90.

34. Testut P, Soubrier F, Corvol P, Hubert C. Functional analysis of the human somatic angiotensin-1 converting enzyme gene promoter. Biochem J 1993; 293:843–848.

35. Jiang C, Poole-Wilson PA, Sarrel PM, Mochizuki S, Collins P, McLeod KT. Effect of 17β-estradiol on concentration, Ca^{2+} current and intracellular free Ca^{2+} in guinea-pig isolated cardiac myocytes. Br J Pharmacol 1992; 106:739–745.

10

SALT SENSITIVITY AND LEFT VENTRICULAR HYPERTROPHY

Antonio Coca and Alejandro De la Sierra

Hypertension Unit
Department of Internal Medicine
Hospital Clinico
University of Barcelona
c/ Villarroel 170
08036-Barcelona, Spain

1. LEFT VENTRICULAR HYPERTROPHY AND CARDIOVASCULAR MORBIDITY AND MORTALITY

Coronary artery disease (CAD), congestive heart failure (CHF) and sudden death remain the most common and major complications of essential hypertension (EH)[1]. The Framingham study[2,3] demonstrated that in 75% of all patients in whom heart failure developed, EH was the underlying disease. Moreover, EH accelerates coronary arteriosclerosis leading to myocardial ischemia in patients with genetic predisposition[4], a phenomenon that exacerbates in the presence of left ventricular hypertrophy (LVH).

One of the most relevant findings in the Framingham study was the demonstration that patients with EH and definite electrocardiographic signs of LVH increased their mortality rates due to all cardiovascular diseases from 3 to 10 times more than hypertensives with no signs of cardiac hypertrophy. The incidence of CAD was 3.2 times higher in the presence of LVH, while the incidence of CHF was approximately 8-fold as high. Of particular interest was the demonstration of a negative prognostic value of LVH even after adjustment for the severity of hypertension, what lend LVH the character of independent risk factor[5]. The confirmation of increased mortality rates due to all cardiovascular diseases among EH with LVH diagnosed by echocardiography[6] strengthens the important prognostic role of LVH in the natural history of hypertensive disease[7].

Indeed, LVH modifies the equilibrium between the oxygen supply and demand by the myocardium. The coronary reserve, which represents the increment by which myocardial blood flow increases in response to maximum vasodilator stimuli, is appreciably reduced in hypertensives with LVH even in the absence of any stenosis of coronary arteries. Thus, in patients with hemodynamically controlled hypertension and normal coronary angiogram, a predisposition toward myocardial ischemia already exists. This process has

Hypertension and the Heart, edited by Zanchetti et al.
Plenum Press, New York, 1997

been associated with the increased prevalence of both frequency and complexity of ventricular arrhythmias in essential hypertensives with LVH[8,9], what could be linked to the increasing risk of sudden death in these patients.

The issue of whether reversal of LVH in EH patients is a desirable therapeutic goal of antihypertensive therapy remains the subject of ongoing debate. Nevertheless, if LVH is judged to be a pathological process, reduction of myocardial hypertrophy would emerge as a desirable therapeutic goal. So far, there is only indirect evidence showing that reduction of LVH reverses the pathologic implications of cardiac hypertrophy in arterial hypertension[10]. Furthermore, clinical studies have shown that not all forms of antihypertensive therapy lead to regression of myocardial hypertrophy, ranging from complete absence of effect, through a largely pressure-related decrease in muscle mass, to a pressure-unrelated reversal of LVH. The discrepancy between the extent of reduction in blood pressure and the regression of myocardial hypertrophy suggests that, apart from arterial blood pressure, the degree of LVH is also determined by other factors.

2. FACTORS INVOLVED IN THE PATHOGENESIS OF LEFT VENTRICULAR HYPERTROPHY

2.1. Blood Pressure and Volume Overload

The expected response of the heart when an increased work load is chronically imposed on the cardiac muscle is myocardial hypertrophy. Thus, it has been generally assumed that the development of LVH constitutes the main physiologic mechanism of adaptation in pressure overload secondary to the increase of peripheral resistance[11]. Although little is known about factors which influence the pattern of hypertrophy in either animals or humans, the classic study performed by Grossman et al[12] provided data suggesting that the left ventricle response to pressure overload was rather different from the observed after a volume overload. Left ventricular wall stress depends on the chamber size and configuration, the thickness of the ventricular wall, and the intraventricular pressure. Thus, for either an ellipsoidal or spherical model, the average meridional systolic wall stress (σm), that is the wall tension supported by the ventricle during systolic ejection, can be calculated throughout the Laplace law from the wall thickness (H), inner chamber radius (R_i) and intraventricular pressure (P):

$$\sigma m = P.Ri/2H \, (1+H/2Ri)$$

When the primary stimulus to hypertrophy is left ventricular pressure overload, the resultant rise in intracavitary pressure (P) leads to a progressive thickening of the ventricular wall (H). Pressure overload resulting in increased peak systolic wall stress leads to a parallel replication of sarcomeres, wall thickening and "concentric hypertrophy" as indicated by the enhanced H/R ratio[12]. When the primary stimulus for hypertrophy is left ventricular volume overload, the enhancement of end left ventricular diastolic pressure results in myocardial fiber elongation and chamber enlargement, thus determining an increase of the internal ventricular diameter but a normal H/R ratio. Volume overload resulting in increased end diastolic wall stress leads to a series replication of sarcomeres, fiber elongation, chamber enlargement and "eccentric hypertrophy."[12]

The structural response of the myocardium to arterial hypertension is heterogeneous in the clinical practice[13]. The Framingham study revealed an important variability in the morphologic patterns of LVH both in the hypertensive patients and their normotensive relatives. On the other hand, LVH is a dynamic process which can develop in the short period of 1 to 2 weeks after experimental hypertension in animals[14]. Conversely, regression of LVH has been demonstrated within few weeks of blood pressure control, both in experimental hypertension[15] and clinical practice[16]. Thus, LVH seems not to be a late and irreversible complication of EH, but an early phenomenon, subject to a dynamic modification in the evolution of the disease[17].

2.2. Genetic Factors

Essential hypertension is genetically determined, and the myocardial growth response to several factors might also be, at least in part, genetically determined. Accordingly, every case of hypertensive cardiac hypertrophy could contain an individually varying genetic component which might help to explain the distinct morphologic patterns as well as the varying responses of the myocardium to antihypertensive treatment.

The variability in the morphologic patterns of LVH both in hypertensives and their normotensive relatives, the simultaneous enlargement of the right ventricle of some hypertensives without concomitant pulmonary hypertension[18], the observation that LVH is more severe in the black hypertensives than in whites, as well as the detection of LVH in animals[19] and in normotensive relatives of hypertensive patients even in the "prehypertensive phase,"[20] support the existence of a genetic predisposition to myocardial growth in essential hypertension. In fact, the demonstration of LVH in normotensive adolescents with high risk of development of hypertension cannot be justified as a hemodynamic compensatory mechanism of adaptation to something that has not been still established. As it happens with blood pressure values, distribution of ventricular mass in the general population is a continuous variable, without a clear defined cut-off level between normality and disease. However, even considering the existence of a bias towards highest values of left ventricular mass index (LVMI) among hypertensives, there is an overlap between hypertensives exhibiting the lowest values of LVMI and normotensives displaying the highest values.

2.3. Non-Hemodynamic Factors

Clinical studies have shown that not all antihypertensive drugs have the same effect with respect to the reversal of LVH, even though when blood pressure control to normotensive levels is achieved. These studies have strengthened the hypothesis that hemodynamic and genetic factors alone are not enough to explain the development of ventricular growth[21,22]. As we previously mentioned, the discrepancy between the extent of reduction in blood pressure and the reversal of LVH implies that, despite blood pressure, other factors such as sympathetic tone and the renin-angiotensin-aldosterone axis are involved in the control of myocardial growth. Norepinephrine stimulates cell growth of isolated cultured myocardial cells[23]. Consequently, if catecholamines play a role in development of LVH, it is possible that the stimulation of the adrenergic tone induced by diuretics and vasodilators had a trophic effect and may be the responsible for the subsistence of an hypertrophied myocardium despite blood pressure reduction. Conversely, the ability of methyldopa to reduce circulating levels of norepinephrine may explain the reversal of cardiac hypertrophy independently of its antihypertensive efficacy[24].

Angiotensin II stimulates protein biosynthesis in the cardiac muscle[25] and may, in addition, enhance catecholamine secretion by the adrenal medulla[26]. It is also highly prob-

Table 1. Factors involved in the pathogenesis of cardiac hypertrophy

Genetic factors: Genetic substrate predisposing to myocardial growth
Hemodynamic factors: Mechanical stretch on the left ventricle
Other factors:
Sympathetic tone (catecholamines)
Renin-angiotensin-aldosterone axis (angiotensin II)
Cardiac angiotensin II
Proto-oncogenes (*c-myc*, *c-fos*, *c*-Ha-*ras*)
Growth factors:
Endothelium derived growth factor (EDGF)
Platelet-derived growth factor (PDGF)
Epidermal growth factor (EPGF)
Insulin-like growth factor (IGF-1)
Fibroblast growth factors (aFGF, bFGF)
Transforming growth factors (αTGF, βTGF)
Growth hormone
Thyroid hormone
Insulin
Endothelin
Arginine-vasopressin
Bradykinin
Thrombin
Prostaglandins
Na$^+$ intake
Caloric intake

(From Coca et al.,[49] with permission.)

able that the local renin-angiotensin-system of the myocardiocyte play an important role inducing cell growth independently of the hyperactivation of the systemic axis. There has been postulated that Angiotensin II synthesized in the myocardial cell could interact with other humoral and growth factors i.e., endothelium derived growth factor, platelet-derived growth factor, epidermal growth factor, insulin-like growth factor and some others, to exert a specific control on cell growth[27].

In addition to factors linked to the adrenergic system and renin-angiotensin-aldosterone system, other vasoactive substances, growth promotors, and several environmental factors such as sodium and caloric intake have been involved in the pathogenesis of LVH (Table 1). All these factors may activate myocardial membrane receptors responsible for a sequence of events, including initiating signals, coupling mechanisms, and regulation of gene expression. As a result of these signals, membrane ion channels and ion transport systems are activated, leading to increased intracellular contents of Na$^+$, Ca^{2+}, inositol phosphates, diacylglycerol, and to greater activity of protein kinases A and C, with increased protein and DNA synthesis.

3. SALT INTAKE AND LEFT VENTRICULAR HYPERTROPHY

Several data suggest a link between salt intake and left ventricular growth in both hypertensive rats[28,29] and EH patients[30]. It has been previously reported that NaCl ingestion is a powerful determinant of left ventricular hypertrophy in patients with essential hypertension[30,31]. Thus, saline overload increases left ventricular mass, and salt restriction in diet determines regression of cardiac hypertrophy. In addition, recent data seem to indicate that LVH is more marked in salt-sensitive than in salt-resistant rats[29]. Similar trends have been observed in salt-sensitive and salt-resistant essential hypertensive patients[32], suggesting a distinct effect of salt-loading on myocardial growth which is dependent on the sensitivity or resistance to the pressor effect of sodium chloride intake.

3.1. Salt Sensitivity and Left Ventricular Hypertrophy in Essential Hypertension

Salt-sensitivity, defined as a significant rise in blood pressure from low to high salt diet is a characteristic of almost 50% of essential hypertensive patients and some strains of hypertensive rats. It has been suggested that salt-sensitive hypertensive subjects might have an increased risk in terms of cardiovascular morbidity[32,33]. In this sense, higher left ventricular mass, increased albumin excretion rate, a worse lipid profile, and impairment of insulin sensitivity have been observed in salt-sensitive when compared with salt-resistant patients[32,33].

We have evaluated echocardiographic characteristics in a group of salt-sensitive EH patients in comparison with salt-resistant patients. Fifty never treated EH patients (23m, 27f), aged 25 to 72 years, with mild-to-moderate hypertension, were included in the study on the basis they had average values of 24-hour DBP above 90 mmHg in ambulatory blood pressure monitoring (ABPM).

After a 4-week unrestricted salt period patients underwent 24-hour ABPM using an automated, noninvasive oscillometric device (SpaceLabs 90207, SpaceLabs Inc., Redmon, WA). The appropriate cuff was placed on the nondominant arm, and blood pressure was registered automatically at 15 minutes intervals for a 24-h period. A fasting venous blood sample was obtained for biochemical measurements and a two-dimensional controlled M-mode echocardiogram was performed. All traced echocardiograms were read by two trained physicians who were not aware of the salt-sensitivity or salt-resistance status of the patient. Measurements were done according to the criteria of the American Society of Echocardiography[34]. Left ventricular mass index was calculated using the Penn convention criteria[35] and divided by the body surface area. The relative wall thickness ratio (WTR) was obtained by dividing the posterior wall thickness by the half of the left ventricular end diastolic diameter (LVEDD)[36].

The diagnosis of salt-sensitivity was based on a previously reported protocol[37]. Briefly, patients followed a two-week period of a low salt diet (20 mmol of NaCl/day) supplemented by placebo tablets during the first seven days and by NaCl tablets (240 mmol/day) during the following seven days. Twenty-four hour urinary Na+ excretion was measured daily in order to assess the scheduled salt intake. ABPM was performed at the end of both periods and compared in each subject by means of the Student's t-test or the Mann-Whitney non-parametric test. Salt-sensitive hypertension was diagnosed in 22 patients (44%), showing a significant rise (p<0.05) in 24-hour mean blood pressure from low to high salt intake. The remaining 28 patients (56%) were considered as having salt-resistant hypertension.

Table 2 shows changes in 24-h SBP and DBP as well as 24-h urinary sodium excretion (measured the last day of both low and high salt periods) in salt-sensitive and salt-resistant hypertensive patients. As can be seen, blood pressure values significantly increased in salt-sensitive patients whereas salt-resistant hypertensives had no change in 24-h blood pressure.

Table 3 shows the comparison of baseline clinical and echocardiographic characteristics between salt-sensitive and salt-resistant hypertensive patients. No significant dif-

Table 2. Mean values (± s.e.m.) of blood pressure and 24-h urinary sodium excretion in salt-sensitive and salt-resistant hypertensive patients during low and high-salt intakes

	Salt-sensitive (n=22)		Salt-resistant (n=28)		Total (n=50)	
	Low-salt	High-salt	Low-salt	High-salt	Low-salt	High-salt
24h SBP	145.1±3.4	154.3±3.7*	147.1±3.1	146.8±3.6	146.3±2.3	150±2.6*
24h DBP	90.6±2.2	95.1±2.4*	89.7±2.1	88.2±2.2	90.1±1.5	91.2±1.7‡
24h UNa⁺	34±4	255±11*	32±2	236±11*	33±2	246±10*

SBP: systolic blood pressure (mmHg)
DBP: systolic blood pressure (mmHg)
UNa⁺: urinary sodium excretion (mmol/24h)
*p<0.001, ‡p<0.05 comparing low vs high-salt intakes
(Adapted from De la Sierra et al.,[38] with permission.)

ferences were observed in clinical parameters, as well as in fasting plasma glucose, creatinine or uric acid. Salt-sensitive patients showed a worse lipid profile with significantly lower HDL-cholesterol with respect to salt-resistant (1.06 ± 0.06 vs 1.25 ± 0.07 mmol/L; p=0.0475). Also total cholesterol/HDL-cholesterol ratio was significantly higher (5.89 ± 0.35 vs 4.74 ± 0.27; p=0.0098).

Salt-sensitive patients exhibited an increased LVMI compared with salt-resistant hypertensives (163.8 ± 8.1 vs 137.9 ± 6.0 g/m²; p=0.0118). This was due to the increased septal (12.7 ± 0.35 vs 11.1 ± 0.34 mm; p=0.0021) and posterior wall thickness (12.0 ± 0.36 vs 10.4 ± 0.32 mm; p=0.0026), with no changes in internal diastolic diameter[38]. The relative WTR was also increased in salt-sensitive patients (0.46 ± 0.02 vs 0.41 ± 0.02; p=0.0427). These results are in agreement with those previously reported by other authors[30,31]. Left ventricular hypertrophy defined by a LVMI higher than 130 g/m² in men or 110 g/m² in women was present in 21 of 22 salt-sensitive patients (95.5%) and only in 17 of the 28 salt-resistant hypertensives (60.7%; p=0.0238). Due to differences (although not significant) in sex distribution between salt-sensitive and salt-resistant patients, the association between LVMI and salt-sensitivity was examined by means of the two-way

Table 3. Comparison of baseline clinical and echocardiographic parameters between salt-sensitive (SS) and salt-resistant (SR) hypertensive patients. Values expressed as mean ± s.e.m.

	SS (n=22)	SR (n=28)	p
Age (years)	54.6 ± 2.1	50.6 ± 2.4	0.2407
Sex (m/f)	12/10	11/17	0.3926
Family history of hypertension (%)	64	57	0.4215
Weight (kg)	78.4 ± 2.7	74.3 ± 2.9	0.3144
Body mass index (kg/m²)	30.2 ± 1.1	28.5 ± 0.9	0.2525
24-h SBP (mmHg)	151.3 ± 3.4	152.2 ± 2.8	0.8325
24-h DBP (mmHg)	93.3 ± 2.4	92.9 ± 2.1	0.8986
Posterior wall thickness (mm)	12.0 ± 0.36	10.4 ± 0.32	0.0026
Septal wall thickness (mm)	12.7 ± 0.35	11.1 ± 0.34	0.0021
LVEDD (mm)	51.5 ± 1.14	51.4 ± 1.59	0.9550
LVMI (g/m²)	163.8 ± 8.1	137.9 ± 6.0	0.0118
WTR	0.46 ± 0.02	0.41 ± 0.02	0.0427

LVEDD: left ventricular end diastolic diameter. LVMI: left ventricular mass index.
WTR: relative wall/thickness ratio.
(Modified from De la Sierra et al.,[38] with permission.)

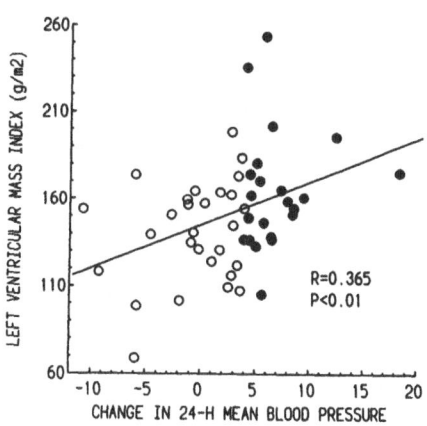

Figure 1. Scatterplot showing a significant direct correlation between changes in 24-hours mean blood pressure induced by high-salt intake and left ventricular mass index. Closed circles represent salt-sensitive patients and open circles represent salt-resistant essential hypertensive patients. (Adapted from De la Sierra et al.,[38] with permission).

analysis of variance, including sex as a grouping factor. The results of this analysis indicated that sex did not influence the association between LVMI and salt-sensitivity. A direct correlation (r=0.365; p<0.01) between LVMI and the change in 24-hour mean blood pressure induced by high-salt intake was observed (Figure 1). This correlation was maintained (r=0.281; p<0.05) after adjustment for age and body mass index[38].

4. MECHANISMS OF SALT-RELATED LEFT VENTRICULAR HYPERTROPHY

The mechanisms of cellular growth after sodium overload are not well understood, but it is believed that high-salt intake activates the sympathetic nervous system in salt-sensitive patients[39]. Salt overload may also lead to stimulation of phospholipase C mediated by platelet-derived growth factors[40]. Finally, salt intake may stimulate myocardial growth throughout hemodynamically mediated mechanisms as blood pressure and volume overload[29].

Nevertheless, it is known that salt-sensitive and salt-resistant hypertensive patients differ in some adaptive responses to changes in dietary salt intake. Among them, the renin-aldosterone axis, the sympathetic nervous system and the intracellular ion composition could play a role in the development of myocardial growth. It has been reported that salt-sensitive patients present a blunted response of the renin-angiotensin axis to the increase in salt intake[41]. We have observed that the decrease in plasma aldosterone in response to high dietary salt is attenuated in salt-sensitive hypertensives compared to salt-resistant patients[42], and experimental studies have demonstrated a trophic effect of aldosterone on myocardial growth[43]. Involvement of sympathetic nervous system in cardiac hypertrophy is supported by the fact that exogenous catecholamines, even in subpressor doses, induce cardiac hypertrophy[44]. Furthermore, basal values of plasma catecholamines seem to be higher in salt-sensitive hypertensives[45], and a further increase in plasma noradrenaline with high salt intake has been observed in salt-sensitive hypertensives[42,46].

On the other hand, abnormalities in sodium and calcium transport have been related with both cardiac hypertrophy[47–49] and salt-sensitivity[50]. Essential hypertensive patients with left ventricular hypertrophy present increased rates of erythrocyte $Na^+–H^+$ *exchange*[47–49]. Likewise, high salt intake induces an acceleration of erythrocyte $Na^+–Li^+$ *countertransport*

Table 4. Different erythrocyte ionic parameters in 40 essential hypertensive patients
classified according to the presence or absence of left ventricular hypertrophy

Parameter	LVH (n = 26)	No LVH (n = 14)
Intraerythrocyte Na$^+$ content (mmol/l.cells)	8.53 ± 0.26*	7.43 ± 0.16
Na$^+$-K$^+$ ATPase		
Vmax (μmol.(l cells.h)$^{-1}$)	8751 ± 392	9334 ± 662
K50% (mmol/l.cells)	18.52 ± 0.85	16.37 ± 1.33
Na$^+$-K$^+$-Cl$^-$ cotransport		
Vmax (μmol.(l cells.h)$^{-1}$)	638 ± 65	760 ± 107
K50% (mmol/l.cells)	13.12 ± 1.13	12.44 ± 1.75
Na$^+$-Li$^+$ countertransport		
Vmax (μmol.(l cells.h)$^{-1}$)	326 ± 27	327 ± 39
K50% (mmol/l.cells)	8.30 ± 1.17	7.23 ± 0.94
Na$^+$-H$^+$ exchanger		
Na$^+$ influx rate (μmol.(l cells.h)$^{-1}$)	10177 ± 772§	7460 ± 773
Passive Na$^+$ leak		
Kp Na$^+$ (10^{-3}.h^{-1})	19.47 ± 0.79	19.06 ± 1.19

Values referred as mean ± s.e.m.; *p= 0.001; §p= 0.0182
(Adapted from Coca et al.,[49] with permission.)

only in salt-sensitive hypertensives[50]. These abnormalities in sodium transport pathways may lead to an increase in intracellular Na$^+$ and Ca^{2+} contents, which has been reported to correlate with left ventricular mass[51]. As it can be seen in Table 4, we previously observed[47–49] that hypertensives with LVH showed a significantly higher intraerythrocyte Na$^+$ content (8.53 ± 0.26 vs. 7.43 ± 0.16 mmol/l.cells; p= 0.0012), and a higher Na$^+$ influx rate dependent of the transmembrane erythrocyte *Na$^+$–H$^+$ exchanger* (10177 ± 772 vs 7460 ± 773 mol.(l cells.h)$^{-1}$; p= 0.0182). Both internal Na$^+$ content (8.54 ± 0.3 vs. 8.52 ± 0.1 mmol/l.cells) and the activity of the *Na$^+$–H$^+$ exchanger* (11837 ± 1252 vs. 9299 ± 933 mol.(l cells.h)$^{-1}$) were identical in patients with concentric or eccentric hypertrophy. The hyperactivity of the *Na$^+$–H$^+$ exchanger* is known to be responsible for a simultaneous net Na$^+$ influx and H$^+$ efflux from the cell. In myocardial cells, this transmembrane ionic movements could lead to either a raise in intracellular Na$^+$ content and alkalinization of the intracellular medium, hence promoting protein synthesis.

Other factor influencing the development of cardiac hypertrophy in salt-sensitive hypertension could be the circadian profile of blood pressure. In this sense, Verdecchia et al[52] reported that essential hypertensive patients who do not have a decrease in nocturnal blood pressure ("non-dipper" profile) showed increased left ventricular mass, compared with those with a decrease in nocturnal blood pressure ("dipper" profile). In agreement with these results, we have recently reported that salt-sensitive patients present a "non-dipper" pattern of the 24-hour blood pressure curve at both low and high salt intakes[37].

Finally, the possible role of some abnormalities of the insulin metabolism in the development of LVH in salt-sensitive essential hypertensives should be considered. It has been reported that glucose tolerance was impaired[53], and insulin-mediated glucose disposal reduced[54] after high salt intake in young normotensive salt-sensitive subjects, with genetic predisposition to hypertension. An association between hyperinsulinemia and salt-sensitivity has been found in young normotensive and borderline hypertensive blacks[55]. Furthermore, Bigazzi et al[56] have recently reported both elevated levels of plasma glucose and insulin, measured after an oral glucose tolerance test, and abnormalities in plasma levels of atherogenic lipoproteins in salt-sensitive essential hypertensives. This cumulative evidence supports a probable pathogenetic link between insulin resistance and salt-sensitivity in essential hypertension[57].

5. SUMMARY AND CONCLUSIONS

Essential hypertensive patients with left ventricular hypertrophy (LVH) increase their mortality rates due to all cardiovascular diseases from 3 to 10 times more than hypertensives without signs of cardiac hypertrophy. LVH modifies the equilibrium between the oxygen supply and demand by the myocardium. The coronary reserve is appreciably reduced in hypertensives with LVH even in the absence of any stenosis of coronary arteries. Thus, in patients with normal coronary angiogram, a predisposition toward myocardial ischemia already exists. This process has been associated with the increased incidence of ventricular arrhythmias in essential hypertensives with LVH, what could be linked to the increasing risk of sudden death in these patients.

In addition to hemodynamic factors (pressure and volume overload) several non-hemodynamic factors have been involved in the pathogenesis of LVH in hypertension. LVH would develop in subjects with a particular genetic substrate by the overlap of high blood pressure values and several factors linked to the adrenergic system, the renin-angiotensin-aldosterone system, other vasoactive substances, and growth factors. It has been previously reported that NaCl ingestion is a powerful determinant of left ventricular hypertrophy in patients with essential hypertension. Furthermore, a relationship between left ventricular mass and abnormalities in intracellular Na^+ or transmembrane Na^+ transport has been observed in several studies.

Salt-sensitive hypertensive subjects seem to exhibit an increased risk in terms of cardiovascular morbidity. We and others have observed a higher left ventricular mass, an increased albumin excretion rate and a worse lipid profile in salt-sensitive compared with salt-resistant patients. The increase in LVMI in salt-sensitive patients is mainly due to the increase in septal and posterior wall thickness, with normal diastolic diameter, suggesting that myocardial growth in these patients is not volume-dependent.

The mechanism of this structural cardiac adaptation is not completely understood. Nevertheless, it is known that salt-sensitive and salt-resistant hypertensive patients differ in some adaptive responses to changes in dietary salt intake. Among them, the renin-aldosterone axis, the sympathetic nervous system and the intracellular ion composition could play a role in the development of myocardial growth.

In conclusion, salt-sensitive hypertensive patients exhibited an increased LVMI and a worse lipid profile, compared with salt-resistant hypertensives, even at the same level of blood pressure. These characteristics may confer to salt-sensitive patients an increased risk in terms of cardiovascular morbidity and mortality.

REFERENCES

1. The 1988 report of the Joint National Committee on Detection, Evaluation and treatment of High Blood Pressure. Arch Intern Med 1988; 148: 1023–1038.
2. Kannel WB. Some lessons,in cardiovascular epidemiology from Framingham. Am J Card 1976; 37: 269–282.
3. Kannel WB, Castelli WP, Mellumara AM, McKee PH, Fernleib M. Role of blood pressure in the development of congestive heart failure. N Eng J Med 1972; 287: 781–787.
4. Chobanian AV, Brecher PI, Haudenschild CC. Effects of hypertension and antihypertensive therapy on atherosclerosis: state of the art lecture. Hypertension 1986; 8(Suppl I): 15–21.

5. Kannel WB. Prevalence and natural history of electrocardiographic left ventricular hypertrophy. Am J Med 1983; 75(Suppl 3A): 4–11.

6. Casalle PN, Devereux RB, Milner M, et al. Value of echocardiographic measurement of left ventricular mass predicting cardiovascular morbid events in hypertensive men. Ann Intern Med 1986; 105: 173–178.

7. Massie BM, Tubau JF, Szlachcic J, O'Kelly BF. Hypertensive heart disease: The critical role of left ventricular hypertrophy. J Cardiovasc Pharmacol 1989; 13(Suppl I): s18–s24.

8. Messerli F, Ventura HO, Elizardi DJ, Dunn FG, Frohlich ED. Hypertension and sudden death: increased ventricular ectopic activity in left ventricular hypertrophy. Am J Med 1984:; 77: 18–22.

9. McLenechan JM, Henderson E, Morris KI, et al. Ventricular arrhythmias in patients with hypertensive left ventricular hypertrophy. N Eng J Med 1987; 317: 787–792.

10. Kannel WB, D'Agostino RB, Levy D, Belanger AJ. Prognostic significance of regression of left ventricular hypertrophy. Circulation 1988; 78(suppl II): 89 (abstract).

11. Tarazi RC. The hemodynamics of hypertension. In: Genest J, Kuchel O, Hamet P, Cantin M Eds. Hypertension: Physiopathology and treatment. New York. McGraw-Hill, 1983; 15–42.

12. Grossman W, Jones D, Mc Laurin LP. Wall stress and patterns of hypertrophy in the human left ventricle. J Clin Invest 1975; 56: 56–64.

13. Tarazi RC. Cardiovascular hypertrophy in hypertension. Hypertension 1986; 8(Suppl II): 187–190.

14. Mulvany MJ, Korsgaard N. Correlation and otherwise between blood pressure, cardiac mass and resistance vessel characteristics in hypertensive, normotensive and hypertensive/normotensive hybrid rats. J Hypertens 1983; 1: 235–244.

15. Sen S. Regression of cardiac hypertrophy: experimental animal model. Am J Med 1983; 75(Suppl 3A): 87–93.

16. Tarazi RC, Fouad FM. Reversal of cardiac hypertrophy by medical treatment. Annu Rev Med 1985; 36: 407–414.

17. Folkow B. Cardiovascular structural adaptation: its role in the initiation and maintenance of primary hypertension. Clin Sci Mol Med 1978; 55(Suppl): 3s–22s.

18. Nuñez BD, Messerli FH, Amadeo C, et al. Biventricular cardiac hypertrophy in essential hypertension. Am Heart J 1987; 114: 813–818.

19. Yamori Y, Mori C, Nishio T, et al. Cardiac hypertrophy in early hypertension. Am J Cardiol 1979; 44: 964–969.

20. Radice M, Alli C, Avanzini F, et al. Left ventricular structure and function in normotensive adolescents with a genetic predisposition to hypertension. Am Heart J 1986; 111: 115–120.

21. Frohlich ED, Tarazi RC. Is arterial pressure the role factor responsible for hypertensive cardiac hypertrophy? Am J Cardiol 1979; 44: 959–963.

22. Frohlich ED. The heart in hypertension, In: Genest J, Kuchel O, Hamet P, Cantin M, Eds. Hypertension: Physiopathology and treatment. New York. McGraw-Hill, 1983; 791–810.

23. Simpson P. Norepinephrine-stimulated hypertrophy of cultured rat myocardial cell is an alpha-1-adrenergic response. J Clin Invest 1983; 72: 732–738.

24. Fouad FM, Nakashima Y, Tarazi RC, Salcedo EE. Reversal of left ventricular hypertrophy in hypertensive patients treated with methyldopa. Lack of association with blood pressure control. Am J Cardiol 1982; 49: 795–801.

25. Schelling P, Fischer H, Ganten D. Angiotensin and cell growth: a link to cardiovascular hypertrophy? J Hypertens 1991; 9: 3–15.

26. Sen S, Tarazi RC, Bumpus FM. Cardiac effects of angiotensin-antagonists in normotensive rats. Clin Sci 1979; 56: 439–444.

27. Ferrario CM. Importance of the renin-angiotensin-aldosterone system (RAS) in the physiology and pathology of hypertension: An Overview. Drugs 1990; 39(Suppl 2): 1–8.

28. Meggs LG, Ben-Ari J, Gummon D, Gordman AA. Myocardial hypertrophy: The effect of sodium and the role of sympathetic nervous activity. Am J Hypertens 1988; 1: 11–15.

29. De Simone G, Devereux RB, Camargo MJF, Wallerson DC, Sealey JE, Laragh JH. Reduction of development of left ventricular hypertrophy in salt-loaded Dahl salt-sensitive rats by angiotensin II receptor inhibition. Am J Hypertens 1996; 9: 216–222.

30. Schmieder RE, Messerli FH, Garaveglia GE, Nuñez BE. Dietary salt intake: a determinant of cardiac involvement in essential hypertension. Circulation 1988; 78: 951–956.

31. Du Cailar G, Ribstein J, Grolleau R, Mimran A: Influence of sodium intake on left ventricular structure in untreated essential hypertensives. J Hypertens 1989; 7(suppl 6): S258–S259.

32. Heimann JC, Drumond S, Rodrigues AT, Guedes AJ, Dichtchekenian V, Marcondes M. Left ventricular hypertrophy is more marked in salt-sensitive than in salt-resistant hypertensive patients. J Cardiovasc Pharmacol 1991; 17(suppl 2): 122–124.

33. Bigazzi R, Bianchi S, Baldari D, Sgherri G, Baldari G, Campese VM: Microalbuminuria in salt-sensitive patients. A marker for renal and cardiovascular risk factors. Hypertension 1994; 23: 195–199.

34. Sahn DJ, De Maria A, Kisslo J, Weyman A: The committee on M-mode standardization of the American society: recommendations regarding quantitation in M-mode echocardiography. Circulation 1978; 58:1071–1083.

35. Devereux RB, Reichek N: Echocardiographic determination of left ventricular mass in man. Anatomic validation of the method. Circulation 1977; 55: 613–618.

36. Koren MJ, Devereux RB, Casale PN, Savage DD, Laragh JH: Relation of left ventricular mass and geometry to morbidity and mortality in uncomplicated essential hypertension. Ann Intern Med 1991; 114: 345–352.

37. De la Sierra A, Lluch MM, Coca A, et al: Assessment of salt-sensitivity in essential hypertension by twenty-four hour ambulatory blood pressure monitoring. Am J Hypertens 1995; 8: 970–977.

38. De la Sierra A, Lluch MM, Paré JC, Coca A, Aguilera MT, Azqueta M. Increased left ventricular mass in salt-sensitive hypertensive patients. J Hum Hypertens 1996; in press.

39. Campese VM, Romoff MS, Levitan D, et al. Abnormal relationship between salt intake and sympathetic nervous system activity in salt-sensitive patients with essential hypertension. Kidney Int 1982; 21: 371–378.

40. Limon I, Blanc J, Koutouzov S, Knorr A, Meyer P, Marche P. Platelet phospholipase C activity in salt-dependent hypertension. Hypertension 1990; 15: 381–387.

41. Campese VM: Salt sensitivity in hypertension. Renal and cardiovacular implications. Hypertension 1994; 23: 531–550.

42. De la Sierra A, Lluch MM, Coca A, et al: Fluid, ionic and hormonal changes induced by high salt intake in salt-sensitive and salt-resistant hypertensive patients. Clin Sci 1996; 91: 155–61.

43. Brilla CG, Weber KT: Mineralocorticoid excess, dietary sodium, and myocardial fibrosis. J Lab Clin Med 1992; 120: 823–825.

44. Simpson P: Norepinephrine-stimulated hypertrophy of culture rat myocardial cell is an alpha-adrenergic response. J Clin Invest 1983; 72: 732–738.

45. Luft FC, Rankin LI, Henry DP, et al: Plasma and urinary norepinephrine values at extremes of Na$^+$ intake in normal man. Hypertension 1979; 1: 261–266.

46. Koolen MI, van Brummelen PV: Adrenergic activity and pheripheral hemodynamics in relation to sodium sensitivity in patients with essential hypertension. Hypertension 1984; 6: 820–825.

47. De la Sierra A, Coca A, Paré JC, Sánchez M, Valls V, Urbano-Márquez A. Erythrocyte ion fluxes in essential hypertensive patients with left ventricular hypertrophy. Circulation 1993; 88: 1628–1633.

48. Navarro F, Coca A, Paré JC, De la Sierra A, Bosch X, Urbano-Márquez A. Left ventricular hypertrophy in asymptomatic essential hypertension: its relationship with aldosterone and the increase in sodium-proton exchanger activity. Eur Heart Journal 1993; 14(Suppl J): 38–41.

49. Coca A, De la Sierra A, Urbano-Márquez A. Ion Transport and left ventricular hypertrophy in essential hypertension. In: A. Coca and R.P. Garay (Eds). Ion Transport in Hypertension. New Perspectives. CRC Press, Boca Raton, Florida (USA), 1994: 247–272.

50. Lluch MM, De la Sierra A, Poch E, Coca A, Aguilera MT, Compte M, Urbano-Márquez A. Erythrocyte sodium transport, intraplatelet pH, and calcium concentration in salt-sensitive hypertension. Hypertension 1996; 27: 919–925.

51. Inoue I, Matsuura H, Shingu T, et al. Role of intracellular cation abnormalities in development of left ventricular hypertrophy. J Cardiovasc Pharmacol 1991; 17(suppl 2): 107–109.

52. Verdecchia P, Porcellati C, Schillaci G, et al: Ambulatory blood pressure. An independent predictor of prognosis in essential hypertension. Hypertension 1994; 24: 793–801.

53. Sharma AM, Ruland K, Spies KP, Distler A: Salt sensitivity in young normotensive subjects is associated with a hyperinsulinemic response to oral glucose. J Hypertens 1991; 9: 329–335.

54. Sharma AM, Schorr U, Distler A: Insulin resistance in young salt-sensitive normotensive subjects. Hypertension 1993; 21: 273–279.

55. Falkner B, Hulman S, Kushner H: Hyperinsulinemia and blood pressure sensitivity to sodium in young blacks. J Am Soc Nephrol 1992; 3: 940–946.

56. Bigazzi R, Bianchi S, Baldari G, Campese VM: Clustering of cardiovascular risk factors in salt-sensitive patients with essential hypertension: role of insulin. Am J Hypertens 1996; 9: 24–32.

57. Weir MR. Insulin resistance and salt sensitivity. A renal hemodynamic abnormality? Am J Hypertens 1996; 9: 193s–199s.

11

VOLUME OVERLOAD, ATRIAL NATRIURETIC PEPTIDE, AND LEFT VENTRICULAR HYPERTROPHY

M. Luque Otero,[1] N. Martell,[1] A. L. Aubele,[1,2] J. L. Rodrigo,[1,2] M. Herrero,[1] J. Moya,[1] I. Egocheaga,[1] A. Fernández-Cruz,[1] and C. Fernandez Pinilla[1]

[1]Hypertension Unit
Hospital Universitario San Carlos
Universidad Complutense
28040 Madrid. Spain
[2]Departamento de Exploración Cardiopulmonar
Hospital Universitario San Carlos
Universidad Complutense
28040 Madrid. Spain

The development of high blood pressure leads to an increased hemodynamic afterload to the heart, wich is compensated by an increase of cardiac mass in order to maintain the cardiac output. However,despite the casual link between high blood pressure and left ventricular hypertrophy (LVH) clinical studies do not show a close correlation between blood pressure level and the degree of LVH (1).

Several explanations for this observation have been suggested, including the inability of casual blood pressure measurements to estimate long-term pressure overload. Highest correlation coefficients with the left ventricular mass (LVM) were found when the mean of the pressures obtained during ambulatory blood pressure monitoring (ABPM) were considered (2). In addition there is a number of non-hemodynamic humoral factors, such as the renin angiotensin system and the adrenergic activity, implicated in the development of LVH.

However it is possible that equal degrees of LVH may be achieved by pure hemodynamic pressure or volume overload, and that LVM may be independently related to arterial pressure and stroke volume.

1. EFFECTS OF ACUTE VOLUME CHANGES IN LVM

Acute changes in extracellular volume modifying the preload may induces changes in the left ventricular end-diastolic diameter (LVID), a parameter included in the Devereux

Hypertension and the Heart, edited by Zanchetti et al.
Plenum Press, New York, 1997

103

formula to calculated the LVM by echocardiogram (3). Small changes of the LVID could be magnified because the cubed effect on LVM calculation.

This have been demonstrated in both acute volumen depletion and acute volumen expansion. Prisant el al (4) studied in normotensive healthy volunteers the effect of acute volumen depletion induced by the intravenous injection 40 mg furosemide on LVM. Echocardiograms were performed before and 2h after the administration of furosemide. No significant modifications of interventricular septum (IVS) or relative wall thickness (RWT) were found after furosemide but significant decreases of both the LVID (from to 51 to 49.2 mm, $p<0.05$) and the LVM index (LVMI) (from 92.8 to 82.7 g/m^2, $p< 0.05$) were observed.

Our group studied the effect of acute volume expansion induced by 2 liter of isotonic saline infused in an antecubital vein in 2 hours in both essential hypertensives and normotensive controls. Patients were maintained at least 4 weeks without antihypertensive treatment before entry in the study. 24-hour urinary sodium was measured the day before the saline infusion. M-mode echocardiograms were performed before and at the end of the saline infusion. Blood samples were obtained to determine plasma levels ot the atrial natriuretic peptide (ANP) by specific radioinmunoassay.

The results are shown in the Table 1. At baseline LVMI was significantly higher in essential hypertensives than in normotensive controls. Saline infusion induced a significant increase of the LVMI in both groups of subjects, due to the increase of the LVID. Neither IVS nor PWT experienced significant modifications during the saline infusion.

Thus, acute volume changes resulted in significant modifications in LVMI. In 1984 Messerli et al (5) identified total blood volume as a determinant of the LVM. The sodium balance is an important determinant of both the intracellular and the extracellular fluid volume state and modifications of the sodium balance may modify the left ventricular dimensions. The variations in left ventricular volume load may induce parallel modifications in left ventricular mass.

2. RELATION BETWEEN SODIUM INTAKE, ATRIAL NATRIURETIC PEPTIDE, AND LVM

The relationship between sodium intake and LVM was demonstrate by Schmieder et al in 1988 (6). They studied 42 untreated essential hypertensive patients on their usual diet. The

Table 1. Mean blood pressure (MBP), atrial natriuretic peptide (ANP) and echocardiographic parameters at baseline and at the end of 2l saline infusion in normotensives and essential hypertensives

	Normotensives		Essential hypertensives	
	Baseline	Post infusion	Baseline	Post infusion
MBP (mmHg)	82 ± 6	85 ± 8	100 ± 9	102 ± 8
ANP (pg/ml)	26 ± 16	78 ± 59**	33 ± 31	73 ± 62**
IVS (mm)	8.1 ± 9	8.1 ± 9	9.6 ± 13[++]	9.6 ± 13
PWT (mm)	8 ± 1	8 ± 0.1	9 ± 1.4	9 ± 1.4
LVID (mm)	46.2 ± 3	47.8 ± 3*	50 ± 4[++]	52 ± 4**
LVMI (g/m²)	80 ± 14	86 ± 15*	104 ± 22[++]	110 ± 24**

IVS: interventricular septum; PWT: posterior wall thickness;
LVID: end-diastolic left ventricular internal diameter; LVMI: left ventricular mass index.
*p<0.05, **p<0.01 as compared with baseline values.
[++]p<0.01 as compared with normotensives.

Table 2. Univariate and multivariate correlations between systolic
blood pressure (SBP), body mass index (BMI), 24 hour urinary sodium
excretion (UNa) and atrial natriuretic peptide (ANP) plasma concentrations
and left ventricular echocardiographic parameters in 23 adolescents

	IVS	PWT	LVID	LVMI
Univariate				
SBP	NS	NS	0.47*	0.41*
BMI	0.56**	0.66**	NS	0.53*
UNa	0.53*	0.53*	0.53*	0.56*
ANP	NS	−0.44*	−0.43*	−0.42*
Stepwise regression				
SBP	NS	NS	NS	NS
BMI	0.31**	0.32**	NS	NS
UNa	NS	NS	0.25**	0.24*
ANP	NS	NS	−0.21*	−0.30**

IVS: interventricular septum; PWT: posterior wall thickness; LVID: end-diastolic left ventricular
internal diameter; LVMI: left ventricular mass index.
*$p<0.05$; **$p<0.01$.

patients collect urine over 24-hours and M-mode echocardiograms were performed. The sodium excretion was found to be the strongest determinant for posterior wall thickness ($r= 0.64$, $p<0.01$), IVS ($r= 0.38$, $p<0.05$), RWT ($r= 0.67$, $p<0.01$) and LVMI ($r= 0.37$, $p<0.05$).

Our group investigate the influence of sodium intake on LVM in a group of 23 adolescents (aged 16.5 ± 2.5 years) selected from an epidemiological survey, the Torrejon Study, on blood pressure in children and adolescents (7). In 15 of the 23 BP levels were persistently above the 95th percentile of the BP distribution according to age and sex. None had ever take antihypertensive therapy. The sodium intake was assessed in urine collected during one 24-hour period on the day before the M-mode echocardiogram. In addition a blood sample was drawn to measure atrial natriuretic peptide (ANP) and plasma renin activity (PRA), two important hormones systems in the control of sodium balance (8).

The results appear in Table 2. Significant univariate positive correlations between the LV size parameters and the urinary sodium excretion were found. The BMI was also a powerful determinant of LV dimensions. In contrast, the correlation between ANP and all left ventricular parameters was negative and statistically significant. Neither diastolic BP nor PRA were correlated with the LV measures. A stepwise multiple regression analysis showed that urinary sodium was the most strong determinant of LVID and of the LVMI, independently of other variables. BMI was the most important determinant of both the IVS and the PWT, but was not correlated with the LVMI. ANP was correlated negatively with the left ventricular internal diameter and with the LVMI.

Our study not only confirms that sodium intake may be an important determinant of the left ventricular size but also shows that ANP had a negative relation with the LVMI. Schmieder (6) had discussed the mechanism to explain the relation between sodium intake and LVM, including the reactivity of the adrenergic system, that increases in parallel with dietary salt intake, and the inadequate supression of the renin-angiotensin system activity when the sodium intake is high, a fact observed in nearly half of the essential hypertensive patients.

Another possibility is that a high sodium intake can increases the intravascular volume thereby increasing preload to the left ventricle. The hemodynamic adaptation to an increase in sodium intake consists of a rise in the cardiac index due to an increase in stroke volume. These changes are due primarily to an increase in end-diastolic left ventricular volume. It seems that as sodium intake increases, both diastolic filling and left ventricular filling dimensions increase. Plasma levels of ANP respond quickly to changes in dietary sodium intake and remain elevated throughout a high sodium intake (8). As sodium intake can increase the LVID and LVMI, the ANP response to sodium intake is negatively correlated with the left ventricular dimensions. A maximal ANP response to sodium intake could facilitate the excretion of sodium, reducing its effects on the left ventricular dimensions.

To extend this observation we studied the modifications of LVMI during an acute intravenous sodium load and its relationship with the changes of ANP plasma levels in both essential hypertensives and normotensive controls. Sixteen patients (9 male) with mild to moderate hypertension were studied. Their age ranged from 16 to 46 years and they were without antihypertensive medication for at least 4 weeks prior the study. The control group consisted of 15 normotensive subjects aged from 20 to 28 years. They do not have a family history of hypertension.

The subjects collected the urine during the day previous to the study. After an overnight pariod of fasting they were placed in the supine position and a catheter was introduced in an antecubital vein to collect blood samples. An M-mode echocardiogram was performed before and at the end of an infusion of 2 liters of saline (300 mmol sodium). ANP was determined at baseline and at the end of the infusion.

The results appears in Table 1. Essential hypertensives were older and had BMI, SBP, DBP and HR significantly higher than the normotensive controls. In contrast 24-hour urinary sodium excretion (Una) and baseline plasma ANP levels were similar in both groups. Both LVMI and ANP plasma concentrations increased significantly after the saline infusion. At baseline a positive significant correlation between 24-hour urinary sodium and LV dimensions in essential hypertensives was observed (LVID $r=0.51$, $p<0.01$); IVS $r=0.47$, $p<0.05$; PWT $r=0.52$, $p<0.01$; LVMI $r=0.56$, $p<0.01$). Again ANP plasma concentrations and LVMI were negatively correlated, being the correlations statistically significants at the end of the saline infusion (normotensives: $r=-0.42$, $p<0.05$; hypertensives: $r=-0.34$, $p<0.05$). The correlations between the variations of both ANP and LVMI during the infusion were negative but not statistically significant. Thus, all these data tend to indicate that the ANP response to saline infusion could be an important mechanism in the control of sodium excretion, reducing the preload, the diastolic diameter and the calculated left ventricular mass.

3. RELATION BETWEEN LVH AND HEMODYNAMIC VARIABLES

The first paper examining the relation between LVH and hemodynamic variables other than BP was published by Devereux and coworkers in 1983 (9). They studied 44 essential hypertensive patients with definite LVH. To evaluate the relation between hemodynamic measurements and echocardiographic parameters they used 2 different indexes of LVH, the LVMI and the relative wall thickness (RWT), that is the ratio between the PWT and the radius of the left ventricle.

Only weak relations between LVMI and BP were observed (SBP: $r=0.32$, $p<0.005$; DBP: $r=0.26$, $p<0.02$ and MBP: $r=0.32$, $p<0.005$) and the correlations between BP and RWT, an index of concentric hypertrophy, were even weaker and non-significants. LVMI had a modest positive significant correlation with the cardiac index ($r=0.26$, $p<0.02$) and was negatively non-significant related with the total peripheral resistance (TPR) ($r=-0.20$,

NS). In contrast RWT exhibited a direct correlation with TPR (r=0.52, p<0.001) and a significant inverse correlation with the cardiac index (r=−0.47, p<0.001). For any level of blood pressure, patients with lower levels of cardiac index tended to have a higher relative wall thickness and vice versa.

These results demonstrate that the relation between hemodynamic variables such as cardiac index or total peripheral resistance, and left ventricular mass is similar or even closer than that of BP with LVM. In addition indicate that concentric LVH is more directly related to peripheral resistance than to blood pressure alone while it is inversely correlated with the cardiac index, perhards because the increased left ventricular stiffness due to increased relative wall thickness may result in an impairment ot the diastolic left ventricular filling and reduction in stroke volume and cardiac index (9).

4. HEMODYNAMIC PROFILE OF THE LEFT VENTRICLE ADAPTATION TO HIGH BLOOD PRESSURE

Although it is generally expected that the adaptation of the left ventricle to sustained hypertension would be concentric hypertrophy, several studies (10,11) had shown this is often not the case, and whereas many patients had normal LVMI and RWT other develop eccentric hypertrophy related to increase cardiac output and preload. High cardiac output and normal total peripheral resistance is the typical hemodynamic profile of the early stages of essential hypertension (12) and it is often seen in patients with renal artery hypertension (13) and in patients with hyperdynamic essential hypertension(14).

In 1992 Ganau et al (15) studied the patterns of ventricular geometric adaptation to high blood pressure, their prevalence and their relations to hemodynamic, left ventricular load and contractile performance in a population of 165 patients with untreated essential hypertension. They divided the patients in four different categories according the values of relative wall thickness and left ventricular mass index (16):

- Normal LV, when both LVMI and RWT within normal limits.
- Concentric remodeling, when the LVMI was normal and the RWT was increased.
- Concentric LVH, characterized by an increase of both LVMI and RWT.
- Eccentric LVH, when the LVMI was increased and the RWT was within normal limits.

The upper limits for LVMI (111 g/m^2 in men and 106 g/m^2 in women) and the partition value for RWT (0.44) were derived from the values obtained in a normotensive population.

In 1995 Shigematsu et al (17) also examined the patterns of left ventricular adaptation to sustained hypertension in a group of 148 patients, 40% of them receiving antihypertensive therapy. In this study the limits for both LVMI and RWT were also derived from the values obtained in a normotensive population (for LVMI they were 108 and 104 g/m^2 in males and females respectively, and for RWT it was 0.44). Our group did the same in a sample of 218 untreated essential hypertensive patients, considering a normal value of LVMI <120 g/m^2 for both sexes and a partition value of 0.44 for RWT.

The Table 3 summarizes the results obtained in the 3 studies. Concentric hypertrophy, the traditional form of adaptation of the left ventricle to high blood pressure was present only in a 8% of the patients studied by Ganau, 14% of those of Shigematsu and 23% of our spanish patients. The prevalence of eccentric hypertrophy was higher than those of concentric hypertrophy in the studies of Ganau and Shigematsu and similar in our study (27%, 27% and 23% respectively). A significant number of the patients, ranging from 13

Table 3. Prevalence (%) of the four different patterns of left ventricular adaptation in 3 different series of essential hypertensive patients

Series (n)	Normal	CR	EH	CH
Ganau (165)	52	13	27	8
Shigematsu (140)	45	14	27	14
Own results (218)	35	19	23	23

CR: concentric remodeling; EH: eccentric hypertrophy; CH: concentric hypertrophy.

to 19% had concentric remodeling and a normal left ventricle was found only in 35 to 52% of the hypertensive patients.

Table 4 shows the hemodynamic characteristics derived from echocardiograms associated with different left ventricular patterns in the patients of Ganau and in those included in our study. In both studies the patients with concentric hypertrophy had higher blood pressures than those included in the other groups. The concentric remodeling group had the highest values of total peripheral resistance observed among the hypertensive groups and the lowest cardiac index. The group with eccentric hypertrophy exhibited opposite findings to those associated with concentric remodeling: cardiac index was increased whereas total peripheral resistance was reduced as compared with the other hypertensive groups.

These findings suggest that the group with concentric remodeling offset the effects of pressure overload by volume underload which may explain the mild blood pressure elevation despite the high peripheral resistance. Eccentric hypertrophy had been usually associated to systolic functional impairment (18) or obesity (19) but in the studies considered here no patients had symptoms or signs of heart failure, and in our study Doppler ultrasound was routinely performed thus excluding some regurgitant valvular lesions that could promote the development of eccentric hypertrophy. In addition BMI did not differ among the four groups of patients in both studies. In our study sodium excretion was similar in the four groups of patients.

The hemodynamic profile of the patients with eccentric hypertrophy suggests an increased ventricular filling as the responsible for the ventricular hypertrophy and the high cardiac index, possibly due to an increase in blood volume (20) or venous tone (21).

Thus volume overload play an important role in determining the pattern and severity of left ventricular hypertrophy in hypertension, and the factors that influence stroke volume (such as blood volume, venous tone or afterload) are able to modulate the cardiac adaptation to high blood pressure.

Table 4. Cardiac index (CI) and total peripheral resistance (TPR) associated with different left ventricular patterns in essential hypertensive patients

	Normal	CR	EH	CH
Ganau				
CI	2.9 ± 0.7	$2.4 \pm 0.5^*$	$3.8 \pm 0.7^{*ao}$	3.1 ± 0.8^{o}
TPR	1741 ± 407	$2217 \pm 637^*$	$1417 \pm 289^{*ao}$	$1992 \pm 513^{*a}$
Own results				
CI	3.5 ± 0.9	$2.4 \pm 0.6^*$	$4.6 \pm 1.1^{*ao}$	3.5 ± 0.9^{ao}
TPR	1471 ± 395	$2289 \pm 712^{*ao}$	$1188 \pm 307^{*ao}$	1829 ± 465^{a}

CR: concentric remodeling; EH: eccentric hypertrophy; CH: concentric hypertrophy.
$^*p<0.05$ vs N; ^{a}vs CR; ^{o}vs CH.

REFERENCES

1. R.B.Devereux, T.G. Pickering, M.H. Alderman, S.Chien, J.S. Borer and J.H. Laragh. Left ventricular hypertrophy in hypertension. Prevalence and relationship to pathophysiologic variables. *Hypertension*, 9(suppl II): II-53–II-60 (1987).

2. J.I.M. Drayer, M.A. Weber and J.L. Young. BP as a determinant of cardiac left ventricular muscle mass. *Arch Intern Med*, 143: 90–92 (1983).

3. R.B. Devereux. Detection of left ventricular hypertrophy by M-mode echocardiography. Anatomic validation, standardization and comparison to other methods. *Hypertension*, 9 (suppl II): II-19–II-26 (1987).

4. L. M: Prisant, D.J. Kleinman, A.A. Carr, P.B. Bottini and C.M. Gross. Assessment of echocardiographic left ventricular mass before and after acute volume depletion. *Am J Hypertens*, 7: 425–428 (1994).

5. F.H. Messerli, K. Sungaard- Ruse, H.O. Ventura, F.G. Dunn, W. Oigmann and E.D. Frohlich. Clinical and hemodynamic determinants of left ventricular dimensions. *Arch Intern Med*, 144: 477–482 (1984).

6. R.E. Schmieder, F.H. Messerli, G.E. Garavaglia and B.D. Nunez. Dietary salt intake. A determinant of cardiac involvement in essential hypertension. *Circulation*, 78: 951–956 (1988).

7. N. Martell, J.L. Rodrigo, C. Fernandez-Pinilla, J. Gutkowska, A. Fernandez-Cruz, F. Vivas, M.C. Ramon, M.J. Pascual and M. Luque-Otero. Sodium intake and atrial natriuretic factor as determinants of left ventricular dimensions: the Torrejon Study. *J Hypertens*, 9 (suppl 6): s258–s259 (1991).

8. G.A. Sagnella, N.D. Markandu, A.C.Shore and G.A. MacGregor. Changes in plasma immunoreactive atrial natriuretic peptide in response to saline infusion or to alterations in dietary sodium intake in normal subjects. *J Hypertens*, 4(suppl 2): s115–s118 (1986).

9. R.B.Devereux, D.D. Savage, I. Sachs and J.H. Laragh. Relation of hemodynamic load to left ventricular hypertrophy and performance in hypertension. *Am J Cardiol*, 51: 171–176 (1983).

10. F. Abi-Samra, F.M. Fouad and R.C. Tarazi. Determinants of left ventricular hypertrophy and function in hypertensive patients: an echocardiographic study. *Am J Med*, 75 (suppl 3A): 26–33 (1983).

11. G. de Simone, L. DiLorenzo, G. Costantino, D. Moccia, S. Buonissimo and O. de Vittiis. Hemodynamic hypertrophied left ventricular patterns in systemic hypertension. *Am J Cardiol*, 60: 1317–1321 (1987).

12. M. Luque Otero, J.L. Rodrigo, J. Alcazar, R. Gabriel, C. Fernandez Pinilla, A. Fernandez-Cruz and N. Martell Claros. Hemodynamic in children with blood pressures in the 95th percentile of the distribution. *J Hypertens*, 5 (suppl 5): s435–s437 (1987).

13. R.C. Tarazi, M.M. Ibrahim, H.P. Dustam and C.M. Ferrario. Cardiac factors in hypertension. *Circ Res*, 34(suppl I): I-213–I-221(1974).

14. M.M. Ibrahim, R.C.Tarazi, H.P. Dustan, E.L. Bravo, R.W. Gifford Jr. Hyperkinetic heart in severe hypertension: a separate clinical hemodynamic entity. *Am J Cardiol*, 35:667–674 (1975).

15. A. Ganau, R.B. Devereux, M.J.Roman, G. de Simone, T.G. Pickering, P.S.Saba, P. Vargiu, Y. Simongini and J.H.Laragh. Patterns of left ventricular hypertrophy and geometric remodeling in essential hypertension. *J Am Coll Cardiol*, 19: 1550–1558 (1992).

16. M.J. Koren, R.B. Devereux, P.N. Casale, D.D. Savage and J.H. Laragh. Relation of left ventricular mass and geometry to morbidity and mortality in uncomplicated essential hypertension. *Ann Intern Med*, 114: 345–352 (1991).

17. Y. Shigematsu, M. Hamada, M. Mukai, H. Matsuoka, T. Sumimoto and K. Hiwada. Clinical evidence for an association between left ventricular geometric adaptation and extracardiac target organ damage in essential hypertension, *J Hypertens*, 13: 155–160 (1995).

18. B.E. Strauer . Hypertensive Heart Disease. Berlin: Springer-Verlag. 1980.

19. C.J. Lavie and F.H. Messerli. Cardiovascular adaptation to obesity and hypertension. *Chest*, 90: 275–279 (1986).

20. A. Ganau, A. Arru, P.S. Saba G. Piga, N. Glorioso, G. Tonolo, G. Madeddu and G. Bianchi. Stroke volume and left heart anatomy in relation to plasma volume in essential hypertension. *J Hypertens*, 9(suppl 6): s150–s151 (1991).

21. M.A. Fitzpatrick, A.L. Hinderliter, B.M. Egan, S. Julius. Decreased venous distensibility and reduced renin responsiveness in hypertension. *Hypertension*, 8(suppl II): II-36–II-43 (1986).

12

THE RENIN-ANGIOTENSIN SYSTEM GENE POLYMORPHISM AND LEFT VENTRICULAR HYPERTROPHY

Laurence Tiret

INSERM U258
Paris, France

Left ventricular hypertrophy (LVH) is a major risk factor for cardiovascular morbidity and mortality, independently of blood pressure. This has been clearly demonstrated in the Framingham Study. On the other hand, inhibitors of angiotensin-converting enzyme (ACE) have been shown to have a beneficial effect on LVH. In the SOLVD trial, treatment by ACE-inhibitors was associated with a reduction of the incidence of myocardial infarction (MI) and unstable angina and of cardiovascular mortality in patients with a low ejection fraction. In the SAVE trial including post-MI patients, treatment by ACE-inhibitors was associated with a decrease of mortality and incidence of re-infarction. These results, together with the fact that angiotensin II is implicated in the modulation of cardiac growth, suggest that polymorphisms of the renin angiotensin system could play a role in the determination of left ventricular mass (LVM) and the genetic predisposition of LVH.

The present talk will focus on ACE which plays a central role in the renin-angiotensin system. The ACE gene has been the most studied so far in relation to LVH. The ACE gene is localized on chromosome 17 and a frequent polymorphism has been identified in intron 16, characterized by an insertion (I)/deletion (D) of a 287 bp sequence. The ACE I/D polymorphism is strongly related to plasma ACE levels, the D allele being associated with increased levels in a codominant fashion. However, the ACE I/D polymorphism has probably no functional role by itself but is only a marker in linkage disequilibrium with a functional variant yet to be identified.

IMPLICATION OF THE ACE I/D POLYMORPHISM IN LVH AND LVM

In Table 1 are summarized the results of studies examining the role of the ACE I/D polymorphism in LVH and LVM[1–9]. The results are conflicting, however it should be

Hypertension and the Heart, edited by Zanchetti et al.
Plenum Press, New York, 1997

111

Table 1. ACE I/D polymorphism and LVH

Author	Year	Country	Population	Phenotype	Sample size	Assoc I/D
Schunkert	1994	Germany	Pop-based	ECG-LVH	LVH+ = 290 LVH - = 290	+
West	1994	Australia	Hypertens	ECHO-LVH	LVH+ = 33 LVH - = 83	-
Iwai	1994	Japan	Outpatient clinic	ECG-LVH	LVH+ = 56 LVH - = 72	+
				ECHO-LVM	N = 142	+
Prasad	1994	UK	Hypertens	ECHO-LVM	N = 85	-
Kupari	1994	Finland	Pop-based	ECHO-LVM	N = 86	-
Lindpaintner	1996	USA	Pop-based	ECHO-LVM	N = 2439	-
Gharavi	1996	USA	Hypertens	ECHO-LVM	N = 64	+
Wong	1996	Australia	Outpatient clinic	ECHO-WT	AS = 54 NBP = 59	+ -
Busjahn	1997	Germany	Twins	ECHO-WT	N = 132	+

LVH: Left ventricular hypertrophy; LVM: Left ventricular mass; WT: Wall thickness

stressed that most of the studies included relatively small sample sizes and had a low statistical power to detect genetic effects of modest magnitude as those expected in the determination of a multifactorial phenotype. Schunkert et al.[4] studied a sample of 717 men and 711 women (aged 45–59 yr) selected from the population covered by the MONICA register of Augsburg (Germany). In this population, 20.3% of subjects had a LVH defined by electrocardiography. These subjects were compared to controls matched for age, sex and blood pressure status. In males, the frequency of the DD genotype was significantly increased in subjects with LVH compared to controls. Such a difference was not observed in females. After dividing up the male population between normotensive and hypertensive subjects, it appeared that the difference of genotype frequency was observed only in normotensive men. However, this difference was due both to an excess of the DD genotype in LVH patients and to a deficit in controls. Lindpaintner et al.[7], in the Framingham Heart Study, reported no association or genetic linkage between the ACE gene and LVM. However, this study had a low power to detect genetic linkage. Moreover, DNA samples were available for only 50% of the subjects having had an echocardiography, which might have induced a selection bias.

IMPLICATION OF THE ACE I/D POLYMORPHISM IN REMODELING AFTER MYOCARDIAL INFARCTION

As shown in Table 2, three studies[10–12] have reported a positive association between the ACE I/D polymorphism and left ventricular dilation after MI. In the CATS study[11], a double blind trial comparing captopril to a placebo in MI patients, end-sytolic and end-diastolic volume indexes did not differ at baseline, but after one year of follow-up, the DD and ID genotypes were associated with a dilation of left ventricular, while no change was apparent in the II genotype. Interestingly, in patients treated with captopril, the deleterious effect associated with the D allele was blunted.

Table 2. ACE I/D and left ventricular remodeling after MI

Author	Year	Country	Population	Method	Phenot	Sample size	Assoc I/D
Pinto	1995	Netherlands	CATS trial	ECHO	ESVI EDVI	N = 96	+
Ohmichi	1995	Japan	PTCA	Catheterization	ESVI EDVI	N = 79	+
Ohmichi	1996	Japan	MI	ECHO	ESVI EDVI	N = 103	+

ESVI: End-Systolic Volume Index; EDVI: End-Diastolic Volume Index

IMPLICATION OF THE ACE I/D POLYMORPHISM IN CARDIOMYOPATHY

The role played in remodeling after MI raised the hypothesis that the ACE I/D polymorphism could act as a modifying factor in pathological conditions. This hypothesis seems also supported by the findings observed in hypertrophic cardiomyopathy (HCM). All studies[13-16] including HCM patients found that the DD genotype was associated with a worse prognosis of the disease (Table 3). This might be explained by the fact that HCM patients having the DD genotype have been found to have a greater extent of LVH compared to patients having the II or ID genotype[14].

By contrast, studies[17-20] examining a possible involvement of the ACE I/D polymorphism in ischemic or idiopathic cardiomyopathy have produced conflicting results (Table 4).

IMPLICATION OF THE ACE I/D POLYMORPHISM IN THE DEVELOPMENT OF PHYSIOLOGICAL LVH

Montgomery et al.[21] recently reported a study based on a sample of 149 male recruits from the British Army who were submitted to a 10-weeks intensive exercise training. Different phenotypes (septal thickness, posterior wall thickness and LVM) were measured before and after the 10-weeks period. Whereas subjects with the II genotype did not exhibit any longitudinal change in the different phenotypes, subjects with the DD

Table 3. ACE I/D and hypertrophic cardiomyopathy

Author	Year	Country	Population	Phenotype	Sample size	Assoc I/D
Marian	1993	USA	HCM families	Disease	HCM = 100 Cont = 106	+
Lechin	1995	USA	HCM fam+spor	ECHO-LVMI	HCM = 183	+
Yonega	1995	Japan	HCM fam+spor	Disease	HCM = 80 Cont= 88	+
Pfeufer	1996	Germany	HCM unrelated	Disease	HCM = 50 Cont = 50	+

Table 4. ACE I/D and ischemic or idiopathic cardiomyopathy

Author	Year	Country	Population	Phenotype	Sample size	Assoc I/D
Raynolds	1993	USA	ISC, IDC	Disease	ISC = 102 IDC =112 Cont = 79	+
Montgomery	1995	UK	IDC	Disease	IDC = 99 Cont = 364	-
Sanderson	1996	Hong-Kong	ISC, IDC	Disease	ISC = 53 IDC = 51 Cont = 18	-
Andersson	1996	Sweden	IHF	5-yr survival ECHO-LVMI	IHF= 193	+ +

ISC: Ischemic cardiomyopathy; ISC: Idiopathic dilated cardiomyopathy;

IHF: Idiopathic heart failure

genotype exhibited an increase for all these parameters. Subjects with the ID genotype were intermediate between II and DD subjects. This result, if confirmed, would suggest that the ACE I/D polymorphism also acts as a modifying factor in physiological conditions.

In conclusion, this review of the literature indicates that large and well-designed studies are still warranted to determine the exact role of the ACE I/D polymorphism, and of other polymorphisms of the renin angiotensin system, in predisposition to LVH in the population at large. Several lines of evidence suggest that the ACE I/D polymorphism could act as a modifying factor in pathophysiological conditions. For these reasons, clinical trials testing the benefits of ACE-inhibitors in complications of different cardiovascular diseases should include the determination of the ACE genotype.

REFERENCES

1. Iwai N, Ohmichi N, Nakamura Y, Kinoshita M. DD genotype of the angiotensin-converting enzyme gene is a risk factor for left ventricular hypertrophy. *Circulation.* 1994;90:2622–2628.
2. Kupari M, Perola M, Koskinen P, Virolainen J, Karhunen P. Left ventricular size, mass and function in relation to angiotensin-converting enzyme gene polymorphism in humans. *Am J Physiol.* 1994;267:H1107–H1111.
3. Prasad N, O'Kane KPJ, Johnstone HA, Wheeldon NM, McMahon AD, Webb DJ, MacDonald TM. The relationship between blood pressure and left ventricular mass in essential hypertension is observed only in the presence of the angiotensin-converting enzyme gene deletion allele. *Q J Med.* 1994;87:659–662.
4. Schunkert H, Hense HW, Holmer SR, Stender M, Perz S, Keil U, Lorell BH, Riegger GAJ. Association between a deletion polymorphism of the angiotensin-converting-enzyme gene and left ventricular hypertrophy. *N Engl J Med.* 1994;330:1634–1638.
5. West M, Summers K, Burstow D, Wong K, Huggard P. Renin and angiotensin-converting enzyme genotypes in patients with essential hypertension and left ventricular hypertrophy. *Clin Exp Pharm Physiol.* 1994;21:207–210.
6. Gharavi A, Lipkowitz M, Diamond J, Jhang J, Phillips R. Deletion polymorphism of the angiotensin-converting enzyme gene is independently associated with left ventricular mass and geometric remodeling in systemic hypertension. *Am J Cardiol.* 1996;77:1315–1319.
7. Lindpaintner K, Lee M, Larson MG, Rao VS, Pfeffer MA, Ordovas JM, Schaefer EJ, Wilson AF, Wilson PWF, Vasan RS, Myers RH, Levy D. Absence of association or genetic linkage between the angiotensin-converting-enzyme gene and left ventricular mass. *N Engl J Med.* 1996;334:1023–1028.

8. Wong K, Summers K, Burstow D, West M. Genetic variants of proteins from the renin angiotensin system are associated with pressure load cardiac hypertrophy. *Clin Exp Pharm Physiol.* 1996;23:587–590.

9. Busjahn A, Knoblauch H, Knoblauch M, Bohlender J, Menz M, Faulhaber H, Becker A, Schuster H, Luft F. Angiotensin-converting enzyme and angiotensinogen gene polymorphisms, plasma levels, cardiac dimensions. A twin study. *Hypertension.* 1997;29[part 2]:165–170.

10. Ohmichi N, Iwai N, Nakamura Y, Izumi M, Kinoshita M. The genotype of the angiotensin-converting enzyme gene and global left ventricular dysfunction after myocardial infarction. *Am J Cardiol.* 1995;76:326–329.

11. Pinto Y, van Gilst W, Kingma J, Schunkert H. Deletion-type allele of the angiotensin-converting enzyme gene is associated with progressive ventricular dilation after anterior myocardial infarction. *J Am Coll Cardiol.* 1995;25:1622–1626.

12. Ohmichi N, Iwai N, Maeda K, Shimoike H, Nakamura Y, Izumi M, Sugimoto Y, Kinoshita M. Genetic basis of left ventricular remodeling after myocardial infarction. *Int J Cardiol.* 1996;53:265–272.

13. Marian AJ, Yu Q, Workman R, Greve G, Roberts R. Angiotensin-converting enzyme polymorphism in hypertrophic cardiomyopathy and sudden cardiac death. *Lancet.* 1993;342:1085–1086.

14. Lechin M, Quinones M, Omran A, Hill R, Yu Q, Rakowski H, Wigle D, Liew C, Sole M, Roberts R, Marian A. Angiotensin-converting enzyme genotypes and left ventricular hypertrophy in patients with hypertrophic cardiomyopathy. *Circulation.* 1995;92:1808–1812.

15. Yoneya K, Okamoto H, Machida M, Onozuka H, Noguchi M, Mikami T, Kawaguchi H, Murakami M, Uede T, Kitabatake A. Angiotensin-converting enzyme gene polymorphism in Japanese patients with hypertrophic cardiomyopathy. *Am Heart J.* 1995;130:1089–1093.

16. Pfeufer A, Osterziel K, Urata H, Borck G, Schuster H, Wienker T, Dietz R, Luft F. Angiotensin-converting enzyme and heart chymase gene polymorphisms in hypertrophic cardiomyopathy. *Am J Cardiol.* 1996;78: 362–364.

17. Raynolds MV, Bristow MR, Bush EW, Abraham WT, Lowes BD, Zisman LS, Taft CS, Perryman MB. Angiotensin-converting enzyme DD genotype in patients with ischaemic or idiopathic dilated cardiomyopathy. *Lancet.* 1993;342:1073–1075.

18. Montgomery H, Keeling P, Goldman J, Humphries S, Talmud P, McKenna W. Lack of association between the insertion/deletion polymorphism of the angiotensin-converting enzyme gene and idiopathic dilated cardiomyopathy. *J Am Coll Cardiol.* 1995;25:1627–1631.

19. Andersson B, Sylven C. The DD genotype of the angiotensin-converting enzyme gene is associated with increased mortality in idiopathic heart failure. *J Am Coll Cardiol.* 1996;28:162–167.

20. Sanderson J, Young R, Yu C, Chan S, Critchley J, Woo K. Lack of association between insertion/deletion polymorphism of the angiotensin-converting enzyme gene and end-stage heart failure due to ischemic or idiopathic dilated cardiomyopathy in the Chinese. *Am J Cardiol.* 1996;77:1008–1010.

21. Montgomery H, Clarkson P, Dollery C, Prasad K, Losi M, Statters D, Jubb M, McEwan J, Humphries S, McKenna W. D polymorphism of the angiotensin converting enzyme gene is strongly associated with the development of physiological left ventricular hypertrophy. *J Am Coll Cardiol.* 1996;27 (suppl A):244A.

13

RENIN-ANGIOTENSIN SYSTEM GENE POLYMORPHISMS AND LEFT VENTRICULAR HYPERTROPHY

The Case against an Association

M. J. West,* K. M. Summers, K. K. Wong, and D. J. Burstow

Departments of Medicine and Cardiology
University of Queensland
Prince Charles Hospital
CHERMSIDE QLD 4032, Australia

SUMMARY

There is accumulating evidence for association between genetic polymorphisms of components of the renin angiotensin system (RAS), especially angiotensin-converting enzyme (ACE), and cardiovascular disease. However, there is lack of agreement that the ACE polymorphism is associated with left ventricular hypertrophy (LVH) in hypertension. A possible paradigm for the development of LVH involves the ACE gene polymorphism influencing cardiac mass by an action on plasma and/or tissue levels of angiotensin II. Such a model has experimental support and provides the basis for examining the lack of agreement between studies. The finding of lack of association between RAS gene polymorphism and LVH may be due to methodological problems, differences in genetic background between populations, interactions between genetic variants of RAS components or to the model being inappropriate.

Low predictability of ACE genotype markers for LVH together with conflicting reports on the influence of RAS genetic variants on angiotensin II production suggests that the simple RAS paradigm may not apply for hypertension. Further information on the nature of the link between the ACE polymorphism and ACE regulation as well as the relation between the RAS and pathophysiology of LVH is needed. At present there is insufficient evidence to accept ACE gene polymorphism as a susceptibility marker for LVH.

---

* Address for Correspondence: Professor MJ West, Department of Medicine, University of Queensland, Level B1, Pathology Building, Prince Charles Hospital, CHERMSIDE QLD 4032. *Telephone*: +61 7 3350 8381, *Fax*: +61 7 3359 2173.

Hypertension and the Heart, edited by Zanchetti et al.
Plenum Press, New York, 1997

1. INTRODUCTION

The finding of association between angiotensin I converting enzyme (ACE) gene polymorphism and myocardial infarction[1] left ventricular hypertrophy (LVH)[2], restenosis after coronary artery angioplasty[3], hypertrophic cardiomyopathy[4], ischaemic and dilated cardiomyopathy[5], renal artery stenosis[6], lacunar stroke[7] and diabetic nephropathy[8] has led to the suggestion that the ACE gene polymorphism is a general marker of susceptibility to cardiac disease. For LVH the view is further supported by studies which show regression of LVH following treatment with ACE inhibitor drugs[9]. Despite such population and individual study findings, the underlying mechanism by which the ACE genotype might influence the pathophysiology of cardiovascular disease is unknown.

2. ASSOCIATION OF ACE GENE POLYMORPHISM AND LVH

Association between ACE gene polymorphism and LVH has been reported in response to physical exertion[17], in subjects randomly selected from the population at large[2] and from hospital outpatient attendees[18], in a group of subjects with modest aortic stenosis[19] and in subjects with hypertrophic cardiomyopathy[4]. In Schunkert's study[2] although the association existed for the population as a whole, the relationship was strongest in normotensive males. In contrast to these results showing association there was an absence of linkage between ACE genotype and left ventricular mass in 2439 subjects selected from the Framingham Heart Study[20]. A smaller study in 86 subjects[21] also failed to find any association. In our own study[22], subjects were recruited from a cardiac outpatient population with a high prevalence of coronary artery disease. No association was found for hypertensive subjects but an association existed in those with aortic stenosis[18].

3. ACE GENE AS A SUSCEPTIBILITY MARKER FOR LVH — THE MODEL

The renin angiotensin system (RAS) is important in the regulation of cardiac mass both in the presence[10] or absence[11] of altered cardiac loading conditions. Cardiac cell growth is modified by the availability of angiotensin II (AII) and its uptake by AII type 1 (AT1) receptors. The action of ACE on degradation of bradykinin and limitation of nitric oxide production may also be important. It is, therefore, possible that genetic variation in the components of the RAS (angiotensinogen (AGT), renin, ACE, ATI receptors) may determine the degree of cardiac cell growth (and as a consequence cardiac mass), during different physiological or pathological states.

Alternatively, it is possible that non-ACE pathways are involved in the generation of AII from AGT directly[12,13] or from AI[14,15]. Chymase, an enzyme in cardiac tissue may also convert either AGT or AI to AII[16]. The significance of these pathways at present is unclear.

A possible explanation for the finding of an association between ACE gene polymorphism and LVH is that the presence or absence of the genetic marker (the ACE deletion (D) allele) influences cardiac cell mass by an action on AII plasma and/or tissue levels. Such a model has experimental support and provides the basis for examining the lack of agreement between studies. The following needs to be considered:

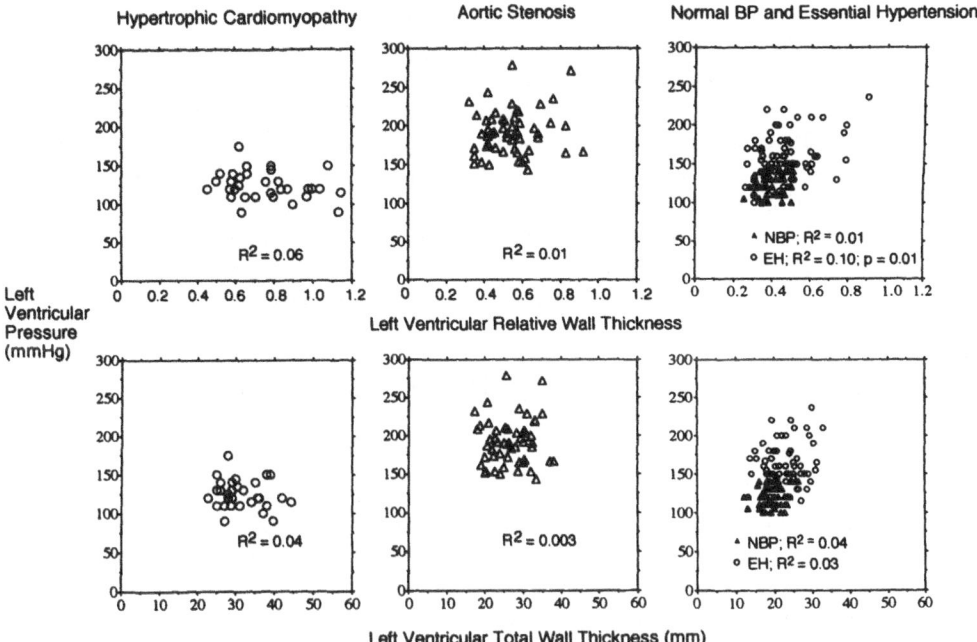

Figure 1. Relation between left ventricular total wall thickness (septum plus free wall) and left ventricular systolic pressure (bottom panel) and between left ventricular relative wall thickness (total wall thickness ÷ left ventricular diastolic diameter) and left ventricular systolic pressure (top panel) in 3 groups of subjects: those with hypertrophic cardiomyopathy (left panels); those with aortic stenosis (centre panels) and those with normal blood pressure or with essential hypertension (right panels).

1. There appears to be no simple relationship between load and increased cardiac mass. A significant relationship was lacking in our own studies (Figure 1), similar to the findings of others. Similarly, the nature of the interaction between load and activation of the RAS in the development of LVH Is unknown. It is possible that a threshold for load exists, above which the RAS modifies the degree of cellular hypertrophy. This, however, seems unlikely since the ACE polymorphism association exists in subjects with normal blood pressure[2], in those undertaking physical exertion[17] and in those with normal blood pressure and hypertrophic cardiomyopathy.[4]

2. Tissue chymase production of AII in the heart or the activation of other non ACE pathways may mask the involvement of ACE. Chymase may have a role in some forms of LVH and not others.

3. The effect of ACE genetic variants in the production of AII may be masked by other RAS variants. For example, there is an association between AGT genetic variants and hypertension[23]. However, there was a failure to demonstrate an association between AGT genetic markers and cardiac hypertrophy in hypertensive subjects[24]. On the other hand, the same group were able to show that the $T^{174}M$ AGT genetic marker predicted left ventricular relative wall thickness in aortic stenosis[19]. Furthermore, the $T^{174}M$ AGT and ACE insertion (I)/deletion genetic polymorphisms acted together to influence the degree of LVH.

4. In experimental hypertension, aldosterone affects cardiac size independently of blood pressure[25], possibly as a result of an increase in fibrous tissue. Plasma

aldosterone levels were not related to LVH in a study of 84 subjects selected according to predisposition for hypertension[26]. The study, however, does not exclude a cardiac tissue effect of aldosterone.

5. Differences in results between studies of subjects with LVH may be due to methodological issues — characterisation of hypertension or LVH, subject selection bias, method of statistical analysis or to differences in genetic background of the population. Significant differences exist in the prevalence of LVH and in the frequency of the ACE gene I/D variants in white compared to black populations[27].

6. It is possible the model proposed does not apply in hypertension, i.e. RAS is not an important determinant of LVH associated with hypertension.

4. EVIDENCE SUGGESTING MODEL IS INADEQUATE

Is there evidence to suggest that the simple RAS paradigm with respect to the development of LVH does not apply?

1. The predictability of the ACE genotype marker for plasma ACE activity and for LVH in an individual is low, indicating that while ACE gene polymorphism accounts for a proportion of the variance, other factors ar acting.

2. The ACE gene polymorphism is due to genetic variation in intron 16 of the ACE gene and as such is unlikely to regulate ACE gene function. Further information regarding the linkage between ACE gene polymorphism and the regulatory function of the gene would assist in understanding the role of the RAS in the pathophysiology of LVH.

3. The relation between ACE gene polymorphism and production of AII in human subjects has not been clarified. Subjects with ACE DD genotype were shown in one study to produce a higher blood pressure response to a given dose of AI[28]. However, in another study the ACE genotype was not found to influence circulating RAS components or blood pressure levels[29], suggesting that the relation between RAS genetic polymorphisms and the level of AII, the level of blood pressure or the degree of LVH is complex. A simple paradigm is unlikely to apply.

5. CONCLUSION

There is accumulating evidence for an association between ACE (and AGT) gene polymorphism and cardiovascular disease. The association between RAS genetic variants (especially the ACE gene) and LVH is conflicting. The association is unpredictable. In the absence of a full understanding of the pathophysiology of the development of LVH, a robust model for testing hypotheses relating to genetic variation is not available. A case for RAS polymorphism as a susceptibility marker for LVH has yet to be made.

REFERENCES

1. Cambien F, Poirier O, Lecerf L, Evans A, Cambou J-P, Arveiler D, Luc G, Bard J-M, Bara L, Ricard S, Tiret L, Amouyet P, Alhenc-Gelas F, Soubrier F. Deletion polymorphism in the gene for angiotensin-converting enzyme is a potent risk factor for myocardial infarction. *Nature* 1992;359:641–644.
2. Schunkert H, Hense H-W, Holmer SR, Stender M, Perz S, Keil U, Lorell BH, Reiger GAJ. Association between a deletion polymorphism of the angiotensin-converting enzyme gene and left ventricular hypertrophy. *N Engl J Med* 1994;330:1634–1638.

3. Ohishi M, Fujii K, Minamino T, Higaki J, Kamitani A, Rakugi H, Zhao Y, Mikani H, Miki T, Ogihara T. A potent genetic risk factor for restenosis. *Nat Genet* 1993;5:324–325.

4. Marian AJ, Yu QT, Workman R, Greve G, Roberts R. Angiotensin-converting enzyme polymorphism in hypertrophic cardiomyopathy and sudden cardiac death. *Lancet* 1993;342:1085–1086.

5. Raynolds MV, Bristow MR, Bush EW, Abraham WT, Lowes BD, Zisman LS, Taft CS, Perryman MB. Angiotensin-converting enzyme DD genotype in patients with ischaemic or dilated cardiomyopathy. *Lancet* 1993;342:1073–1075.

6. Missouris CG, Barley J, Jeffery S, Carter ND, Singer DRJ, MacGregor GA. Genetic risk for renal artery stenosis: association with deletion polymorphism in angiotensin 1-converting enzyme gene. *Kidney Int* 1996;49:534–537.

7. Markus HS, Barley J, Lunt R, Bland J, Jeffery S, Carter N, Brown M. Angiotensin-converting enzyme gene deletion polymorphism: a new risk factor for lacunar stroke but not carotid atheroma. *Stroke* 1995;126:1329–1333.

8. Doria A, Warram JH, Krolewski AS. Genetic predisposition to diabetic nephropathy. *Diabetes* 1994;43:690–695.

9. Dahlof B, Pennert K, Hansson L. Reversal of left ventricular hypertrophy in hypertensive patients: meta-analysis of 109 treatment studies. *Am J Hypertens* 1992;5:95–100.

10. Schunkert H, Dzau VJ, Tang SS, Hirsch AT, Apstein CS, Lorell BH. Increased rat cardiac angiotensin-converting enzyme activity and mRNA expression in pressure overload left ventricular hypertrophy. *J Clin Invest* 1990;86:1913–1920.

11. Baker KM, Aceto JF. Angiotensin II stimulation of protein synthesis and cell growth in chick cells. *Am J Physiol* 1990; 259(Heart Circ Physiol 28):H610–H618.

12. Dzau VJ, Sasamura H, Hein L. Heterogeneity of angiotensin synthetic pathways and receptor subtypes: physiological and pharmacological implications. *J Hyptertens* 1993;11 Suppl 3:S13–8.

13. Phillips MI, Speakman EA, Kimura B. Levels of angiotensin and molecular biology of the tissue renin angiotensin systems. *Regul Pept* 1993;43:1–20.

14. Klickstein LB, Kaempfer CE, Wintraub BU. The granulocyte-angiotensin system. Angiotensin 1-converting activity of cathepsin G. *J Biol Chem* 1982;257:15042–6.

15. Tang SS, Loscalzo J, Dzau VJ. Tissue plasminogen activator activates renin angiotensin *in vitro. J Vasc Med Biol* 1989;1:67–74.

16. Urata H, Nishimura H, Ganten D. Chymase-dependent angiotensin II forming system in humans. *Am J Hypertens* 1996;9:277–84.

17. Montgomery H, Clarkson P, Dollery C, Prasad K, Losi M-A, Statters D, Jubb M, McEwan J, Humphries S, McKenna W. D polymorphism of the angiotensin-converting enzyme gene is strongly associated with the development of physiological left ventricular hypertrophy. (Abstract.) *J Am Coll Cardiol* 1996;27(Suppl A):244A.

18. Iwai N, Ohmichi N, Nakamura Y, Kinoshita M. DD genotype of the angiotensin-converting enzyme gene is a risk factor for left ventricular hypertrophy. *Circulation* 1994;90:2622–2628.

19. Wong KK, Summers KM, Burstow DJ, West MJ. Genetic variants of proteins from the renin angiotension system are associated with pressure load cardiac hypertrophy. *Clin Exptl Pharmacol Physiol* 1996;23:587–590.

20. Lindpaintner K, Lee M, Larson MG, Rao S, Pfeffer MA, Ordovas JM, Schaefer EJ, Wilson AF, Wilson PWF, Vasan RS, Myers RH, Levy D. Absence of association or genetic linkage between angiotensin-converting enzyme gene and left ventricular mass. *N Engl J Med* 1996;334:1023–1028.

21. Kupari M, Perola M, Koskinen P, Virolainen J, Karhunen P. Left ventricular size and function in relation to angiotensin-converting enzyme gene polymorphism in humans. *Am J Physiol* 1994;267(Heart Circ Physiol 36):H1107–H1111.

22. West MJ, Summers KM, Burstow DJ, Wong KK, Huggard PR. Renin and angiotensin-converting enzyme genotypes in patients with essential hypertension and left ventricular hypertrophy. *Clin Exptl Pharmacol Physiol* 1994;21:207–210.

23. Jeunemaitre X, Soubrier F, Kotelvtsev YV, et al. Molecular basis of human hypertension: role of angiotensinogen. *Cell* 1992;71:169–80.

24. West MJ, Wong KK, Summers KM, Burstow DJ. Inability to demonstrate association between markers of angiotensinogen or angiotensin-converting enzyme in hypertensive subjects with different phenotypes of cardiac hypertrophy (abstract). *7th Europ Meeting on Hypertension* 1995, P206.

25. Brilla CG, Pick R, Tan LB, Janicki JS, Weber KT. Remodeling of the rat right and left ventricles in experimental hypertension. *Circ Res* 1990;67:1355–1364.

26. Harrap SB, Dominiczak AF, Fraser R, Lever AF, Morton JJ. Plasma angiotensin II, predisposition to hypertension and left ventricular size in healthy young adults. *Circulation* 1996;93:1148–1154.

27. Barley J, Blackwood A, Carter ND, Crews DE, Cruickshank JK, Jeffery S, Ogunlesi AO, Sagnella GA. Angiotensin-converting enzyme insertion/deletion polymorphism: association with ethnic origin. *J Hypertens* 1994;12:955–957.
28. Ueda S, Elliot HL, Morton JJ, Connell JMC. Enhanced pressor response to angiotensin I in normotensive men with the deletion genotype (DD) for angiotensin-converting enzyme. *Hypertension* 1995; 25:1266–1269.
29. Lachurie ML, Azizi M, Guyennne TT, Alhenc-Gelas F, Menard J. Angiotensin-converting enzyme gene polymorphism has no influence on the circulating renin angiotensin aldosterone system or blood pressure in normotensive subjects. *Circulation* 1995; 91:2933–2942.

LEFT VENTRICULAR HYPERTROPHY AND ARTERIAL HYPERTROPHY

Jean-Michel Mallion, Jean-Philippe Baguet, Jean-Philippe Siché, F. Tremel, and R. De Gaudemaris

Medécine Interne et Cardiologie
CHU de Grenoble
BP 217-38043 Grenoble Cedex 9
France

INTRODUCTION

In the most recent WHO recommendations of 1996 (1) it has been clearly stated that the definition of hypertension (HT) depends on diastolic and/or systolic blood pressure (BP) values. The measurement of BP using classical methods in the doctor's surgery with a mercury manometer and using the auscultatory method remains the method of reference. This measure of BP in the surgery can be complemented in certain cases by other measurements such as recording in the patient's home or ambulatory measures. The WHO also notes that the classification of HT still remains based on BP values but also on the extent of organic lesions and the cause of the HT. The severity of organic lesions is often correlated with the level of BP values but this is not always the case. Furthermore the rate of progression of lesions varies from one person to another in relation to many factors most of which are unknown. Therefore the BP and the organic effects should be evaluated separately. Thus study of the cardiac and vascular function and in particular, the presence of hypertrophy or remodeling in these areas should be studied.

For many years investigators have focused separately on cardiac or vascular function and there are very few simultaneous studies of cardiac status and vessel disease. Obviously the first hurdle is the justification for such studies. In the first instance is the fact that there is an anatomic continuity between the heart and the vessels. This anatomical continuity does not, however, imply anatomo-pathological similarity. Cardiac muscle and in particular the left ventricle consists of myocytes or muscle cells. At arterial level one must distinguish conductance-compliance vessels vessels which are predominantly of elastic fibers from resistance-distribution vessels which are predominantly composed of muscle fibers (2). These facts imply study of more than one vascular territory and the need to integrate the data in the correlations which need to be examined.

There is also a haemodynamic continuity between the cardiac and vascular systems. but if one examines the variations in pressure as well as in flow emanating from the heart

Hypertension and the Heart, edited by Zanchetti et al.
Plenum Press, New York, 1997

to the periphery all the haemodynamic data are far from being identified. Thus the mean BP varies progressively from the heart to the periphery but in contrast the BP pulse increases. Likewise the pressure waves recorded between the ascending aorta and femoral artery in the adult human are very different (3).

According to O'Rourke (4) the major factors contributing to change in wave contour are cardiac (pattern and duration of ventricular ejection) and vascular: velocity of wave propagation in large arteries, and the degree of vasomotor tone and of wave reflection in peripheral beds. Moreover, different patterns are seen in different arteries and in the same artery at different ages and in the same artery under different physiological conditions (4). All these points need to be taken into account if one wishes to compare structural, cardiac and vascular modifications.

The different hormonal systems directly or indirectly implicated in the regulation of BP have very important roles in cardiac and vascular remodeling as for example the renin-angiotensin-aldosterone system. Initially it had been thought that angiotensin II intervened in BP regulation in an autocrine manner only. Recent studies have established that this hormone also has effects on cell proliferation, cardiac and vascular remodeling and an effect on growth factors as well. The transformation of angiotensin I to angiotensin II is mediated by the angiotensin converting enzyme (ACE) but we now know that in certain vascular territories other enzyme systems can intervene with their own specificity. Thus glycoprotein chymases have a specific affinity for angiotensin I in cardiac tissue. In vascular tissues chymase-like substances (chymostatin sensitive angiotensin II generating enzyme (CAGE)) are likewise substantially responsible for the formation of angiotensin II which probably varies according to the vascular territory (5). For these different reasons the results of parallel measures at cardiac and different arterial levels should be interpreted with caution.

PARAMETERS MEASURED

It needs to be constantly kept in mind that the type, and kind of measure needs to take account of its reliability and the reproducibility and the normal and reference values established.

At cardiac level the parameters measured are well defined and include intraventricular septal thickness, left ventricular internal diameter, relative wall thickness and the index of LVM.

At the vascular and particular at carotid level the indices of interest are arterial wall thickness, endiastolic diameter, relative wall thickness and cross sectional area. It is possible to compare intraventricular septal thickness with arterial wall thickness or the left ventricular internal diameter with arterial endiastolic diameter or the cross sectional area with mass index, but these comparisons need to be interpreted with great caution.

The introduction and the development in the last 20 years of ultrasound imaging has permitted a qualitative and quantitative approach to the definition of the above parameters. However if one is investigating the cardiac or vascular system then the ultrasound probes used and their frequencies differ as well as the image resolution; for instance, at vascular level, the data recorded are not the same depending on whether one use B mode ultrasonography or radiofrequency signals (wall track or nius 0,2) (6).

These different modes of approach explain that the reproducibility of the measures are not the same at cardiac level compared to vascular level and in particular are less good at cardiac level, the difference being 15 to 20% for the measure of the LVM (7) compared to 3 to 10% (8) for measures of the parietal wall thickness in the common carotid artery. Even the technical feasibility of measuring is poorest at cardiac level compared to vascular.

Reference values have evolved with time. For example the reference values for LVM were initially inferior to 125 g/m^2 for men and 110 g/m^2 for women (9). These values have changed with time and in recent large series are inferior to 111 g/m^2 for men and 106 g/m^2 for women (10). Note, however, that factors such as race and age are not taken into account.

At the vascular and particularly at carotid level the reference values for such measures as the wall dimensions are still under discussion and vary according to the technique and the level at which the measures are taken be it in the common carotid, bifurcation, or internal carotid, and vary from 0.6 to 1 mm (11). One must not use a localized thickening in the area of a plaque. It has become increasingly clear of the necessity of integrating with these morphological data the haemodynamic data such as BP of course but more so the arterial strain or the Peterson elastic modulus (12) for example.

Thus it is clear that according to different studies the terms vascular and cardiac hypertrophy do not correspond to the same adaptive mechanism. At the vascular level it seems more logical to speak of intimal media thickness than hypertrophy.

RELATIONSHIPS BETWEEN LVH AND VASCULAR HYPERTROPHY

If by means of these different developments one can justifiably compare the vascular and cardiac systems, that it is logical to proceed by examining the prevalence of such associations and their relationships and correlations, distinguishing the compliance and resistance vessels.

COMPLIANCE VESSELS (CAROTID ARTERY)

Roman et al. (13) studied 172 healthy normotensive subjects and noted a prevalence of both left ventricular and arterial hypertrophy of 5,2%. In 172 asymptomatic untreated hypertensive subjects they found a prevalence of left ventricular hypertrophy (LVH) of 12.2% and a similar level of arterial hypertrophy of 11%. These authors also found that in hypertensive subjects with LVH an arterial hypertrophy was observed in 24% of cases while arterial hypertrophy was found in only 9% of hypertensive subjects without LVH.

Baguet et al. (14) studied 50 hypertensive subjects who had never been treated and who were selected on the basis of ambulatory BP measurements with a mean systolic BP and diastolic BP of 147/96 mmHg respectively. They used the criteria of Devereux (9) to define LVH with an index of left ventricular (LVM) ≥ 125 g/m^2 for men and ≥ 110 g/m^2 in women. Their criteria for vascular hypertrophy were a IMT ≥1 mm (15). They found a prevalence of LVH of 30% and thickening of the common carotid of 8%. In this same population the prevalence of vascular hypertrophy was greater in subjects with LVH (20%) than in subjects without LVH (2.9%). Thus depending on the reference values the prevalence may differ.

The left ventricular geometric pattern is also an element to be considered. According to Roman et al. (18), only patients with concentric hypertrophy demonstrated significant increases in carotid artery size as shown by diastolic diameter and IMT and cross sectional

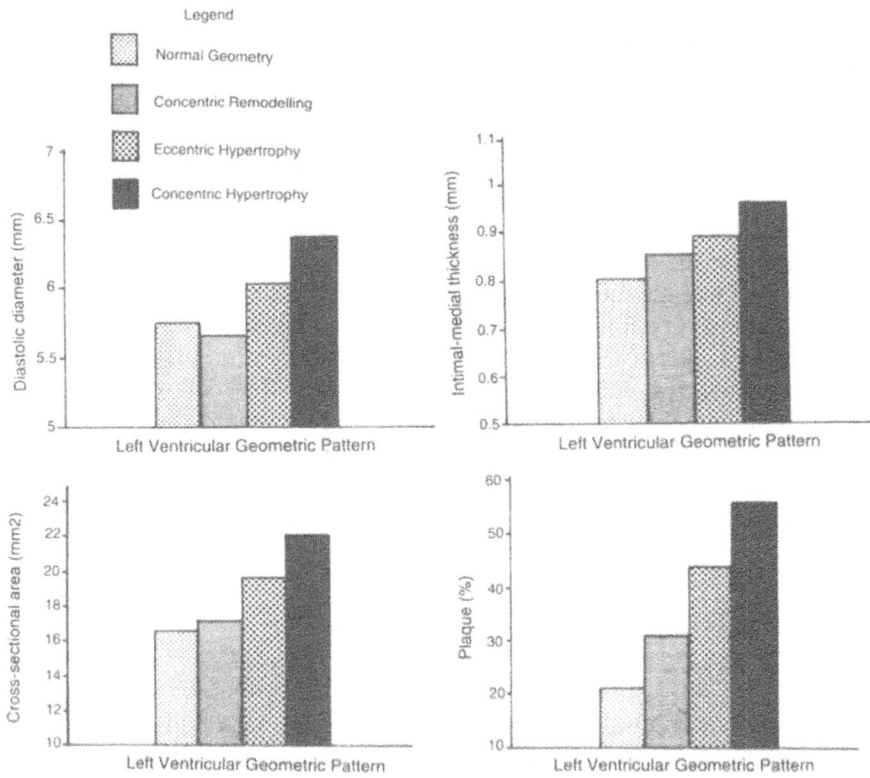

Figure 1. Relationship of left ventricular geometric pattern to the common carotid artery structure and the prevalence of atherosclerosis (Roman et al., JACC 1996, 28: 751–756).

atea. Patients with concentric hypertrophy had significant increases in arterial diameter and cross sectional area compared with those with concentric remodeling (Fig. 1).

Cuspidi et al. studied 62 hypertensives who had never been treated and who had a normal LVM (less than 125 g/m^2 in men and 110 g/m^2 in women) They reported also that the posterior wall of the common carotid artery at end-diastole was significantly thicker in subjects with concentric remodeling defined by a relative wall thickness ≥ 0,45.

More recently, Baguet et al. (14) confirm the presence of a statistical difference in IMT for the subjects who had a normal LV geometry and those with concentric LVH (Mean IMT respectively 0,70 mm and 0,84 mm).

Besides the presence of cardiac hypertrophy, Cuspidi et al. (17) reported a prevalence of carotid plaque significantly higher in subjects with concentric remodeling (34%) than in subjects with normal geometry (19%).

In another study performed on 486 subjects with 267 normotensive and 209 untreated hypertensives, Roman et al. (18) noted that the presence of atherosclerotic plaque within the extracranial carotid arteries increase significantly from the lowest quintile of LVM index to the highest. They reported that absolute and relative left ventricular and common carotid wall thickness were greater in the group with carotid atherosclerosis and that the prevalence of plaques was highest in the group with concentric hypertrophy (56%) in reference to normal geometric and concentric remodeling group despite similarities between groups in age, serum lipids and smoking histories. It is too soon to conclude that there is a relationship between remodeling and atherosclerosis in hypertension.

The existence of an association between the presence of LVH and vascular hypertrophy does not necessarily imply a correlation. As regards LVH, it is no longer questioned that its frequency is augmented in HT. The left ventricular wall thickness and its mass are strongly related to body surface, area systolic BP and to a lesser degree with age. For reasons probably related to technical difficulties it is only recently that a relationship has been established between the presence of VH and the existence of HT. In the Kuopio ischemic heart study, in 120 men hypertension was not associated with the presence of an increase in intimal media thickness (19).

As a result of a number of studies (16,20,21), it is now established one can now retain that common carotid IMT and the cross sectional area are strongly related to age and blood pressure. These results can be further examined by multivariate analysis.

Roman et al. (20) studied 43 untreated hypertensive patients and found that the relations between carotid and cardiac wall thickness and internal dimension remained significant after consideration of age and blood pressure. Later in a study of 172 untreated hypertensive patients they confirmed that the carotid cross sectional area is related to LVM (r=0,33 p<0,0005) (13). Cuspidi et al. (16) also found a significant correlation between the LVM and the common carotid artery IMT (r=0,43 p<0,01) in a cohort of 62 hypertensive subjects. This relationship between carotid wall thickening and LVH appears to be independent of age, blood pressure and serum lipid level.

However, Tices et al. (22), using multivariate analysis in 20 newly diagnosed non treated hypertensives and 81 treated hypertensives, found that only age, systolic arterial pressure and Murgo class were independent predictors of carotid artery intimal media thickness. Thus in a univariate analysis, the strongest univariate relations to carotid artery thickness were age, systolic arterial pressure, Murgo class, LVM and sex.

Baguet et al. (14) found in addition a significant correlation between LVM and IMT of the common carotid artery (r=0.30 p<0.05) (Fig. 2).

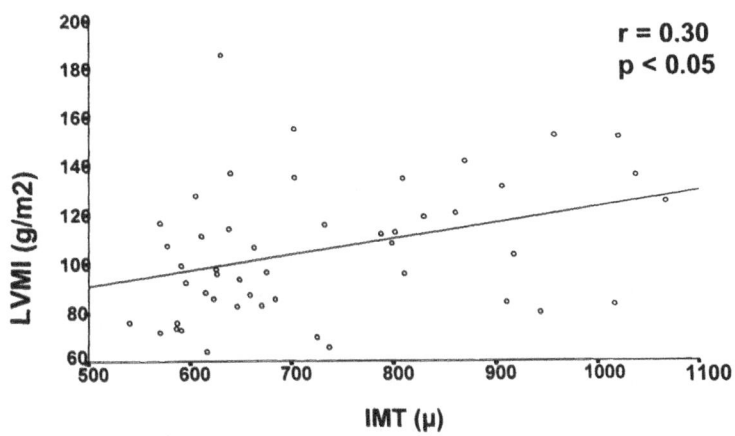

Figure 2. Correlation between left ventricular mass index (LVMI) and intima media thickness (IMT) (common carotid artery) independant of age, blood pressure. Fifty never treated hypertensive subjects (mean ABPM values 145/96).

RESISTANCE ARTERIES (RADIAL ARTERY)

Few studies have been carried out in this area. Siché et al. (23) studied the radial artery intimal media thickness (IMT) and the media lumen ratio (MLR) to describe the radial artery structure in 83 essential hypertensive subjects who had never been treated. Twenty-six subjects had LVH (normal LVM was defined as a mass <125g/m2 in men and <110g/m2 in women). In subjects with or without LVH, they did not find any significant difference for IMT or diameter. In contrast, they did note an increase in the MLR which is an expression of concentric remodeling in the group with LVH (Fig. 3).

Boutouyrie et al. (24), in a study of 86 hypertensives of which 31 were untreated, 31 had stopped treatment and 24 were on anti-hypertensive treatment, analyzed vessel wall motion by a pulsed ultrasound echo-tracking system (wall track system). They observed a highly significant correlation between left ventricular mean wall thickness and common carotid artery distensibility and compliance. They also noted that the LVM index was positively correlated to carotid and diastolic luminal cross sectional area (LCSA) (r=0.23 p=0.02).

Siche et al. (23) found a significant correlation between the radial medial lumen ratio and the relative wall thickness, but this correlation disappeared when one took into account age and systolic BP.

DETERMINING ELEMENTS OF THESE STRUCTURAL CHANGES

One can conclude that in compliance vessels such as the carotid there is an association between the presence of remodeling or LVH and the presence of corresponding modifications at vessel wall level. Depending on the reference values used to differentiate the presence or absence of modification or anomaly the prevalence rate may vary substantially. Such conclusions are not available for the radial artery.

It is logical to consider that these structural changes in arteries and in the heart which occurred in hypertension may be in response to similar factors but one must not confuse large arteries and resistant arteries. In this context both haemodynamic and humoral influences should be taken into account. The parallel increase of left ventricular and carotid dimensions among hypertensive patient are in part the result of an increased level of blood pressure. That additional hemodynamic abnormalities may contribute to the observed parallels between cardiac and vascular hypertrophy is probable. Thus changes in arterial properties such as vascular hypertrophy or atherosclerosis may cause earlier return of reflected pressure waves to the central circulation. An elevation of effective arterial compliance may thereby stimulate increases in LVM and relative wall thickness without a detectable alteration in systolic or diastolic arterial pressure (25,26).

The association between carotid atherosclerosis and increasing LVM may be explained by higher levels of both distending pressure and pulsatile force resulting in greater susceptibility to endothelial damage (16,18).

The observations of Boutouyrie et al. (24) that left ventricular mean wall thickness and mass volume ratio were inversely related to carotid artery distensibility and compliance, are consistent. Nonetheless one cannot exclude the possibility of other factors: humoral, genetic, etc., which may be importants in determining cardiac and vascular hypertrophy in hypertension.

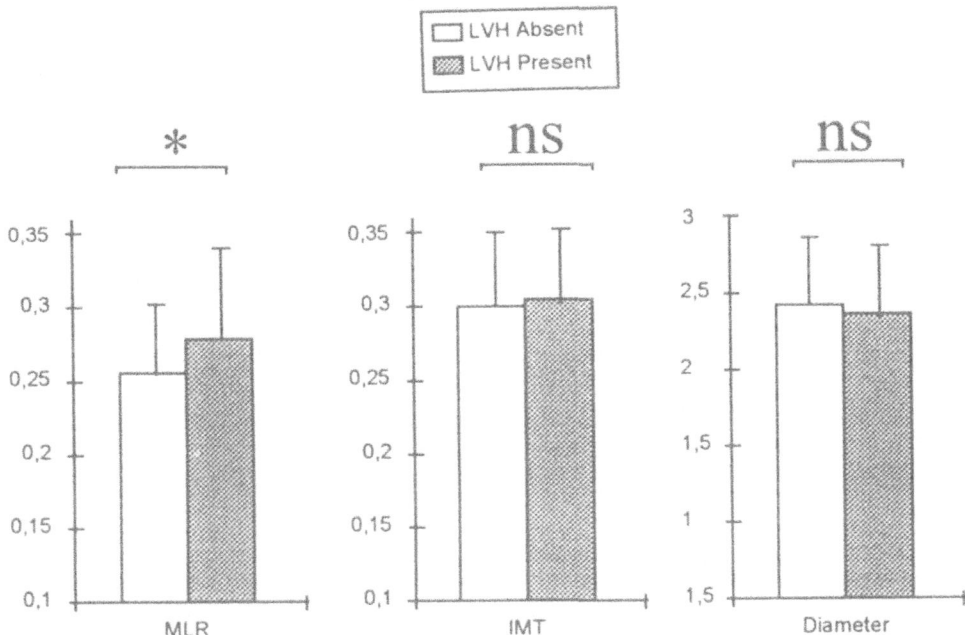

Figure 3. Bar graph shows comparison of radial artery structure of hypertensive subjects in whom left ventricular hypertrophy (LVH) is present or absent. IMT = intima media thickness in mm, MLR = media lumen ratio, diameter = internal diastolic diameter in mm. Data presented are mean values ± sd in mm. *p.01 ANOVA (with cofactors of age, sex, and ambulatory systolic BP).

CLINICAL IMPLICATIONS

At Diagnostic Level

The observation of a remodeling of the vessel wall and of hypertrophy of that wall at a relatively early stage of hypertension even before cardiac hypertrophy and when only cardiac remodeling exists may justify in itself the systematic practice of this examination in hypertensive subjects (16).

In the future the determination of simultaneous alterations such as hypertrophy in the heart and the vasculature should allow better estimation of the systemic effects and severity of HT. However these extra investigations would not be justified unless there are prognostic or therapeutic implications.

Prognostic Data

The prognostic usefulness of studying LV function in HT is now well established. Thus the presence of ventricular hypertrophy and in particular LVH is an indisputable risk factor both for acute or chronic coronary artery disease, for risk of sudden death and the development of cardiac failure. The mechanisms implicated include an augmentation of cardiac arythmia. The relative roles of atherosclerosis, myocardial fibrosis, alteration of coronary reserve or other factors to explain these outcomes remain to be established (27,28,29,30,31,32,33,34,35).

An association between the presence of LVH and the risk of cerebrovascular accidents (CVA) has been reported. Likewise more severe retinopathy and increased proteinuria have been shown in patient with LVH and in particular concentric hypertrophy (37).

As regards vascular changes, Bonithon-Kopp in a recent review of the literature (38), showed that intimal media thickening is clearly associated with an atherogenic profile suggesting it may be a marker of early atherosclerosis. This risk is expressed by an increased number of myocardial infarctions and rates of coronary insufficiency, cerebrovascular accidents and peripheral vascular disease (39,40,41).

In these studies HT is a relative limited risk factor in the absence of increased IMT.

The question arises as to whether the simultaneous presence of LVH and IMT in the carotid is a cumulative risk. To date there is no epidemiological answer available. For some authors (17) the association of an increased frequency of carotid plaques in the context of concentric LVH and perhaps the increased frequency of carotid plaques in the presence of IMT could possibly explain the increased risk of CVA and concentric LVH. In fact to consider the presence of carotid lesions together with LVH as an increased cumulative risk is premature and further long-term studies are needed.

Therapeutic Data

The expected result of well conducted anti-hypertensive treatment is not only to reduce to normal the BP values but also to cause regression or disappearance of lesion in target organs. As regards LVH two meta-analyses by Dahlöff (42), and by Schmieder (43) have shown that not all classes of anti-hypertensive have a similar effect and it seems that angiotensin converting enzyme (ACE) inhibitors have a greater effect in reducing LVH than beta blockers or diuretics in particular.

The effects of anti-hypertensive treatments on remodeling of vascular hypertrophy has been very little studied. Safar et al. (26) examined the wall thickness, and reported the radial artery mass and the radial thickness ratio are significantly higher in an untreated hypertensive group than in a control group. The MIDAS study whose objective was to investigate the regression of atherosclerotic plaques did not reach such conclusions (44).

In relation to the data available to date it seems logical to take into account the state of the vasculature in the same manner as the cardiac status in order to properly appreciate the effect of an anti-hypertensive. This is all the more important as there seems to be a correlation between vascular and cardiac hypertrophy and also because there are also independent factors acting on one or other area.

Depending on the haemodynamic modifications which they can induce a particular type of anti-hypertensive could have a positive or negative effect on one or other target organ. It seems logical to expect that anti-hypertensive treatment would have identical effects on the cardiac and vascular systems but this remains to be established.

ABSTRACT

In the most recent WHO recommendations of 1996 it was reiterated that the classification of HT still remains based on the actual BP figures but also on the importance of target organ lesions. Thus the study of cardiac and vascular function and in particular the presence of hypertrophy or remodeling is of importance.

A limited number of studies have examined the prevalence, the association and the correlation between modifications and remodeling in the heart and in the vasculature. It is important to distinguish compliance vessels such as the carotid from resistance vessels such as the radial. For compliance vessels the prevalence of cardiac and vascular hypertrophy are nearly identical being around 5% for normotensive subjects and around 12% for hypertensive subjects. This prevalence of thickening in the intima-media is more evident in subjects with left ventricular hypertrophy (LVH). The left ventricular geometric pattern is also an element to take into account. The presence of concentric remodeling of the left ventricle without LVH has already been associated with an increase in intima-media thickness (IMT). When there is an LVH this IMT is similar in severity to the LVH and in particular concentric. For resistance vessels such as the radial artery the number of studies is limited but a significant correlation between left ventricular mean wall thickness and common carotid artery distensibility and compliance has been found. There is also a significant correlation between the radial median lumen ratio and the relative wall thickness but this correlation disappears when age and systolic BP are taken into account. Thus for this type of vessel it is too early to conclude the elements contributing to structural changes. The determinant factors for these structural changes in the heart and the carotid arteries associated with hypertension are certainly multiple be they haemodynamic, hormonal or genetic. The observation establishing an association between anomalies at cardiac and vascular level may have undoubted diagnostic, prognostic and therapeutic implications which are all intimately related and which require refinement and confirmation.

REFERENCES

1. La lutte contre l'hypertension. Rapport d'un Comité d'Experts. Genève, Organisation Mondiale de la Santé 1996. (OMS, série de Rapports techniques, N°862).
2. Orcel L, Chomette G. Anatomie pathologique vasculaire. Ed; Flammarion Médecine Sciences, Paris 1978.
3. Nichols WW, O'Rourke MF. McDonald's blood flow in arteries. Third Edition,. Edt Lea & Febiger, Philadelphia, London, 1990.
4. O'Rourke MF, Kelly R, Avolio A. The Arterial Pulse. Edt Lea & Febiger, Philadelphia, London, 1992.
5. Urata H, Nishimura H, Ganten D. Mechanisms of angiotensin II formation in humans. European Heart J. 1995, 16 (Sup N): 79–85.
6. Girerd X, Botouyrie P, Pannier B, Mourad JJ, Safar M, Laurent S. Noninvasive ultrasound methods for the measurement of arterial wall thickness. Touboul P.J. Intima-Media thickness and atherosclerosis. Predicting the Risk? Ed. Parthenon Publishing Group, NY USA & Lancs UK, 1997: 45–57.
7. De Simone G, Ganau A, Verdecchia P, Devereux RB. Echocardiography in arterial hypertension: when, why and how? J Hypertens 1994; 12: 1129–1136.
8. Salonen R, Haapanen A, Salonen JT. Measurement of intima-media thickness of common carotid arteries with high-resolution B-mode ultrasonography: inter and intra-observer variability. Ultrasound Med Biol 1991; 17: 225–230.
9. Devereux RB, Lutas EM, Casale PN, Kligfield P, Eisenberg RR, Hammond IW et al. Standardization of M-mode echocardiographic left ventricular anatomic measurements. J Am Coll Cardiol 1984; 4: 1222–1230.
10. Ganau A. Devereux RB, Roman MJ, De Simone G, Pickering TG, Saba PS et al. Patterns of left ventricular hypertrophy and geometric remodeling in essential hypertension. J Am Coll Cardiol 1992; 19: 1550–1558.
11. Päivänsalo M, Rantala A, Kauma H, Lilja M, Reunanen A, Savolainen M, et al. Prevalence of carotid atherosclerosis in middle-aged hypertensie and control subjects. A cross-sectional systematic study with duplex ultrasound. J hypertens 1996; 14: 1433–1439.
12. Botouyrie P, Laurent S, Girerd X, Benetos A, Lacolley P, Abergel E, et al. Common carotid artery stiffness and patterns of left ventricular hypertrophy in hypertensive patients. J hypertens 1995; 25: 651–659.
13. Roman MJ, Pickering TG, Schwartz JE, Pini R, Devereux RB. Prevalence and Determinants of Cardiac and Vascular Hypertrophy in Hypertension. J hypertens 1995; 26: 369–373.
14. Baguet JP, Mallion JM, Moreau-Gaudry A, Siché JP, Cinquin P, Tremel F. Cardiac and vascular remodelling in never treated hypertensive subjects selected on ABPM data. To be published.
15. Salonen TJ, Salonen R. Ultrasonographic B-mode imaging in observational studies of atherosclerotic progression. Circulation 1993, 87 (suppl. 3); 56–65.

16. Roman MJ, Pickering TG, Schwartz JE, Pini R, Devereux RB. Relation of Arterial Structure and Function to Left Ventricular Geometric Patterns in Hypertensive Adults. J Am Coll Cardiol 1996; 28: 751–6.
17. Cuspidi C, Lonati L, Sampieri L, Pelizzoli S, Pontiggia G, Leonetti G, et al. Left Ventricular concentric remodelling and carotid structural changes in essential hypertension. J Hypertens 1996; 14: 1441–1446.
18. Roman MJ, Pickering TG, Schwartz JE, Pini R, Devereux RB. Association of Carotid Atherosclerosis and Left Ventricular Hypertrophy. J Am Coll Cardiol 1995; 25: 83–90.
19. Salonen JT and Salonen R. Ultrasonographically assessed carotid morphology and the risk of coronary heart disease. Arterioscler Thromb 1991; 11: 1245–1249.
20. Roman MJ, Saba PS, Pini R, Spitzer M, Pickering G, Rosen S, et al. Parallel Cardiac and Vascular Adaptation in Hypertension. Circulation 1992; 86: 1909–1918.
21. Hughes AD, Sinclair AM, Geroulakos G, Mayet J, Mackay J, Shahi M, et al. Structural changes in the heart and carotid arteries associated with hypertension in humans. J Hum Hypertens 1993; 7: 395–397.
22. Tice FD, Peterson JW, Orsinelli DA, Binkley PF, Cody RJ, Guthrie R, et al. Vascular hypertrophy is an early finding in essential hypertension and is related to arterial pressure waveform contour. Am Heart J 1996; 132: 621–7.
23. Siché JP, Naarouf N, Baguet JP, Tremel F, Degaudemaris R, Mallion JM. 24 H ambulatory pulse pressure is an independant predictor of the cardiac and vascular radial artery structural adaptation. Poster presentation. Eighth European Meeting on Hypertension, Milan 1997. To be published.
24. Boutouyrie P, Laurent S, Girerd X, Benetos A, Lacolley P, Abergel E et al. Common Carotid Artery Stiffness and Patterns of Left Ventricular Hypertrophy in Hypertensive Patients. Hypertens 1995; 25: 651–659.
25. Gariepy J, Massonneau M, Levenson J, Heudes D, Simon A. Evidence for in vivo carotid and femoral wall thickening in human hypertension. Hypertens 1993; 22: 111–8.
26. Safar ME, Girerd X, Laurent S. Structural changes of large conduit ateries in hypertension. J hypertens 1996; 14: 545–555.
27. Houghton JL, Frank MJ, Carr AA, Von Dohlen TW, Prisant LM. Relations among impaired coronary flow reserve, left ventricular hypertrophy and thallium perfusion defects in hypertensive patients without obstructive coronary artery disease. J Am Coll Cardiol 1990; 15: 43–51.
28. Treasure CB, Klein JL, Vita JA, Manoukian SV, Renwick GH, Selwyn AP et al. Hypertension and left ventricular hypertrophy are associated with impaired endothelium-mediated relaxation in human coronary resistance vessels. Circulation 1993; 87: 86–93.
29. Anthony I, Nitenberg A, Foult JM, Aptear E. Coronary vasodilatator reserve in untreated and treated hypertensive patients with and whithoud left ventricular hypertrophy. J Am Coll Cardiol 1993; 22: 514–520.
30. Schwartzkopff B, Motz W, Frenzel H, Vogt M, Knauer S, Strauer BE. Structural and functional alterations of the intramyocardial coronary arterioles in patients with arterial hypertension. Circulation 1993; 88: 993–1003.
31. Young W, Gofman JW, Tandy R. The quantitation of atherosclerosis. Quantitative aspects of the relationship of blood pressure and atherosclerosis. Am J Cardiol 1960; 6: 294–299.
32. Levy D, Anderson KM, Savage DD, Balkus S.A., Kannel WB, Castelli WP. Risk of ventricular arrhythmias in left ventricular hypertrtophy; the Framingham Heart Study. Am J Cardiol 1987; 60: 560–565.
33. McLenachan JM, Henderson E, Morris KI, Dargie HJ. Ventricular arrhythmias in patients with hypertensive left ventricular hypertrophy. N Engl J Med; 1987: 317: 782–792.
34. Ghali JK, Kadakia S, Cooper RS, Liao Y. Impact of left venticular hypertrophy on ventricular arrhythmias in the absence of coronary artery disease. J Am Coll Cardiol 1991; 17: 1277–1282.
35. Koyanagi S, Eastham CL, Harrison DG, Marcus ML. Increased size of myocardial infarction in dogs with chronic hypertension and left ventricular hypertrophy. Circ Res 1982; 50: 55–62.
36. Bikkina M, Levy D, Evans JC, Larson MG, Benjamin EJ, Wolf PA et al. Left ventricular mass and risk of stroke in an elderly cohort: The framingham Heart Study. JAMA 1994; 272: 33–36.
37. Blake J, Devereux RB, Herrold E McM, Jason M, Fisher J, Borer L. et al. Relation of concentric left ventricular hypertrophy and extracardiac target organ damage to supranormal left ventricular performance in established essential hypertension. Am J Cardiol 1988; 62: 246–252.
38. Bonithon-Kopp C; Prevalence of and risk factors for intima-media thickening: a literature review. Touboul P.J. Intima-Media thickness and atherosclerosis. Predicting the Risk? Ed. Parthenon Publishing Group, NY USA & Lancs UK, 1997: 27–44.
39. Salonen TJ and Salonen R. Arterial wall thickness, carotid atherosclerosis and the risk of myocardial infarction and cerebrovascular stroke. Touboul P.J. Intima-Media thickness and atherosclerosis. Predicting the Risk? Ed. Parthenon Publishing Group, NY USA & Lancs UK, 1997: 97–104.
40. Crouse JR. Association of arterial wall thickning and coronary disease. Touboul P.J. Intima-Media thickness and atherosclerosis. Predicting the Risk? Ed. Parthenon Publishing Group, NY USA & Lancs UK, 1997: 105–115.

41. Bots ML, Grobbee DE. Carotid intima-media thickness and atherosclerosis in the lower extremities. Touboul P.J. Intima-Media thickness and atherosclerosis. Predicting the Risk? Ed. Parthenon Publishing Group, NY USA & Lancs UK, 1997: 117–126.

42. Dahlöf B, Pennert K, Hansson L. Reversal of Left Ventricular Hypertrophy in Hypertensive Patients. A Metaanalysis of 109 Treatment studies. Am J Hypertens 1992; 5: 95–110.

43. Schmieder RE, Martus P, Klingbeil A. Reversal of left Ventricular Hypertrophy in Essential Hypertension. Jama 1996; 275: 19.

44. Borhani NO, Mercuri M, Borhani PA, Buckalew VD, Canossa-Terris M, Car AA, et al. Final outcome results of the multicenter isradipine diuretic atherosclerosis study (MIDAS). JAMA 1996; 276: 785–791.

RELATIONSHIP BETWEEN CARDIAC HYPERTROPHY AND MICROALBUMINURIA

Luis M. Ruilope

Insalud, Unidad de Hipertensión
Hospital "12 de Octubre"
Carretera de Andalucia Km. 5,400
28041 Madrid, Spain

INTRODUCTION

The term microalbuminuria was coined in 1982 at Guy's Hopsital in London (1) to define an abnormally elevated urinary albumin excretion (UAE) in absence of clinical proteinuria as measured by standard laboratory methods. A positive standard test for proteinuria appears when the quantity of proteins in urine exceeds 300 mg/day (2). Table 1 contains the definition of microalbuminuria as excretion rate in 24 hours or overnight urine collection, as albumin/creatinine ratio and as albumin concentration in morning or random urine sample. Determination of UAE in morning urine sample constitutes the ideal test for screening and overnight urine collection might be the best choice for monitoring microalbuminuria.

The normal urinary excretion of albumin oscillates between 1 and 22 mg/day and varies with posture, exercise, and blood pressure; the day-to-day variation is in the range of 31% to 52% (4,5). Therefore, a mean of three urine collections has been recommended to determine the UAE level of a given subject (1).

Different assays, recently reviewed (3), can be used to measure UAE including radioimmunoassay, enzyme-linked immunoassay, radial immunodiffusion, nephelometry and immunoturbidimetry. The two last are readily automated and allow a large number of samples to be processed in a minimum amount of time. Several semi-quantitative tests are also available, with the advantage of bringing the test closer for general practitioners (3). The Micral-test, is a test-strip method in which the colour reaction is mediated by an antibody-bound enzyme. Nycocard U-albumin is a three drop test based on a solid phase enzyme-linked immunosorbent assay. Both methods have shown good correlations with radioimmunoassay and can be readily used for screening.

MICROALBUMINURIA IN THE GENERAL POPULATION

It is now apparent that between 5 and 10 percent of nondiabetic individuals have a UAE within the microalbuminuric range (6). Initial studies (7,8,9,10) indicated that micro-

Hypertension and the Heart, edited by Zanchetti et al.
Plenum Press, New York, 1997

135

Table 1. Definition of microalbuminuria

Excretion rate
20-200 ug/min (valid for overnight urine collection)
30-300 mg/24 h
Albumin/creatinine ratio
2.5-25 mg/mmol (Europe)
30-300 mg/g (USA)
Albumin concentration
30-300 mg/L

(early morning urine)

albuminuria may be a strong predictor of mortality of cardiovascular origin. Nevertheless, it could not be concluded whether microalbuminuria is a predictor in its own value, or whether it is the association with other risk factors that is of importance. In this sense, elevated UAE has been shown to be related to elevated serum triglycerides and low high-density lipoprotein cholesterol, obesity and glucose intolerance (11,12,13). Association between smoking, alcohol intake and microalbuminuria also seem to exist (14,15). Finally, a correlation between systemic blood pressure and UAE has been found in the general population (16,17). Interestingly, the recent data of Jiang et al (17), indicate that the association between blood pressure and UAE is stronger in blacks than in whites, which supports the notion that blacks may be more susceptible to renal damage from relatively low levels of blood pressure increase.

The finding of an elevated UAE in non-diabetic individuals usually reflects the existence of an elevated glomerular passage of albumin that cannot be reabsorbed by the proximal tubule. Increased UAE could be the consequence of an augmented intraglomerular capillary pressure, it could reflect the existence of intrinsic glomerular damage that causes changes in glomerular barrier filtration, or it could be the consequence of a tubular alteration that impedes the normal reabsorption of filtered albumin. It has been suggested that microalbuminuria may represent the renal manifestation of a generalized, genetically conditioned vascular endothelial dysfunction, which may underlie the link between an increased UAE and an elevated risk for cardiovascular disease (18,19). A recent observation, has led to the hypothesis that microalbuminuria could also be the consequence of non-genetically conditioned influences affecting renal growth or vascularization. In this sense, subjects presenting microalbuminuria are significantly shorter in stature than normoalbuminuric ones (6). Adverse nutritional and other enviromental influences operating *in utero* have been shown to be associated with hypertension, impaired glucose tolerance and diabetes, and other cardiovascular risk factors (20,21) and could facilitate the development of proteinuria in adult life.

MICROALBUMINURIA IN INSULIN-DEPENDENT DIABETES MELLITUS (IDDM)

In Type I Diabetes the presence of microalbuminuria is an early marker of renal disease and decreased glomerular filtration rate and also a marker for increased risk of cardiovascular morbidity and mortality (1,3,22). Clinical nephropathy in insulin-dependent diabetics is defined by the presence of albuminuria in excess of 300 mg/day. Before this advanced stage of nephropathy is reached, UAE increases slowly from the normal range to values within the range of microalbuminuria and eventually progresses to values above 300 mg/day. The knwoledge of the natural history of diabetic nephropathy has led to consider that the presence of microalbuminuria can be considered as "incipient nephropathy."

On the other hand microalbuminuria is also a marker for increased cardiovascular morbidity and mortality. Six years after the onset of clinical nephropathy in patients with IDDM, the cumulative incidence of coronary heart disease is 8 times higher than in diabetics with normal UAE matched for age, duration of diabetes and sex (24). After 25 years of diabetes at age 40–45, cardiovascular mortality in albuminuric patients is 50 times higher than in the background population and 10 times higher than in a comparable group of diabetic patients without nephropathy (25).

The reasons for the association between albuminuria and cardiovascular risk are not totally clear. One reason, might be the frequent coexistence with other cardiovascular risk factors such as hyperlipidemia, coagulation abnormalities and hypertension in patients with incipient and clinical nepropathy in type 1 diabetes (1,3,22,24). However, these factors cannot fully account for the higher cardiovascular mortality in these patients, and this discrepancy points to the action of additional factors. It has been hypothesized that the simultaneous development of similar structural defects within the glomeruli and the large vessel wall could account for the coincidence of albuminuria and coronary heart disease in diabetic patients (26). In this sense in type I diabetics, microalbuminuria is accompanied by elevated generalized albumin leakage from the vessels (26). Recently, the existence of a decreased concentration of heparan sulphate within the extracellular matrix of patients with IDDM has been invoked as the explanation for an increased albuminuria and premature atherosclerosis (27). Other factors proposed to account for a simultaneous defect in the glomeruli and in the vessels have been the genetic predisposition to essential hypertension (28) and the presence of reduced insulin sensitivity (29). It has also been proposed that an angiotensin-converting enzyme (ACE) gene insertion or deletion polymorphism could be the basis for genetic predisposition to diabetic nephropathy (30,31) as it can be for myocardial infarction (32).

Attempts have been made to assess factors that might predict the development of microalbuminuria in insulin-dependent diabetics (see Table 2). In a recent prospective study the main baseline that predicted the development of microalbuminuria in normoalbuminuric patients were mean blood pressure, initial albumin excretion rate, smoking and blood glucose control (33). Ambulatory blood pressure monitoring (ABPM) has recently stressed the relationship between blood pressure levels and UAE. In microalbuminuric insulin-dependent diabetics with casual blood pressure within the normotensive range,

Table 2. Factors predicting the development of microalbuminuria in insulin-dependent diabetics

Initial blood pressure levels (33,34,35,36)
  • absence of nocturnal blood pressure fall in ABPM (34,36)
Initial albumin excretion rate (33)
Smoking (33)
Blood glucose control (33)
Family history of arterial hypertension (28)
Reduced insulin sensitivity (29)
Insertion or deletion polymorphism of ACE gene (30)
Elevated levels of plasma renin activity (42)
Elevated levels of plasma prorenin (43)

ambulatory blood pressure monitoring has showed higher blood pressure values when compared to normoalbuminuric patients (34,35,36); higher nocturnal blood pressure levels could be particularly relevant for the appearance of elevated UAE levels in IDDM (34,65). Once microalbuminuria is present, blood pressure may rise by 3–4 mmHg per year in contrast to 1 mmHg per year in healthy controls and normoalbuminuric patients (16).

It has also been described that in young insulin-dependent diabetics UAE is associated with cardiovascular changes consisting of increased left ventricular mass, and performance and contractility indexes (37). Microalbuminuria may also be a marker of future proliferative retinopathy (38) and has been shown to correlate with diabetic neuropathy (39).

Primary prevention for the development of the micro and macrovascular consequences of type 1 diabetes has been shown to occur with intensified insulin treatment leading to an improved glucose control in the Diabetes Control and Complications Trial (40). In this study the risk to develop microalbuminuria and proteinuria was decreased by 40%. Secondary prevention of the development of diabetic nephropathy has also been shown to occur in insulin-dependent diabetics with microalbuminuria and normotension (41). This European multicenter Study showed that the ACE inhibitor Captopril prevented the development of overt proteinuria when compared to placebo. The good effect of ACE inhibitors could depend on the fact that in youth-onset IDDM persistently elevated levels of plasma renin activity are associated with continued abnormal microalbuminuria, while declining plasma renin activity levels are significantly associated with low levels of UAE (42). Recently, the presence of microalbuminuria has been shown to correlate well with a rise in plasma prorenin (43); this finding also strengthens the possibility of a link between diabetic nephropathy and certain genetically controlled renal hemodynamic factors.

MICROALBUMINURIA IN NON-INSULIN-DEPENDENT DIABETES MELLITUS (NIDDM)

Elevated UAE levels are found in 20–25% of type II diabetics, including both newly-diagnosed and patients with established diabetes (44). As in type I diabetics, microalbuminuria predicts premature mortality (45,46) due mainly to coronary heart disease, cardiac failure or stroke (47) rather than to uremia.

Subsequent proteinuria can also be predicted by early microalbuminuria in NIDDM (45), but this finding is obscured by the premature death of many patients (22,45).

Some of the abnormalities and correlations related to the metabolic syndrome and albuminuria documented in the background population and in type I diabetics are also present in type II diabetics. This includes poor metabolic control, blood pressure elevation, male sex, older age, use of insulin, alcohol consumption and a history of cardiovascular disease (22,48,49,50).

High blood pressure is frequently present when type II diabetes is diagnosed and frequently develops in previously normotensive patients with established disease (22,45–50). A positive correlation between UAE and blood pressure has been described in NIDDM (16,22,48,49,50). In fact, prediabetic blood pressure levels have been shown to predict the development of microalbuminuria in NIDDM (51).

Insulin resistance in extrahepatic tissues seems to precede the onset of hypertension and microalbuminuria in NIDDM (52) and higher levels of insulin resistance seem to persist when elevated UAE is found in NIDDM (53). Recently, it has been suggested that in NIDDM microalbuminuria may be a feature of the prediabetic state and that the increase in UAE may be the consequence of increases in glucose and insulin concentrations (54).

This possibility was previously suggested by the significant association of parental history of both diabetes and impaired glucose tolerance with microalbuminuria in non-diabetic subjects (55).

As in type I diabetes, secondary prevention of diabetic nephropathy in patients with NIDDM treated with an ACE inhibitor has also been shown by Ravid et al (56). Patients with NIDDM, normotension and microalbuminuria treated with enalapril maintained a stable UAE, while those receiving placebo had significant progression of UAE, accompanied by a fall in renal function.

MICROALBUMINURIA IN ESSENTIAL HYPERTENSION — RELATIONSHIP BETWEEN MICROALBUMINURIA AND TARGET ORGAN DAMAGE

In 1974 Parving et al (57), reported the finding of elevated UAE levels in insufficiently treated essential hypertensives. They also reported that UAE correlated significantly with blood pressure levels and fell after blood pressure control. This finding has been amply confirmed and it is now recognized that microalbuminuria can be found in up to 40% of untreated hypertensive population (58,59,60). In treated patients prevalence can be as high as 25% when diuretics and beta-blockers are used (61,62).

Different mechanisms could be implicated in the appearance of elevated urinary albumin excretion in arterial hypertension. Such mechanisms include: renal hemodynamic changes due to the direct transmission of increased systemic pressure to the glomeruli (57,58,62), permselectivity changes of the glomerular filter and/or insufficient tubular reabsorption of albumin (58,63), and structural damage to the glomeruli and arterioles (62).

A significant positive correlation between office blood pressure levels and UAE has been shown by most groups (16,57,59,64,65). The correlation is more pronounced when UAE values are plotted against ambulatory blood pressure values (65,66,67). Higher levels of UAE have been described in those patients not exhibiting the nocturnal fall in ABPM (non-dippers), indicating that a greater degree of renal involvement could be present in this particular group of patients (66,67).

Hypertensive target organ damage is more common in microalbuminuric patients (61). Patients with elevated UAE have higher left ventricular mass (68,69,70), and a higher prevalence of hypertensive retinopathy (71). However, the correlation between left ventricular mass and and UAE does not seem to exist in the initial phases of hypertension according to recently published data (72) Furthermore, the presence of microalbuminuria in essential hypertensive patients has been interpreted as a marker of early intrarenal vascular dysfunction in essential hypertension (73,74). An absence of the capacity of the renal vasculature to vasodilate in response to an iv aminoacid infusion (73) or to an ACE inhibitor (74) has been described in patients with microalbuminuria. These findings could be of great relevance for two reasons, first because the existence of functional renal vasoconstriction since the very early stages of essential hypertension contributes to the development of high blood pressure (75); second because microalbuminuria could be a marker of the presence of nephrosclerosis (62).

Elevated UAE and proteinuria, are also independent predictors cardiovascular morbidity and mortality in patients with essential hypertension (2,7,70,76).

As can be seen in Table 3, microalbuminuria has been shown to be associated to a series of alterations that could facilitate the accompanying risk for atherosclerosis and car-

Table 3. Factors known to be associated to microalbuminuria in essential hypertension

Endothelial dysfunction (18,19)
Insulin resistance (61,77)
Altered lipid levels (77,78)
Higher body mass index (75)
Salt-sensitivity (79)

diovascular disease and also contribute to consider that microalbuminuria in essential hypertension has a genetic origin.

Antihypertensive therapy of any kind is able to lower UAE in essential hypertensives by simply lowering blood pressure (2). Nevertheless, ACE inhibitors have been shown to exhibit a higher capacity to decrease microalbuminuria in hypertensive patients that goes beyond their capacity to decrease renal perfusion pressure (2,80).

Interestingly, UAE could be elevated in the during the prehypertensive state, according to the finding by Fauvel et al (81) of elevated UAE values in the normotensive offspring of hypertensive parents and to the description of Hoegeholm et al (65) of higher UAE rate in white coat hypertensive patients when compared to a normotensive control group. Should these data be confirmed, they stress the relevance of screening microalbuminuria in subjects at risk of developing essential hypertension.

Whether or not gains can be obtained from screening of microalbuminuria in essential hypertension remains to be seen. Stratification of cardiovascular risk is needed to identify the patients at the highest risk to suffer cardiovascular events or death. Microalbuminuria, due to their close relationship with the most significant associated risk factors and in particular left ventricular hypertrophy, could become one of the best methods to evaluate the global cardiovascular risk in a hypertensive patient. The simplicity and low-cost of semi-quantitative methods will probably speed the answer to this question.

REFERENCES

1. Viberti GC, Mackintosh D, Bilous RW, Pickup JC, Keen H. Proteinuria in diabetes mellitus: role of spontaneous and experimental variations of glycemia. Kidney Int 1982, 21: 714–720.
2. Ruilope LM, Rodicio JL. Clinical relevance of proteinuria and microalbuminuria. Curr Opin Nephrol Hypertens 1993, 2: 962–967.
3. Poulsen PE. Microalbuminuria-techniques of measurement. In Microalbuminuria a marker for organ damage. Edited by CE Mogensen. London. Science Press Ltd. 1993: 10–19.
4. Mogensen CE. Microalbuminuria as a predictor of clinical diabetic nephropathy. Kidney Int 1987, 31: 673–689.
5. Pedersen EB, Mogensen CE, Larsen JS. Effects of exercise on urinary excretion of albumin and beta2-microglobulin in young patients with mild essential hypertension without treatment and during long-term propranolol treatment. Scand J Clin Lab Invest 1981, 41: 493–498.
6. Yudkin JS. Microalbuminuria in vascular disease. In Microalbuminuria a marker for organ damage. Edited by CE Mogensen. London. Science Press Ltd. 1993: 69–80.
7. Yudkin JS, Forrest RD, Jackson CA. Microalbuminuria as predictor of vascular disease in non-diabetic subjects. Islington Diabetes Survey. Lancet 1988, ii: 530–533.
8. Damsgaard EM, Froland A, Jorgensen OD, Mogensen CE. Microalbuminuria as predictor of increased mortality in elderly people. Br Med J 1990, 300: 297–300.
9. Hahhner SM, Stern MP, Gruber MKK. Microalbuminuria-potential marker for increased cardiovascular risk factors in nondiabetic subjects?. Arteriosclerosis 1990, 10: 727–731.
10. Winocour PH et al. Microalbuminuria and associated cardiovascular risk factors in the community. Atherosclerosis 1992, 93: 71–81.

11. Ferrannini E. The Metabolic Syndrome. In Target Organ Damage in the Mature Hypertensive. Part 2. Edited by Mogensen CE. London. Science Press Ltd. 1993: 31–49.

12. Metcalf P, Baker J, Scott A, Wild C, Scragg R, Dryson E. Albuminuria in people at least 40 years old: effect of obesity, hypertension and hyperlipidemia. Clin Che 1992, 38: 1802–1808.

13. Vestbo E, Damsgaard EM, Froland A, Mogensen CE. Microalbuminuria in a population based cohort. J Diab Compl 1994, (in press).

14. Ticket J, Vol S, Hallab M, Caces F, Marre M. Epidemiology of microalbuminuria in a french population. J Diab Compl 1994, 8: 294–295.

15. Metcalf PA, Baker JR, Scragg RKR, Dryson E, Scott AJ, Wild CJ. Albuminuria in people at least 40 years old: effect of alcohol consumption, regular exercise and cigarrette smoking. Clin Che 1993, 39: 1793–1797.

16. Mogensen CE. Systemic blood pressure and glomerular leakage with particular reference to diabetes and hypertension. J Int Med 1994, 235: 297–316.

17. Jiang X, Srinivasan SR, Radhakrishnamurthy B, Dalferes ER, Bao Weihang B, Berenson GS. Microalbuminuria in young adults related to blood pressure in a biracial (black-white) population. Am J Hypertens 1994, 7:794–800.

18. Stehouwer CD, Nauta JJ, Zeldenrust GC, Hackeng WH, Donker AJ, den Ottolander GJ. Urinary albumin excretion, cardiovascular disease, and endothelial dysfunction in non-insulin-dependent diabetes mellitus. Lancet 1992, 340: 319–323.

19. Pedrinelli R, Giampietro O, Carmassi F, Melillo E, Dell'Olmo G, Catapano G, Matteucci E, Talarico L, Morale M, De Negri F, Di Bello V. Microalbuminuria and endothelial dysfunction in essential hypertension. Lancet 1994, 344: 14–18.

20. Hales CN, Barker DJ, Clark PM, Cox LJ, Fall C, Osmond C, Winter PD. Fetal and infant growth and impaired glucose tolerance at age 64. Br Med J 1991, 303: 1019–1022.

21. Barker DJP, ed. Fetal and infant origins of adult disease. British Medical Journal Press. London. 1992.

22. Mogensen CE, Hansen KW, Sommer S, Klebe J, Christensen CK, Marshall S, Schmitz A, Pedersen MM, Christiansen JS, Pedersen EB, Jespersen B, Petersen RS, Schmitz O, Damsgaard EM, Froland A. Microalbuminuria: studies in diabetes, essential hypertension and renal diseases as compared with a background population. Adv Nephrol 1991, 20: 191–228.

23. Hostetter TH. Diabetic nephropathy. In The Kidney. Edited by Brenner BM & Rector FC. Philadelphia. WB Saunders Company. 1991: 1695–1727.

24. Jensen T, Borch-Johnsen K, Kofoed-Enevoldeen A, Deckert T. Coronary heart disease in young type 1 (insulin-dependent) diabetic patients with and without diabetic nephropathy: incidence and risk factors. Diabetologia 1987, 30: 144–148.

25. Borch-Johnsen K, Kreiner S. Proteinuria: value as predictor of cardiovascular mortality in insulin dependent diabetes mellitus. Br Med J 1987, 294: 1651–1654.

26. Deckert T, Feldt-Rasmussen B, Borch-Johnsen K, Jensen T, Kofoed-Enevoldeen A. Albuminuria reflects widespread vascular damage. The Steno hypothesis. Diabetologia 1988, 32: 219–226.

27. Deckert T. Nephropathy and coronary death-the fatal twins in diabetes mellitus. Nephrol Dial Transplant 1994, 9: 1069–1071.

28. Mangili R, Bending JJ, Scott G, Lil K, Gupta A, Viberti GC. Increased sodium-lithium countertransport activity in red cells of patients with insulin-dependent diabetes and nephropathy. N Eng J Med 1988, 318: 146–150.

29. Yip J, Mattock M, Morocutti A, Sethi M, Trevisan R, Viberti GC. Insulin resistance in insulin-dependent diabetic patients with microalbuminuria. Lancet 1993, 342: 883–887.

30. Marre M, Bernadet P, Gallois Y, Savagner F, Guyenne TT, Hallab M, Cambien F, Passa Ph, Alhenc-Gelas F. Relationships between angiotensin I converting enzyme gene polymorphism, plasma levels, and diabetic retinal and renal complications. Diabetes 1994, 43: 384–388.

31. Doria A, Warram JH, Krolewski AS. Genetic predisposition to diabetic nephropathy. Evidence for a role of the angiotensin I-converting enzyme gene. Diabetes 1994, 43: 690–695.

32. Cambien F, Poirier O, Lecerf L, Evans A, Cambou JP, Arveiler D, Luc G, Bard JM, Bara L, Ricard S, Tiret L, Amouyel Ph, Alhenc-Gelas F, Soubrier F. Deletion polymorphism in the gene for angiotensin converting enzyme is a potent risk factor for myocardial infarction. Nature 1992, 359: 641–644.

33. Microalbuminuria Collaborative Study Group, United Kingdom. Risk factors for development of microalbuminuria in insulin dependent diabetic patients: a cohort study. Br Med J 1993, 306: 1235–1239.

34. Lurbe A, Redon J, Pascual JM, Tacons J, Alvarez V, Batlle D. Altered blood pressure during sleep in normotensive subjects with type I diabetes. Hypertension 1993, 21: 227–235.

35. Hansen KW, Poulsen PL, Mogensen CE. Ambulatory blood pressure and abnormal albuminuria in type I diabetic patients. Kidney Int 45 (suppl 45): S-134–S-140.

36. Berrut G, Hallab M, Bouhanick B, Chameau AM, Marre M, Fressinaud Ph. Value of ambulatory blood pressure monitoring in type I (insulin-dependent) diabetic patients with incipient diabetic nephropathy. Am J Hypertens 1994, 7: 222–227.

37. Kimball TR, Daniels SR, Khoury PR, Magnotti RA, Turner AM, Dolan LM. Cardiovascular status in young patients with insulin-dependent diabetes mellitus. Circulation 1994, 90: 357–361.

38. Cruickshanks KJ, Ritter LL, Klein R, Moss SE. The association of microalbuminuria with diabetic retinopathy: the Wisconsin Epidemiologic Study of Diabetic Retinopathy. Ophtalmology 1993, 100: 862–867.

39. Bell DSH, Ketchum CH, Robinson CA, Wagenknecht LE,, Williams BT. Microalbuminuria associated with diabetib neuropathy. Diab Care 1992, 15: 528–531.

40. The Diabetes Control and Complications Trial Research Group. The effect of intensive treatment on long-term complications in insulin-dependent diabetes mellitus. N Eng J Med 1993, 329: 977–986.

41. Viberti GC, Mogensen CE, Groop LC, Pauls JF, for the European Microalbuminuria Study Group. Effect of captopril on progression to clinical proteinuria in patients with insulin-dependent diabetes mellitus and microalbuminuria. JAMA 1994: 271: 275–279.

42. Paulsen EP, Burke BA, Vernier RL, Mallare MJ, Innes Jr DJ, Sturgill BC. Juxtaglomerular body abnormalities in youth-onset diabetic subjects. Kidney Int 1994, 45: 1132–1139.

43. Daneman D, Crompton CH, Balfe JW, Sochett EB, Chatzilias A, Cotter BR, Osmond DH. Plasma prorenin as an early marker of nephropathy in diabetic (IDDM) adolescents. Kidney Int 1994, 46: 1154–1159.

44. Mogensen CE, Poulsen PL. Epidemiology of microalbuminuria in diabetes and in the background population. Curr Opin Nephrol Hypertens 1994, 3: 248–256.

45. Mogensen CE. Microalbuminuria predicts clinical proteinuria and early mortality in maturity-onset diabetes. N Eng J Med 1984, 310: 356–360.

46. Jarrett RJ, Viberti GC, Argyropoulos A, Hill RD, Mahmud U, Murrels TJ. Microalbuminuria predicts mortality in non-insulin-dependent diabetics. Diabet Med 1984, 1: 17–19.

47. Mattock MB, Morrish NJ, Viberti GC, Keen H, Fitzgerald AP, Jackson G. Prospective study of microalbuminuria as predictor of mortality in NIDDM. Diabetes 1992, 41: 736–741.

48. Klein R, Klein BEK, Moss SE. Prevalence of microalbuminuria in older-onset diabetes. Diab Care 1993, 16: 1325–1329.

49. Groop L, Ekstrand A, Forsblom C, Widen E, Groop PH, Teppo AM, Briksson J. Insulin resistance, hypertension and microalbuminuria in patients with type 2 (non-insulin-dependent) diabetes mellitus. Diabetologia 1993, 36: 642–647.

50. Olivarius NF, Andreasen AH, Keiding N, Mogensen CE. Epidemiology of renal involvement in newly-diagnosed middle-aged and elderly diabetic patients. Cross-sectional data from the population-based study "Diabetes Care in General Practice". Denmark. Diabetologia 1993, 36: 1007–1016.

51. Nelson RG, Pettitt DJ, Baird HR, Charles MA, Liu QZ, Bennett PH, Knowler WC. Pre-diabetic blood pressure predicts urinary albumin excretion after the onset of type (non-insulin-dependent) diabetes mellitus in Pima indians. Diabetologia 1993, 36: 998–1001.

52. Nosadini R, Solini A, Velussi M, Muollo B, Frigato F, Sambataro M, Cipollina MR, de Riva F, Brocco E, Crepaldi G. Impaired insulin-induced glucose uptake by extrahepatic tissue is hallmark of NIDDM patients who have or will develop hypertension and microalbuminuria. Diabetes 1994, 43: 491–494.

53. Niskanen L, Laakso M. Insulin resistance is related to albuminuria in patients with type II (non-insulin-dependent) diabetes mellitus. Metabolism 1993, 42: 1541–1545.

54. Mykkänen L, Haffner SM, Kuusisto J, Pyorälä K, Laakso M. Microalbuminuria precedes the development of NIDDM. Diabetes 1994, 43: 552–557.

55. Haffner SM, Gonzales C, Valdez RA, Mykkänen L, Hazuda HP, Mitchell BD, Monterrosa A. Is microalbuminuria part of the prediabetic state?. Diabetologia 1993, 36: 1002–1006.

56. Ravid M, Savin H, Jutrin I, Bental T, Katz B, Lishner M. Long-term stabilizing effect of angiotensin-converting enzyme inhibition on plasma creatinine and on proteinuria in normotensive type II diabetic patients. Ann Intern Med 1993, 118: 577–581.

57. Parving HH, Jensen HAE, Mogensen CE, Evrin PE. Increased urinary albumin excretion rate in benign essential hypertension. Lancet 1974, i: 1190–1192.

58. Ljungman S. Microalbuminuria in essential hypertension. Am J Hypertens 1990, 3: 956–960.

59. Gerber LM, Shmukler C, Alderman MH. Differences in urinary albumin excretion rate between normotensive and hypertensive, white and nonwhite subjects. Arch Intern Med 1992, 152: 373–377.

60. Bigazzi R, Bianchi S, Campese V, Baldari G. Prevalence of microalbuminuria in a large population of patients with mild to moderate essential hypertension. Nephron 1992, 61: 94–97.

61. Agewall S, Persson B, Samuelsson O, Ljungman S, Herlitz H, Fagerberg B, on behalf of The Risk Factor Intervention Study Group. Microalbuminuria in treated hypertensive men at high risk of coronary disease. J Hypertens 1993, 11: 461–459.

62. Ruilope LM, Alcazar JM, Rodicio JL. Renal consequences of arterial hypertension. J Hypertens 1992, 10 (suppl 7): S85–S90.

63. Cottone S, Cerasola G. Microalbuminuria fractional clearance and early renal permselectivity changes in essential hypertension. Am J Nephrol 1992, 12: 326–329.

64. Redon J, Pascual JM, Miralles A, Sanz C, Gutierrez M, Ros MJ, Baldo E, Michavila J, Sanchez C, Alegre B. Microalbuminuria in essential hypertension (in spanish). Med Clin (Barc) 1991, 96: 525–529.

65. Hoegholm A, Bang LE, Kristensen KS, Nielsen JW, Holm J. Microalbuminuria in 411 untreated individuals with established hypertension, white coat hypertension and normotension. Hypertension 1994, 24: 101–105.

66. Bianchi S, Bigazzi R, Baldari G, Sgherri G, Campese VM. Diurnal variations of blood pressure and microalbuminuria in essential hypertension. Am J Hypertens 1994, 7: 23–29.

67. Redon J, Liao Y, Lozano JV, Miralles A, Pascual JM, Cooper RS. Ambulatory blood pressure and microalbuminuria in essential hypertension: role of circadian variability. J Hypertens 1994, 12: 947–953.

68. Cerasola G, Cottone S, D'Ignoto G, Grasso L, Mangano MT, Carapelle E, Nardi E, Andronico G, Fulantelli MA, Marcellino T, Seddio G. Microalbuminuria as a predictor of cardiovascular damage in essential hypertension. J Hypertens 1989, 7 (suppl 6): S332–S333.

69. Redon J, Gomez-Sanchez MA, Baldo E, Casal MC, Fernandez ML, Miralles MA, Gomez-Pajuelo C, Rodicio JL, Ruilope LM. Microalbuminuria is correlated with left ventricular hypertrophy in male hypertensive patients. J Hypertens 1994, 9 (suppl 6): S148–S149.

70. Agrawal B, Berger A, Wolf K, Luft FC. Microalbuminuria screening by reagent strip predicts cardiovascular risk in hypertension. J Hypertens 1996, 14:223–228

71. Biesenbach G, Zazgornik J. High prevalence of hypertensive retinopathy and coronary heart disease in hypertensive patients with persistent microalbuminuria under short intensive antihypertensive therapy. Clin Nephrol 1994, 41: 211–218.

72. Palatini P, Graniero GR, Mormino P, Mattarei M, Sanzuol F, Cignacco GB, Gregori S, Garavelli G, Pegoraro F, Maraglino G, Bortolazzi A, Accurso V, Dorigatti F, Graniero F, Gelisio R, Businaro R, Vriz O, Dal-Follo M, Camarotto A, Pessina AC. Prevalence and clinical correlates of microalbuminuria in stage I hypertension. Results from the Hypertension and Ambulatory Recording Venetia Study (HARVEST Study). Am J Hypertens 1996, 9:334–341

73. Losito A, Fortunati F, Zampi I, del Favero A. Impaired renal functional reserve and albuminuria in essential hypertension. Br Med J 1988, 296: 1562–1564.

74. Minram A, Ribstein J, DuCalair G. Is microalbuminuria a marker of early intrarenal vascular dysfunction in essential hypertension? Hypertension 1994, 23 (part 2): 1018–1021.

75. Ruilope LM, Lahera V, Rodicio JL, Romero JC. Are renal hemodynamics a key factor in the development and maintenance of arterial hypertension in humans. Hypertension 1994, 23: 3–9.

76. Cerasola G, Cottone S, Mule G, Nardi E, Mangano MT, Andronico G, Contorno A, Galione P, LaMilia D, Renda F, Piazza G, Volpe V, Lisi A, Ferrara L, Panepinto N. Relationship between microalbuminuria, blood pressure and cardiovascular changes in essential hypertension. Contrib-Nephrol 1996, 119: 130–134.

77. Bianchi S, Bigazzi R, Valtriani C, Chiapponi I, Sgherri G, Baldari G, Natali A, Ferrannini E, Campese VM. Elevated serum insulin levels in patients with essential hypertension and microalbuminuria. Hypertension 1994, 23 (part 1): 681–687.

78. Redon J, Liao Y, Lozano JV, Miralles A, Baldo E, Cooper RS. Factors related to the presence of microalbuminuria in essential hypertension. Am J Hypertens 1994, 7: 801–807.

79. Bigazzi R, Bianchi S, Baldari D, Sgherri G, Baldari G, Campese VM. Microalbuminuria in salt-sensitive patients: marker for renal and cardiovascular disease. Hypertension 1994, 23: 195–199.

80. Ruilope LM, Alcazar JM, Hernandez E, Praga M, Lahera V, Rodicio JL. Long-term influences of antihypertensive therapy on microalbuminuria in essential hypertension. Kidney Int 1994, 45 (suppl 45): S-171–S-173.

81. Fauvel JP, Hadj-Aissa A, Laville M, Fadat G, Labeeuw M, Zech P, Pozet N. Microalbuminuria in normotensives with genetic risk of hypertension. Nephron 1991, 57: 375–376.

16

PHYSIOLOGICAL VERSUS PATHOLOGICAL HYPERTROPHY

The Athlete and the Hypertensive

Cesare Cuspidi,[1] Laura Lonati,[1] Lorena Sampieri,[1] Gastone Leonetti,[1,2] and Alberto Zanchetti[1]

[1]Istituto di Clinica Medica Generale e Terapia Medica
Università di Milano
Centro di Fisiologia Clinica e Ipertensione
Ospedale Maggiore, IRCCS, Milano
[2]Centro Auxologico Italiano
IRCCS, Milano, Italy

1. INTRODUCTION

Left ventricular hypertrophy (LVH) in humans is a common adaptive process induced by different physiological and pathological stimuli.

Arterial hypertension and long term athlete training are the most frequent causes of pathological and physiological LVH, respectively (1,2). Hypertension induced LVH is considered to be an adaptive process intended to normalize or attenuate the increased wall stress induced by high blood pressure (3,4). Therefore this compensatory change, even in early phases, has a negative prognostic relevance; LVH in fact is an important and independent risk factor for cardiovascular complications (5,6).

The mechanisms which may account for the increased cardiac risk in hypertensive patients with LVH include an increased vulnerability of the myocardium to ischemia enhanced arrhythmogenesis and abnormal diastolic function (7). In contrast, physiological LVH in athletes is associated with normal coronary reserve, diastolic function and properties of arterial vessels (8). This paper will discuss differences and similarities in hypertensive's and athlete's heart considering the following points: 1) left ventricular structure, 2) right ventricular structure, 3) left ventricular function, 4) coronary arteries, 5) left ventricular hypertrophy regression and 6) large arteries structure.

2. LEFT VENTRICULAR STRUCTURE

LVH diagnosed by electrocardiographic or echocardiographic criteria is associated with increased risk of cardiovascular disease and death in patients with arterial hyperten-

Hypertension and the Heart, edited by Zanchetti et al.
Plenum Press, New York, 1997

145

Table 1. Left ventricular (LV) structural
changes induced by arterial hypertension

---

1. Concentric LV remodelling
   normal LV mass, increased relative wall thickness (RWT)
   (ratio of twice of the LV posterior wall thickness to LV
   cavity dimension in diastole ≥0.45)
2. Concentric LV hypertrophy
   increased LV mass and RWT
3. Eccentric LV hypertrophy
   increased LV mass, normal RWT
   A) non dilated (LVIDd/BSA)
      <3.2 cm/m^2 women;
      <3.1 cm/m^2 men
   B) dilated (LVIDd/BSA)
      ≥3.2 cm/m^2 women;
      ≥3.1 cm/m^2 men
4. Asymmetric LV hypertrophy
   septal/posterior wall thickness ratio ≥1.5 in diastole

---

sion and in the general population. Epidemiologic prospective studies have demonstrated that the increase in left ventricular mass and the abnormal LV geometry, even in absence of definite LVH, characterize a subgroup of hypertensive patients with high cardiovascular risk profile (9,10).

Four different types of LV changes have been shown by echocardiography in hypertensive patients: 1) concentric LV remodelling (normal LV mass and increased relative wall thickness), 2) concentric LVH (increased LV mass and relative wall thickness), 3) eccentric LVH (increased LV mass and normal relative wall thickness), 4) asymmetric LVH (septal/posterior wall thickness ratio ≥1.5 in diastole) (3,4) (Tab. 1). This wide spectrum of cardiac changes suggests that a complex relationship exists between high blood pressure and heart (11). The most important factor inducing pathological LVH is increased blood pressure although several other factors, including non-hemodynamic variables, may contribute to the development of cardiac hypertrophy (12).

A rise in LV wall stress determined by high systolic intraventricular pressure represents a potent stimulus for the development of LVH which in turn reduces the wall stress. In fact, according to the Laplace law the stress on the LV wall is directly proportional to the intraventricular pressure and squared radius and is inversely correlated with wall thickness. The increase in wall thickness, intended to normalize or attenuate the wall stress is secondary to cardiac muscle cell hypertrophy, characterized by a significant rise in the number of sarcomers arranged in parallel in concentric LVH and longitudinally in eccentric LVH.

The mechanisms by which cardiac hypertrophy increases the risk of cardiovascular events are not fully understood. There are some major alterations in cardiac structure and function that may contribute to the increased incidence of cardiovascular complications. Reduced coronary reserve, diastolic and systolic dysfunction and arrhythmias are the most frequent negative consequences of the pathological increase in left ventricular mass. There are many factors influencing LV geometry and type of LVH in arterial hypertension. Age, race, severity of hypertension, hemodynamic patterns, etiology of hypertension and humoral factors may play an important role in determining the adaptive response of the heart. Concentric LVH is normally associated with moderate to severe hypertension and is more common in middle aged and in older patients than in young ones. Concentric and eccentric non

Table 2. Factors influencing cardiac geometry and type of LVH in arterial hypertension

	Concentric LVH	Eccentric non-dilated LVH
Age	old patients	young patients
Race	blacks	—
Severity of hypertension	moderate–severe	mild
Hemodynamic patterns	normal or low cardiac output	high cardiac output
Umoral factors	high renin patients (?)	low or normal renin patients (?)

dilated LVH are characterized by different hemodynamic patterns: cardiac output is normal or low in concentric LVH and elevated in the eccentric one. The influences of humoral factors and etiology of hypertension on LVH patterns are not so well defined (13,14), so far (Tab. 2).

The prevalence of LVH is dependent on clinical and demographic variables of the hypertensive patients considered and of course on methodologic diagnostic approach. When echocardiographic criteria for LVH are used the prevalence of hypertrophy is much higher than when electrocardiographic (ECG) criteria are employed. The prevalence of LVH determined by echocardiography in hypertensive patients has been reported to range from 20 to 90%.

In the Treatment of Mild Hypertension Study (THOMS) performed in borderline or mild hypertensives the prevalence of LVH was 15% and eccentric LVH was the most common type of LV change. In the Hypertension Optimal Treatment (HOT) study based on patients with more sustained hypertension the prevalence of LVH resulted 62% and concentric LVH was the most prevalent type of cardiac change (15,16). LV hypertrophic process related to high blood pressure involves uniformly the interventricular system and the other free walls. Only a small percentage (4–5%) of hypertensives shows a predominant involvement of interventricular septum (asymmetric hypertrophy with septal posterior wall ratio > 1.3 or 1.5). LVH in hypertension includes mild, moderate and marked or severe forms depending on clinical, racial and social circumstances. In mild to moderate hypertensives with LVH the myocardial acoustic properties seem to be normal and this suggests that in early phases of cardiac hypertrophy dysproportionate connetive tissue growth does not accompany this compensatory response (17).

Long term athletic training is known to produce physiological changes in cardiac structure that have commonly been referred to as the "athletic heart" (18). This cardiac adaptation to intense physical exercise consists of an increase either in the cavity size or in the ventricular wall thickness or both. The modifications in cardiac structure in athletes may differ depending on the type of training activity (19). Dynamic exercise (such as running or swimming) induces an increase in volume load on left ventricle and the main circulatory change observed is a marked increase in cardiac output (20). Static exercise (such as weight-lifting, shot putting, wrestling) causes a significant pressure overload on left ventricle and the main circulatory change is a large increase in systolic and diastolic pressure (Tab. 3).

Two different morphological types of LV changes have been described in athletes: concentric and eccentric LVH. Eccentric LVH, usually found in athletes with dynamic activities, is characterized by an increased LV mass and chamber size, whereas wall thickness is normal (21). Concentric hypertrophy occurs in sports with high static component, is characterized by a significant increase in LV mass with normal or reduced cavity dimensions (22). A combination of eccentric and concentric LVH is found in several sports with mixed dynamic and static demands (cycling, rowing) (23).

Table 3. Exercise and cardiovascular system

Dynamic exercise ($\uparrow$volume load on LV)		Static exercise ($\uparrow$pressure load on LV)	
Involves changes in muscle length and joint movement with rhythmic contractions that develop a relatively small intramuscular force.		Involves development of a relatively large intramuscular force with little or no change in muscle length or joint movement.	
Effects		Effects	
Increase in	cardiac output heart rate systolic pressure	Increase in	systolic pressure diastolic pressure mean pressure
Decrease in	diastolic pressure total peripheral resistance	Small changes in	cardiac output stroke volume total peripheral resistance

Echocardiographic studies have demonstrated that LVH in athletes is usually mild and the differences in LV anatomical parameters between athletes and sedentary subjects are statistically significant but generally small. In the majority of elite athletes absolute LV wall thickness is normal or only mildly increased ($\leq$12 mm). Pelliccia and coworkers have recently documented that only a small percentage (1.7%) of 947 male elite athletes involved in 27 different types of sport show LV wall thickness greater than 13 mm (24).

The mild LV thickening in athletes is almost always symmetrically distributed with a septal/free wall ratio <1.3. Between the determinants of cardiac changes in athletes, the level of training is the most important factor: in fact professional athletes have larger LV mass than recreational sportsmen (Tab. 4). It would appear that increased cardiac dimensions and thickness of these individuals are truly a direct response to training. However, it is also possible that such cardiac changes are not induced only by intense and prolonged physical exercise, but are due in part to genetic predisposition and to bradycardia. In particular, the increase in LV internal dimensions is partially related to the prolongation of the diastolic filling phase, as consequence of the marked bradycardia.

Gender has a significant impact on cardiac adaptation to sport activities. It has been demonstrated that only 1% of elite female athletes have LV wall thickness exceeding the normal range ($\geq$11 mm) (25).

Cardiac morphofunctional changes in athletic individuals are related also to age and duration of training. Nishimura reported that older bicyclists with lifelong activity show LV wall thicknesses and mass significantly higher than younger bicyclists with the same level of training (26). Finally, in physiological hypertrophy myocardial acoustic properties, studied with quantitative analysis of ultrasound backscatter, have been found normal. The normal cardiac reflectivity in athletes is in agreement with the lack of abnormal

Table 4. Factors influencing cardiac dimensions and LVH in athletes

Level of training:	Professional athletes have larger LV mass than recreational sportsmen.
Type of sport:	Sports differ greatly regarding their effects on cardiac morphology.
Gender:	Male gender is associated with larger cardiac dimensions than female gender.
Age:	Older age is associated with larger LV diastolic cavity dimension and thickness.
Body surface area:	Larger BSA is associated with larger LV diastolic cavity dimension and wall thickness.

fibrous tissue deposition and the absence of myocardial tissue disorganization that seem to characterize this type of hypertrophy (27).

3. RIGHT VENTRICULAR STRUCTURE

It has been shown that pressure, vascular resistance and reactivity of the pulmonary circulation in essential hypertensive patients are significantly higher than in normotensive subjects (28). These observations indicate that a parallelism may exist between the vascular tone of the pulmonary and systemic circuits. A small number of echocardiographic studies have been performed in hypertensive patients to explore the possibility of the right ventricular involvement secondary to hemodynamic alterations of the pulmonary circulation. These reports, limited in number because of the difficulties in measuring anatomic and functional parameters of the RV, have documented that right ventricular wall thickness is slightly greater in hypertensive patients than in normotensive controls (Fig. 1). A significant correlation was found between left and right wall thickness and diastolic

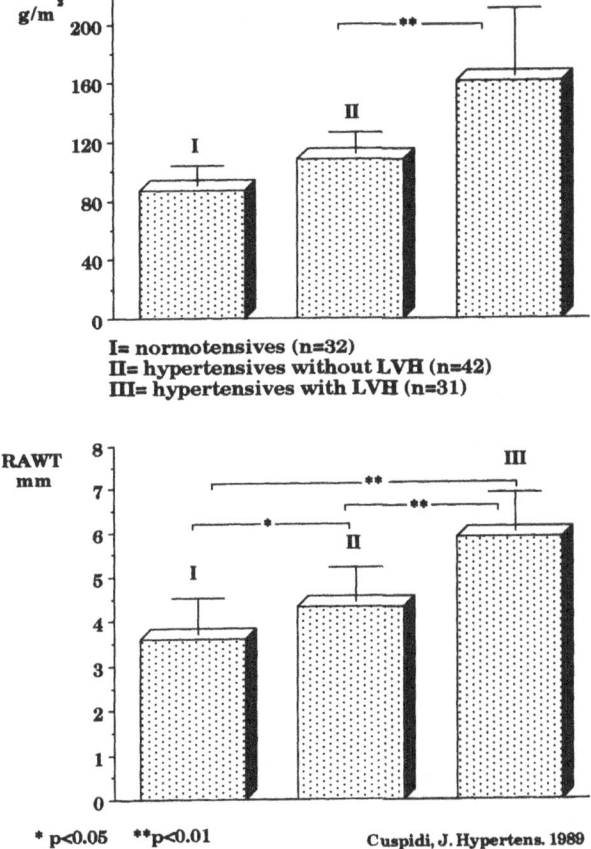

Figure 1. Left and right ventricular structure in hypertension. Left ventricular mass index (LVMI) and right anterior wall thickness (RAWT) in normotensive and hypertensives with or without LVH.

parameters of both ventricles (29,30). These data suggest that the effects of hypertension are not limited to the left section of the heart but involve also the right one.

A considerable number of studies exists concerning physical adaptation of the left ventricle to athletic training but little is available for the right ventricle. Some authors have reported that cardiac enlargement occurs symmetrically in both right and left sections in endurance athletes, reflecting increased hemodynamic volume load related to high cardiac output during exercise (31). A mild thickening of right ventricular free walls have been also observed in some but not in all studies addressed to this argument.

4. LEFT VENTRICULAR FUNCTION

Left ventricular systolic dysfunction at rest is not a frequent echocardiographic finding in patients with arterial hypertension and LVH, but impaired systolic function during exercise may be more common (1). It has been demonstrated that the ejection fraction response to exercise is impaired in a significant percentage of hypertensive patients without concomitant coronary artery disease, although the mechanisms responsible for this finding have not been fully elucidated (32).

LVH reduces systolic wall stress and preserves normal systolic performance under basal conditions. However this compensatory mechanism may be inadequate to support an additional increase in wall stress, such as that developing during physical exercise or stress. Also impaired left ventricular filling might predispose to the reduced systolic function during exercise because both ejection fraction and fractional shortening of left ventricle depend on adequate relaxation and diastolic filling (33). Some recent studies reported a reduction in LV fractional shortening at rest in hypertensive patients when this parameter is measured at mid-wall level rather than at endocardial level (34).

LVH in hypertensives is more commonly associated with an altered diastolic function, although abnormalities of the diastolic process may often develop even in patients with normal LV mass (35,36). Pulsed Doppler echocardiography and radionuclide angiography have been used to investigate and describe abnormal diastolic characteristics in hypertensive patients (37,38). These abnormalities consist of a prolongation of the isovolumic relaxation time, a decrease in early filling velocity and an increase in atrial velocity; altogether they may represent early markers of LV diastolic dysfunction that lead to clinical manifestations of heart failure.

The mechanisms of abnormal diastolic function are not fully understood, although several possible explanations for the impaired LV diastolic process in arterial hypertension may exist. Increase in myocardial collagen content, structural and functional abnormalities in the large and small coronary vessels and high blood pressure levels could contribute to impair LV diastolic filling. Reduction in myocardial adenosine triphosphate (ATP) related to pressure overload may impair relaxation due to reduced calcium uptake by the sarcoplasmatic reticulum. It is evident that alterations in diastolic function of pathological LV are not dependent on a pure increase in LV mass.

Echocardiographic assessments of left ventricular systolic parameters in athletes has shown that these indexes are within normal limits in most athletes. Percent fractional shortening (and ejection fraction) is usually normal in athletes because long term conditioning induces increases of similar magnitude in left ventricular end-diastolic and end-systolic dimensions.

Recent studies have investigated diastolic function in trained athletes using different noninvasive techniques, including digitized M-mode echocardio-graphy, Doppler echo-

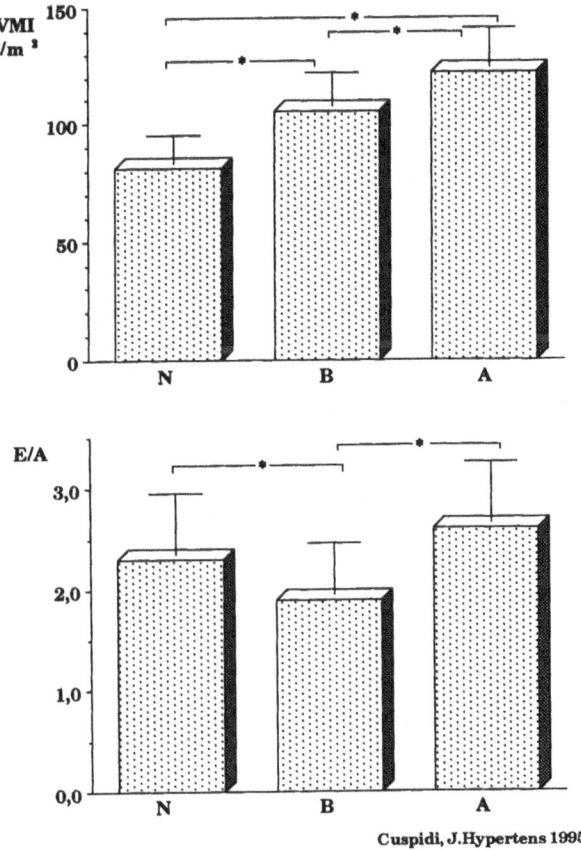

Figure 2. Left ventricular structure and diastolic function in normotensive controls (N), borderline hypertensives (B), and athletes (A).

cardiography and radionuclide angiography (39–41). These reports uniformly have shown various indexes of diastolic function to be within normal limits under basal conditions with two possible exceptions: athletes taking steroids and older athletes. Moreover, there is a number of comparison studies performed in athletes and in hypertensives. In one of them we have demonstrated that young borderline hypertensives with mild increase in LV mass show reduced E/A mitral ratio (normalized by heart rate) with respect to normal controls and athletes (judokas) (42) (Fig. 2). This observation, in agreement with the results of other authors, suggests that diastolic properties are different in pathological and physiological cardiac hypertrophy.

5. CORONARY ARTERIES

Many mechanisms may induce myocardial ischemia in hypertensive patients with LVH (43,44). High blood pressure can accelerate atherosclerosis of epicardial coronary arteries with consequent reduction in coronary blood flow and myocardial oxygen supply. However, in hypertensive patients with LVH, coronary reserve is reduced even in the absence of stenosis of epicardial coronary arteries. Several mechanisms may cause myocardial ischemia in hypertension in the absence of lesions of extramural coronary arteries: 1) the increase in myocardial oxygen demand related to elevation in arterial pressure and in wall tension and to LVH per se, 2) relative vascular rarefaction resulting from inadequate increase in capillary bed with respect to augmented LV mass, 3) functional and morphological changes in intramural arterioles.

In this chapter we will, discuss briefly a particular finding: the relationship between LVH and the diameter of extramural coronary arteries in hypertensives and in athletes. We measured by transthoracic echocardiography the internal diameter of left coronary artery (LCA) main trunk in 26 hypertensive patients (14 with and 12 without LVH) (45). The two groups had similar demographic characteristics and blood pressure levels. In patients with LVH the diameter of LCA main trunk was not different when compared to hypertensives without LVH. In the whole group studied we found that the correlation between LCA main trunk diameter and LV mass index was not statistically significant (Fig. 3). The lack of this correlation observed also in a transophageal echocardio-graphic study by Palombo et al, means that the increase in LV mass in hypertensives is not associated with simultaneous increase in lumen of coronary arteries and it may contribute, in part, to impairment of coronary reserve. On the contrary some echocardiographic studies in athletes have shown that they have larger coronary arteries than in sedentary controls. These findings underline the different response of extramural coronary arteries in presence of pathological and physiological LVH.

6. LEFT VENTRICULAR HYPERTROPHY REGRESSION

The aim of the antihypertensive treatment should be not only to normalize blood pressure but also to induce regression of the structural changes related to the increased blood pressure, such as LVH in order to reduce cardiovascular complications.

In hypertensive patients numerous studies have examined the effect of non pharmacologic and pharmacologic treatment on LVH. It has been possible to show a relevant reduction in LVH mass only after two or three months of treatment, because a shorter period usually is not sufficient to induce significant changes in LV structure. Many factors influence the reversal of LVH in humans: pretreatment LV mass, blood pressure control (efficacy and duration) patients-related factors (age, sex, race, concomitant cardiac and non cardiac diseases) drug related factors (activation or blocking of cardiac trophic factors).

To obtain maximum information on the effects of various antihypertensive agents on LVH regression three important meta-analysis of all relevant studies have been performed in the recent years (46–48). In the first by Dahlöf et al, including 109 studies with a total of 2357 patients, arterial blood pressure was reduced by 15% and LV mass by 12%. ACE-inhibitors (−16%) were the most effective drugs in reducing LV mass followed by calcium antagonists (−10%), beta-blockers (−9%) and diuretics (−7%). The ACE-inhibitors, beta-blockers and calcium antagonists exerted their effect by reducing the wall thickness while the diuretics mainly by decreasing left ventricular volume. Cruickshank et al, analizing 104 published papers with 2107 patients, found a similar trend as of Dahlöf et al: ACE-inhibitors induced a more significant reversal of LVH than other drugs. In the third meta-analysis by Schmieder et al, based on 39 studies of high scientific quality for a similar fall in blood pressure, LV mass decreased with ACE-inhibitor by 13%, with calcium antagonists by 9%, with beta-blockers by 6% and with diuretics by 7%. The reduction of LV

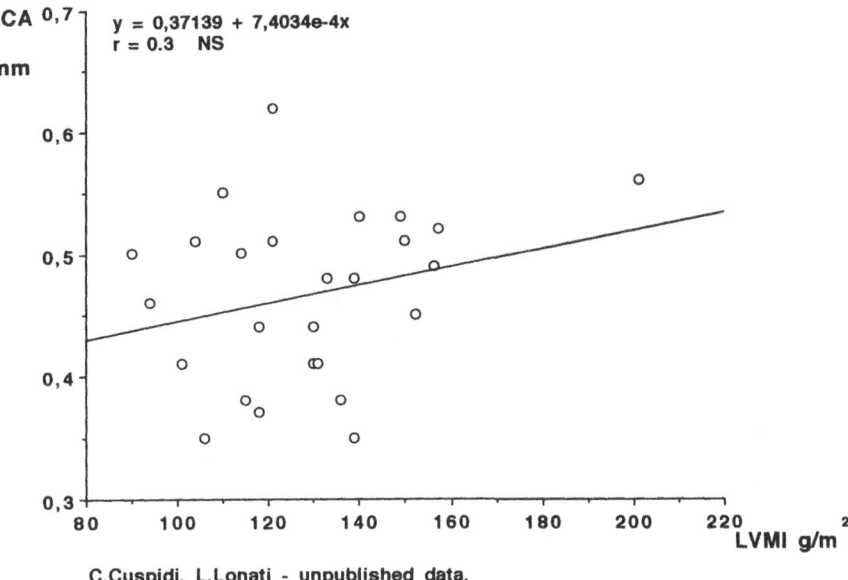

C.Cuspidi, L.Lonati - unpublished data.

Figure 3. Correlation between LCA (left coronary artery) main trunk diameter and LVMI (left ventricular mass index) in hypertensives.

mass does not influence negatively the systolic function while the effects of LVH regression on diastolic function are unclear.

Many clinical studies show that LVH is not fully reversible in a significant number of hypertensive patients despite a good control of blood pressure, even if the main reason of persistence of LVH is related to sub-optimal anti-hypertensive therapy and compliance. LVH regression in athletes may be analyzed from two different points of view. The first concerns the seasonal variations of LV structure induced by training and detraining. The second point concerns the complete interruption of athletic activity; LVH usually is fully reversible in young athletes but residual LVH, associated with diastolic abnormalities may persist in some older athletes.

Several studies have observed that a significant increase in LV mass can develop quite rapidly (within weeks or months) in response to activation of an intense physical conditioning program. Reports on the structural cardiac changes after a period of deconditioning also underline the dynamic nature of LVH present in trained athletes. Ehsani et al showed a substantial decrease in LV mass (27%) within a week of total cessation of training. Pelliccia et al demonstrated a significant reduction in LV wall thickness and mass in six olympic athletes with substantial ventricular septal thickening, which resembled that of hypertrophic cardiomyopathy, after 6–34 weeks (mean 13 weeks) of deconditioning (50). The findings of this study suggest that a brief period of forced deconditioning may be useful in distinguishing by serial echocardiography between physiological and pathological LVH in athletes with marked cardiac hypertrophy.

The complete interruption of athletic activity is usually accompanied by normalization of morpho-functional cardiac parameters, with the possible exception of older athletes with life long training. Our group documented that former athletes, studied after 3–5 years of complete cessation of their professional activity, show LV mass index and early to late mitral peak velocity ratio similar to sedentary controls (51) (Fig. 4).

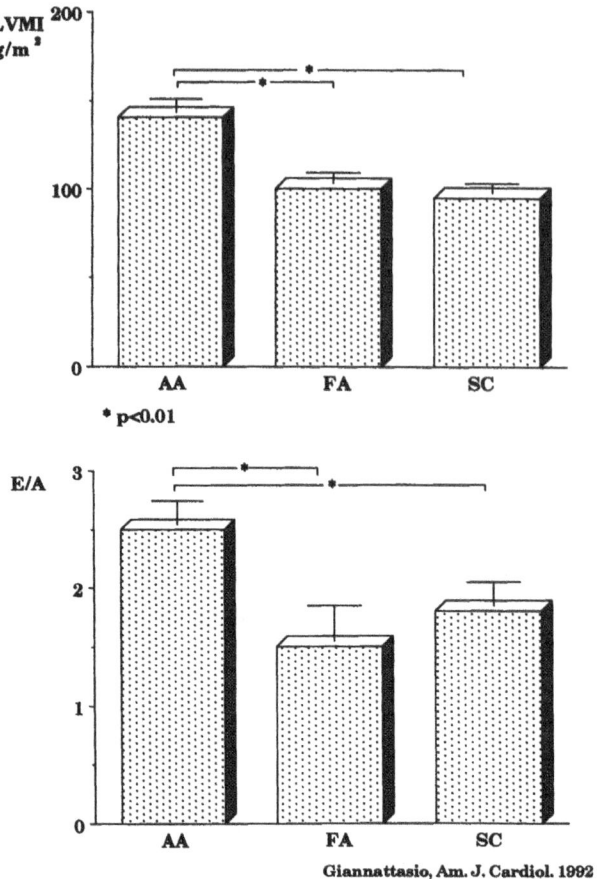

Figure 4. Left ventricular structure and diastolic function in sedentary controls (SC), active athletes (AA), and former athletes (FA).

7. CAROTID STRUCTURE IN HYPERTENSIVES AND IN ATHLETES

In recent years, ultrasound techniques have been developed that allow to evaluate the thickness of superficial arteries in humans (52). With ultrasonographic techniques, arterial thickness is measured non invasively and directly in-vivo conditions. Because of the resolution and the limitations of this non invasive approach, the findings can only be analyzed in terms of intima-media complex. The extracranial carotid arteries have been studied most intensively. Recent studies showed that a significant increase in carotid thickness paralleles cardiac hypertrophic changes in patients with sustained hypertension (53). In these studies the relationship between carotid wall thickening and LVH was found to be independent of age, blood pressure or serum lipid levels.

In animal studies elevated blood pressure has been shown to promote the growth of smooth muscle cells, leading to a thickening of the conduit artery wall. There is increasing evidence that the abnormal wall thickening both of the heart and of the arteries in hypertension involves common pressure-related and non pressure-related mechanisms. Carotid intima-media thickening and uncomplicated plaques in hypertensives without other significant cardiovascular risk factors may be considered a marker of vascular damage directly related to high blood pressure.

Several studies have shown a significant increase in intima media thickness in essential hypertensive patients compared with age-matched normotensive controls, indicating that both systolic and diastolic blood pressure (or even pulse pressure) are significantly correlated to the degree of carotid thickness (54–56). Little information exists about the conduit vessel properties in athletes. Experimental data indicate that long term endurance training of rats induced an increased wall thickness of their conductance arteries without modifications in the number of smooth muscle cells. Cameron et al reported that mild non competitive exercise training increases total systemic compliance in humans (57).

We recently demonstrated that the thickness of the carotid artery wall is significantly greater in athletes than in sedentary subjects and that the mean intima-media thickness is similar to that found in young borderline hypertensives in spite of the fact that athletes have normal blood pressure values (42). The thickening of the arterial wall related to long-term athletic training might result from vascular hypertrophy in response to an increase in vessel wall stress during exercise.

During athletic activity blood flow and transmural pressure are elevated simultaneously; both of these forces increase shear and tangential stress on the arterial wall. Therefore, vascular hypertrophy could represent a structural autoregulation process to reduce hemodynamic stress during exercise. Frequent activation of the sympatho-adrenergic system and of the renin-angiotensin system during regular and competitive physical activity might also play a role in inducing or facilitating a hypertrophic response of conduit arteries in athletes. A pure increase in the muscle component of the arterial wall might also explain the increased arterial compliance in athletes at difference from hypertensive patients in whom carotid compliance is reduced. This observation demonstrates the different nature of carotid intima-media thickening in athletes and in hypertensives.

8. CONCLUSIONS

The increase in LV mass in hypertensive patients is a pathologic process associated with systolic and diastolic dysfunction, abnormal myocardial tissue properties, impaired

Table 5. Physiological and pathological LVH

Differences	Similarities
Degree	LV geometry
• usually mild (A)	• eccentric–concentric (A)
• mild–severe (H)	• eccentric–concentric (H)
Function	Cardiac reflexes
• normal (A)	• impaired? (A)
• impaired (H)	• impaired (H)
Coronary reserve	
• normal (A)	
• reduced (H)	
LVH regression	
• fully reversible (A)	
• fully reversible? (H)	
Tissue properties	
• normal (A)	
• altered (H)	

A: athletes; H: hypertensives

coronary reserve, enhanced arhythmogenesis and arterial wall thickening; moreover LVH induced by hypertension is not in all cases fully reversible. These findings differentiate the hypertensive LVH from physiological athlete's LVH characterized by normal cardiac function, coronary reserve, myocardial tissue and vascular properties and by complete normalization of LV mass after cessation of athletic activity (see Tab. 5).

In conclusion the two types of LVH show more differences than similarities, they are limited to increase in LV mass only and probably to impairment of cardiac reflexes.

REFERENCES

1. E.D.Frohlich, C.Apstein, A.M.Chobanian, R.B.Ducreux, H.P.Dustan, V.Dzau, F.Fouad Tarazi, M.J.Horan, M.Marcus, B.Massie, M.R.Pfeffer, R.W.Re, E.J.Roccella, D.Savage and C.Shub. The heart in hypertension. N Engl J Med 1992;327:998–1008.
2. L.M.Shapiro. Physiological left ventricular hypertrophy. Br Heart J 1984;52:130–135.
3. G.Leonetti and C.Cuspidi. The heart and vascular changes in hypertension. J Hypertens 1995;13 (suppl 2):S29–S34.
4. J.E. Otterstad, O. Smireth and S.E. Kjeldsen. Hypertension left ventricular hypertrophy: pathophysiology assessment and treatment. Blood Pressure 1996;5:5–15.
5. D.D.Savage. Overall risk of left ventricular hypertrophy secondary to systemic hypertension. Am J Cardiol 1987;60:81–121.
6. P.N.Casale, R.B.Devereux. M.Milner, G.Zullo, G.A.Harshfield and T.G.Pickering. Value of echocardiographic left ventricular mass in predicting cardiovascular morbid events in hypertensive men. Ann Intern Med 1986;105:173–178.
7. B.Dahlöf, J.M.Cruickshank and P.R.Danby. Managing left ventricular hypertrophy in primary care. Science Press, London, 1993.
8. U.Sechtem. The athlete's heart revisited. Eur Heart J 1996;17:1138–1140.
9. D.Levy, R.J.Garrison, D.D.Savage, W.B.Kannel and W.P.Castelli. Left ventricular mass and incidence of coronary heart disease in an elderly cohort: the Framingham Heart study. Ann Intern Med 1989;110:101–107.
10. D.Levy, R.J.Garrison, D.D.Savage, W.B.Kannel and W.P.Castelli. Prognostic implications of echocardiographically determined left ventricular mass in the Framingham Heart study. N Engl J Med 1990;332:1561–1566.
11. D.D.Savage, R.J.Garrison and W.B.Kannel. The spectrum of left ventricular hypertrophy in a general population sample: the Framingham study. Circulation 1987;75 (suppl I):26–33.
12. G.Parati, G.Pomidossi, F.Albini, D.Malaspina and G.Mancia. Relationship of 24-hour blood pressure mean and variability to severity of target organ damage in hypertension. J Hypertens 1987;5:93–98.
13. K.T.Weber and C.G.Brilla. Pathological hypertrophy and cardiac interstitium: fibrosis and renin-angiotensin-aldosterone system. Circulation 1991;83:1849–1865.
14. F.M.Fouad Tarazi, M.Imamura, E.L.Bravo, G.Rossi, H.K.Nagi, W.W.Lin, M.Cressman and P.Wicker. Differences in left ventricular structural and functional changes between pheochromocytoma and essential hypertension. Role of elevated circulating catecholamines. Am J Hypertens 1992;5:134–140.
15. P.R.Liebson, G.Grandits, R.Prineas, S.Dianzumba, J.M.Flack, J.A.Cutler, R.Grimm and J.Stamler. Echocardiographic correlates of left ventricular structure among 844 mildly hypertensive men and women in the treatment of mild hypertension study (THOMS). Circulation 1993;87:476–486.
16. M.Zabalgoitia. Left ventricular mass and function in primary hypertension. Am J Hypertens 1996;9:55S–59S.
17. G.Gigli, F.Lattanzi, A.R.Lucarini, E.Picano, A.Genovesi-Ebert, C.Marabotti, R.Zunino, A.Mazzarisi, L.Landini, M.Iannetti and D.Distante. Normal ultrasonic myocardial reflectivity in hypertensive patients. A tissue characterization study. Hypertension 1993;20:329–334.
18. B.J.Maron. Structural features of the athlete heart as defined by echocardiography. JACC 1986;7:190–203.
19. R.Fagard, A.Aubert, J.Staessen, E.V.Eynde, L.Vanhees and A.Amery. Cardiac structure and function in cyclists and runners. Comparative echocardiographic study. Br Heart J 1984;52:124–129.
20. J.Morganroth, B.J.Maron, L.W.Hentry and S.E.Epstein. Comparative left ventricular dimensions in trained athletes. Ann Intern Med 1975;82:521–524.
21. J.C.Longhurst, A.R.Kelly, W.J.Gonyee and J.H.Mitchell. Chronic training with static and dynamic exercise cardiovascular adaptation and response to exercise. Circ Res 1981;48 (suppl I):171–178.

22. J.C.Longhurst, A.R.Kelly, W.J.Gonyee and J.H.Mitchell. Echocardiographic left ventricular masses in distance runners and weight lifters. J Appl Physiol 1980;48:154–162.

23. T.Miki, Y.Yokota, T.Seo and M.Yokoyama. Echocardiographic findings in 104 professional cyclists with follow-up study. Am Heart J 1994;127:898–905.

24. P.Spirito, A.Pelliccia, M.A.Proschass, M.Granata, A.Spataro, P.Bellone, G.Caselli, A.Biffi, C.Vecchio and B.M.Maron. Morphology of the athlete's heart assessed by echocardiography in 947 elite athletes representing 27 sports. Am J Cardiol 1994;74:898–905.

25. A.Pelliccia, B.J.Maron, F.Culasso, A.Spataro and G.Caselli. Athlete's heart in women. JAMA 1996;276: 211–215.

26. T.Nishimura, Y.Yamada and C.Kawai. Echocardiographic evaluation of long term effects of exercise on left ventricular hypertrophy and function in professional bicyclists. Circulation 1980;61:832–840.

27. F.Lattanzi, U.Di Bello, E.Picano, M.T.Caputo, L.Talarico, C.Di Muro, L.Landini, G.Santoro, C.Giusti and A.Distante. Normal ultrasonic myocardial reflectivity in athletes with increased left ventricular mass: a tissue characterization study. Circulation 1992;85:1828–1834.

28. C.Fiorentini, C.Galli, G.Tamborini, P.Moruzzi, M.Berti, S.Riva and M.D.Guazzi. Combined hemodynamic overload of the left and right ventricles as a possible cause of interventricular septum preponderance in high blood pressure. Am Heart J 1988;116:509–514.

29. C.Cuspidi, L.Sampieri, L.Angioni, L.Boselli, R.Bragato, G.Leonetti and A.Zanchetti. Right ventricular wall thickness and function in hypertensive patients with and without left ventricular hypertrophy: echo-Doppler study. J Hypertens 1989;7 (suppl 6):S108–S109.

30. B.D.Nunez, F.H.Messerli, C.Amodeo, G.E.Garavaglia, R.E.Schmieder and E.D.Frohlich. Biventricular cardiac hypertrophy in essential hypertension. Am Heart J 1987;114:813–818.

31. E.Enriksen, J.Landelins, L.Wesslen, H.Arnell, C.Nyström-Rosander, T.Kangro, T.Jonason, C.Rolf, C.Liddel, E.Hammarstrom, I.Ringqvist and G.Friman. Echocardiographic right and left ventricular measurements in male elite endurance athletes. Eur Heart J 1996;17:1121–1128.

32. A.Cuocolo, F.L.Sax, J.E.Brush, B.J.Maron, S.Bacharach and R.O.Borrow. Left ventricular hypertrophy and impaired diastolic filling in essential hypertension. Circulation 1990;81:978–986.

33. E.Grossman, S.Oren and F.Messerli. Left ventricular filling and stress response pattern in essential hypertension. Am J Med 1991;97:502–506.

34. G.De Simone, R.B.Devereux, M.J.Roman, A.Ganau, P.S.Saba, M.H.Alderman and J.H.Laragh. Assessment of left ventricular function by midwall fractional shortening end systolic stress relation in human hypertension. JACC 1994;23:1444–1451.

35. P.Verdecchia, G.Schillaci, M.Guerrieri, F.Boldrini, C.Gatteschi, G.Benemio and C.Porcellati. Prevalence and determinants of left ventricular diastolic filling abnormalities in an unselected hypertensive population. Eur Heart J 1990;11:679–691.

36. R.C.Harizi, J.A.Bianco and J.S.Alpert. Diastolic function of heart in clinical cardiology. Arch Intern Med 1988;148:99–109.

37. A.W.De Maria, T.W.Wisenbaugh, M.D.Smith, M.R.Harrison and M.R.Berk. Doppler echocardiographic evaluation of diastolic dysfunction. Circulation 1991;84 (suppl I):288–295.

38. M.J.Lim and A.J.Buda. Doppler echocardiography in the evaluation of left ventricular diastolic function. Curr Opinion Cardiol 1991;6:937–945.

39. C.B.Granger, M.K.Karimeddini, V.E.Smith, H.R.Shapiro, A.M.Katz and A.L.Riba. Rapid ventricular filling in left ventricular hypertrophy: I. Physiologic hypertrophy. JACC 1985;5:862–868.

40. S.D.Colan, S.P.Sanders, D.MacPherson and K.M.Borrow. Left ventricular diastolic function in elite athletes with physiologic cardiac hypertrophy. JACC 1985;6:545–549.

41. C.Cuspidi, L.Sampieri, L.Boselli, L.Angioni, R.Bragato, G.Leonetti and A.Zanchetti. Left ventricular diastolic function in athletes and hypertensives with mild cardiac hypertrophy. Cardiology 1991;78:278–281.

42. C.Cuspidi, L.Lonati, L.Sampieri, G.Leonetti and A.Zanchetti. Similarities and differences in structural and functional changes of left ventricle and carotid arteries in young borderline hypertensives and in athletes. J Hypertens 1996;14:759–764.

43. F.G.Dunn and S.D.Pringle. Left ventricular hypertrophy and myocardial ischemia in systemic hypertension. Am J Cardiol 1987;60:191–221.

44. A.Zanchetti, P.Sleight and W.H.Birkenhager. Evaluation of organ damage in hypertension. J Hypertens 1993;11:875–882.

45. L.Lonati, C.Cuspidi, L.Sampieri, T.Zaro, S.Pelizzoli, G.Pontiggia, G.Leonetti and A.Zanchetti. Lack of correlation between left ventricular mass and diameter of extramural coronary arteries in hypertensive patients: a transthoracic echocardiographic study. Eight Eur Meeting on Hypertension, Milan 1997 (abstract).

46. J.M.Cruickshank, J.Lewis, E.U.Moor and C.Dodd. Reversibility of left ventricular hypertrophy by different types of antihypertensive therapy. J Human Hypertens 1992;6:85–95.

47. B.Dahlöf, K.Pennert and L.Hansson. Reversal of left ventricular hypertrophy in hypertensive patients: a meta-analysis of 109 treatment studies. Am J Hypertens 1992;5:95–110.
48. R.E.Schmieder, P.Martus and R.Klingheil. Reversal of left ventricular hypertrophy in essential hypertension: a meta-analysis of randomized double blind studies. JAMA 1996;275:1507–1513.
49. A.A.Ehsani, J.M.Hagberg and R.C.Hickson. Rapid changes in left ventricular dimensions and mass in response to physical conditioning and deconditioning. Am J Cardiol 1978;42:52–56.
50. B.J.Maron, A.Pelliccia, A.Spataro and M.Granata. Reduction in left ventricular wall thickness after deconditioning in highly trained olympic athletes. Br Heart J 1993;69:125–128.
51. C.Giannattasio, G.Seravalle, B.M.Cattaneo, C.Cuspidi, L.Sampieri, G.B.Bolla, G.Grassi and G.Mancia. Effect of detraining on the cardiopulmonary reflex in professional runners and hammer throwers. Am J Cardiol 1992;69:677–680.
52. M.E.Safar, X.Girerd and S.Laurent. Structural changes of large conduit arteries in hypertension. J Hypertens 1996;14:545–555.
53. M.J.Roman, T.G.Pickering, J.C.Schwartz, R.Pini and R.B.Devereux. Association of carotid atherosclerosis and left ventricular hypertrophy. JACC 1995;25:83–90.
54. C.Cuspidi, L.Boselli, R.Bragato, L.Lonati, L.Sampieri, M.Bocciolone, G.Leonetti and A.Zanchetti. Echocardiographic and ultrasonographic evaluation of cardiac and vascular hypertrophy in patients with essential hypertension. Cardiology 1992;80:305–311.
55. A.P.Hughes, A.M.Sinclair, G.Geroulakos, J.Mayet, J.Mackay, M.Shahi, S.Thoen, A.Nicolaides and P.J.Sever. Structural changes in the cardiovascular system of untreated essential hypertensives. Blood Pressure 1995;4:42–47.
56. C.Cuspidi, M.Marabini, L.Lonati, L.Sampieri, G.Comerio, S.Pelizzoli, G.Leonetti and A.Zanchetti. Cardiac and carotid structure in patients with established hypertension and white-coat hypertension. J Hypertens 1995;13:1707–1711.
57. J.D.Cameron and A.M.Dart. Exercise training increases total systemic arterial compliance in humans. Am J Physiol 1994;266:H693–H703.

17

BRADYKININ AND CARDIAC PROTECTION

Peter Gohlke,[1] Carsten Tschöpe,[1,2] and Thomas Unger[1]

[1]Department of Pharmacology
University of Kiel
Hospitalstraße 4
D-24105 Kiel, Germany
[2]Department of Cardiology and Pneumology
Universiy Hospital Benjamin Franklin
Free University of Berlin
Hindenburgdamm 30
D-12220 Berlin, Germany

1. INTRODUCTION

Administration of bradykinin to humans and several animal species engenders a variety of effects, including blood pressure reduction through endothelium-dependent vasorelaxation, changes in renal blood flow and tubular function, inflammatory reactions, vasoconstriction via direct effects on smooth muscle cells, alteration in vascular permeability and activation of sensory pain fibres[1-3]. Since circulating concentrations of bradykinin are usually too low to cause systemic effects[4,5], autocrine and paracrine actions of kinins have increasingly received scientific attention.

Kinins are rapidly degraded by a number of enzymes including aminopeptidase P, neutral endopeptidase 24.11, carboxypeptidase N (Kininase I) and angiotensin-converting enzyme (ACE) which is identical to kininase II. ACE is found predominantly on the luminal surface of endothelial cells. The enzyme belongs to the tissue-bound inactivating system of kinins and is the major contributor to the degradation of bradykinin in peripheral organs such as the lung and the heart[6]. Inhibitors of ACE exert numerous actions on the cardiovascular system, some of which have been attributed to a decreased kinin degradation. These actions include the prevention of neointima formation after endothelial denudation in rats[7], preservation of endothelial function in experimental atherosclerosis in rabbits[8], reduction of postischemic reperfusion arrhythmias in isolated working rat hearts[9] and of infarct size in dogs[5,10-12] cats[13] and rats[14-18], or prevention of development of left ventricular hypertrophy (LVH) in rats with aortic banding[19] and improvement of cardiac function and metabolism in spontaneously hypertensive rats (SHR)[20]. Furthermore, we have shown that chronic ACE inhibitor treatment can induce myocardial capillary growth in SHR and SHRSP even at doses too low to prevent the development of hypertension and

Hypertension and the Heart, edited by Zanchetti et al.
Plenum Press, New York, 1997

LVH[21,22]. Since this effect could be prevented by bradykinin B_2 receptor blockade capillary growth may be related to chronic kinin potentiation[22].

In the following we will outline some of the experiments investigating the contribution of bradykinin to the cardioprotective actions of ACE inhibitors

2. THE KALLIKREIN-KININ-SYSTEM IN THE HEART

An independent tissue kallikrein-kinin system, which may participate in the regulation of cardiac function, has recently been demonstrated in the heart[23]. In rat artria and ventricles glandular kallikrein, its mRNA and kininogen could be detected. Coronaries also contain and release kallikrein. Binding sites for bradykinin have been described in myocytes as well as in cardiac fibroblasts. Additionally, cardiac kinin levels are reportedly much higher than blood kinin levels[24]. Thus, cardiac kinins may be generated continuously by a local kallikrein-kinin system. The biological effects of kinins are mediated by stimulation of specific kinin receptors, classified as B_1- and B_2 receptors. B_2 receptors mediate most of the known effects of BK[1]. B_1 receptors are more sensitive to the bradykinin metabolite, des-Arg[9]-bradykinin and have been reported to be expressed mainly under pathological conditions such as tissue injury[25]. Important tools to study the actions of bradykinin are selective bradykinin receptor antagonists. The development of the first B_2 receptor antagonist through substitution of D-phenylalanine for -Pro[7] of BK by Stewart and Vavrek in 1985[26] was a breakthrough in the investigation of the physiological role of kinins. More recently, a new B_2 receptor antagonist, icatibant (Hoe 140; D-Arg, [Hyp[3], Thi[5], D-Tic[7], Oic[8]]-bradykinin), has been developed. At present, it is one of the the most potent, stable and long-acting specific kinin antagonist at the B_2 receptor[27–29]. This compound has greatly facilitated the studies on the effects of B_2 receptor-mediated actions even under chronic conditions[20,30,31].

3. CONTRIBUTION OF KININS TO THE CARDIOPROTECTIVE ACTIONS OF ACE INHIBITION

3.1. Myocardial Ischemia and Infarction

Several studies have shown an induction of ACE activity and ACE mRNA synthesis in experimental heart failure[32,33]. In order to identify the role of ACE in ventricular remodeling after myocardial infarction we studied the cellular distribution of ACE in human and rat hearts[34]. Three weeks after myocardial infarction, ACE expression was markedly increased in the repairing scar. Macrophages and capillary endothelial cells were ACE positive, while vascular smooth muscle cells, cardiomyocytes and fibroblasts did not stain for ACE. These findings suggest a role of ACE related to tissue repair and remodeling after myocardial infarction.

Although in some experimental studies ACE inhibitors failed to reduce cardial ischemic damage after permanent coronary occlusion or in models of coronary occlusion and reperfusion[35–37], the beneficial effects of ACE inhibitors in the prevention of heart failure following myocardial infarction have recently been demonstrated in large clinical intervention trails[38,39]. However, the role of the kallikrein-kinin system is still matter of discussion in this respect.

While several authors reported an acute increase in bradykinin or its metabolites in the coronary effluent in different models of cardiac ischemia with and without ACE-inhibition[40-42], Duncan et al. did not find a significant increase in cardiac tissue bradykinin levels during ACE inhibitor-treatment started 48h after induction of myocardial infarction[18]. Under regional ischemic conditions or after ACE inhibition, bradykinin outflow of isolated working rat hearts was found to be markedly increased compared to normoxic or untreated rat hearts[41]. However, in this study concentrations of immunoreactive kinins were measured in the nanogram range, which appears extremely high. Probably, the presence of kinin precursors and/or kinin-forming enzymes in the perfusate interferred with the assay. Similarly, Lamontagne et al.[42] did not detect any change in bradykinin and in des-Arg[9]-bradykinin levels in untreated globally ischemic rat hearts following reperfusion. However, in ACE-inhibitor treated hearts an increase of des-Arg[9]-bradykinin levels was observed following reperfusion[42].

These discrepancies may be due to different designs of the studies and methods used. Theoretically, an increased bradykinin outflow in hypoxic conditions could be part of a compensatory mechanism since bradykinin has been demonstrated to exert positive inotropic actions[43,44] and to increase coronary flow[45-47].

The infarct size limiting actions of many cardioprotective drugs was thought to be mainly mediated by lowering afterload, heart rate, and cardiac contraction. The first evidence that ACE inhibitors might be cardioprotective in the setting of acute coronary artery occlusion was provided by Ertl et al.[48] In anaesthetized dogs, captopril or vehicle were continuously infused from 30 min to 6h after the onset of ischemia. Infarct size assessed at 6h postocclusion averaged 57% of the occluded coronary artery bed in ACE inhibitor-treated animals, which were significantly smaller than the value of 75% obtained in controls. This initial observation was followed by reports of cardioprotection with other ACE inhibitors in different animal models[13,14]. Although Ertl et al. concluded initially that the reduction in infarct size after ACE-inhibitor treatment was most probably due to the increase in collateral perfusion to the ischemic zone[48] they demonstrated in a subsequent study that in ACE inhibitor-treated dogs the area at risk and the infarcted area after coronary artery ligation were smaller than predicted from the concomitant augmentation of coronary blood flow[11]. This points to additional effects of ACE inhibitor with respect to myocardial metabolism independently of the improvement in coronary flow. Martorana et al.[12] demonstrated that low-dose intracoronary infusion of ramipril or bradykinin significantly reduced infarct size in anesthetized dogs. In this instance, the protective effects of ACE inhibitor treatment were not a consequence of hemodynamic alterations. Since these effects were abolished by coadministration of icatibant, the authors concluded that the benefits of ramipril in this model were due in large part to inhibition of kinin metabolism.

In contrast, some studies failed to document a cardioprotective effect of ACE inhibitor treatment following permanent coronary occlusion[35,37]. An intriguing explanation for this discrepancy was recently provided by de Lorgeril et al.[37], who have shown that in a subgroup of animals with severe ischemia during coronary occlusion ACE inhibitor treatment tended to reduce infarct size but increased infarct size in the subgroup of animals with high collateral blood flow during ischemia. The worsening of myocardial injury in the high-flow subgroup was attributed to coronary vasodilation and a subsequent decrease in collateral perfusion to the ischemic tissue, comparable to a coronary steal phenomenon. Accordingly, Przyklenk and Kloner[49] speculated that ACE inhibitors might be cardioprotective in models characterized by low native collateral perfusion (i.e. rat, pig, rabbit) and in models of highly variable collateral flow (i.e canine), and in subgroups of animals with a paucity of native collateral vessels.

Comparing captopril and the AT_1 receptor antagonist, losartan, Smits et al. reported that the acute beneficial hemodynamic effects of ACE-inhibition after coronary occlusion might not depend on AT_1 receptor mechanisms. However, they found an inhibition in heart weight during treatment with losartan or captopril, started 3 to 5 weeks after myocardial infarction[50]. In contrast, Raya et al. reported that treatment with captopril or losartan in rats with chronic heart failure after myocardial infarction reduced left ventricular end-diastolic pressure without significant changes in left ventricular/body weight ratio[51].

We also have recently investigated the contribution of bradykinin potentiation versus ANG II reduction to the effects of ACE inhibition after myocardial infarction in a rat model. One week pretreatment and subsequent 6-week treatment post-myocardial infarction with the ACE inhibitor, moexipril, reduced infarct size and improved ventricular function. Cotreatment with the B_2 receptor antagonist, icatibant, prevented the beneficial effects of moexipril. Losartan was ineffective under these treatment conditions[16].

In another part of this study we investigated the effects of late-onset 6-week treatment with moexipril and losartan beginning six weeks after myocardial infarction. ACE inhibitor-treatment reduced heart weight, but had no significant influence on end-diastolic pressure. The effect on heart weight could be prevented by cotreatment with icatibant. Treatment with losartan improved cardiac function by a significant reduction on end-diastolic pressure, but had no influence on heart weight and, similar to the results during the ACE inhibitor-treatment, no influence in infarct size[17,52]. The differences between the studies described earlier and our observations might be due to the variable extent of myocardial infarction between studies differing from 39% to 55% of left ventricular mass.

However, in this experimental model of myocardial infarction the kinin-mediated cardioprotective effects produced by ACE inhibition in heart failure after a large transmural infarction seem to be more significant, when treatment is commenced early, in this case before myocardial infarction. When treatment is started later after myocardial infarction, i.e. when remodeling is in process, ACE expression is stimulated and congestive heart failure is developing, the beneficial effects of ACE inhibition seems to be more related to a reduced ANG II production.

To further investigate the mechanism underlying the infarct size limiting action of ACE inhibitors, we used a laser doppler flow meter to measure tissue blood flow in the marginal zone of area at risk after in rats. One-week pretreatment with ramipril increased tissue blood flow in the marginal flow zone of the infarcted area 15 min after left coronary artery ligation. Treatment was withdrawn after myocardial infarction. Three weeks later, the infarct size was found to be reduced. Both effects were abolished by coadministration with icatibant. Losartan had no significant effects on blood flow and infarct size[53]. These findings suggest that ACE inhibitors improve collateral myocardial blood flow in the acute ischemic zone after left coronary artery ligation by potentiation of endogenous kinins and that this mechanism contributed to the reduction of infarct size.

Recently, Groves et al. reported that under basal conditions intracoronary administration of icatibant lead to an increase in vasomotor tone in human epicardial vessels and a corresponding reduction in coronary blood flow[45]. These findings, together with similar observations of studies in animals[46,47] imply a role for endogenous bradykinin in mediating a vasomotor response in the coronary circulation.

3.2. Left Ventricular Hypertrophy

Cardiac LVH, a frequent consequence of arterial hypertension, is an independent cardiovascular risk factor giving rise to cardiac failure, arrhythmias and ischemia[47].

Hypertension-induced pathophysiological changes in cardiac and vascular structure are partly triggered by the blood pressure rise itself and represent a compensatory response to the increased cardiac output and elevated wall stress. On the other hand, there is evidence from in vivo and in vitro studies that ANG II exerts trophic actions and may accelerate cardiovascular hypertrophy and chronic vascular disease by directly inducing cellular growth in addition to its systemic actions in hypertension[54–57]. Regression of left ventricular mass after ACE inhibitor treatment was demonstrated in normal rats[58] and in hypertensive patients[59–61] and in different forms of experimental hypertension[62,63]. Linz et al.[64] demonstrated that chronic treatment with a subantihypertensive dose ramipril prevented left ventricular hypertrophy in rats with renal hypertension due to aortic banding (pressure overload hypertrophy), suggesting that in this form of hypertension, early-onset treatment with ACEI can induce structural changes of the heart independently of the blood-pressure lowering actions of these drugs. These effects were abolished by coadministration of icatibant, demonstrating a participation of kinins in the antihypertrophic effects of ramipril[19]. However, Rhaleb et al.[65] could not confirm these data, using the same model and experimental protocol. Only at antihypertensive doses ramipril possessed antihypertrophic activity, and kinins were not involved in this effect. These discrepancies cannot be explained so far and need further investigation. In contrast, in SHR and stroke prone SHR (SHRSP) we demonstrated that the reduction in LVH by chronic ACE inhibitor treatment strongly correlates with the reduction in blood pressure. Antihypertensive treatment with an ACE inhibitor prevented the development of LVH while subantihypertensive doses of the ACE inhibitor failed to affect the development of cardiac hypertophy[20,21]. Furthermore, the effects of the ACE inhibitor on LVH were not influenced by cotreatment with icatibant, suggesting that kinins are not the dominant factor in the antihypertrophic effects of ACE inhibitors in SHR and SHRSP, i.e. in animal models with to low to normal plasma renin levels[20].

3.3. Myocardial Capillary Supply

The development of hypertension-induced cardiac hypertrophy is characterized by a preferential growth of cardiac myocytes when compared to capillaries[66]. Therefore, in hypertrophied hearts, the capillary supply is diminished. An objective three-dimensional parameter of capillarization, the capillary length density, has been determined recently in non-hypertrophied hearts from normotensive rats of different age[67]. The authors demonstrated that cardiac capillarization was highest in young, 5 week old rats and decreased gradually with age as well as with increasing heart weight. It has also been shown that capillary length density in non-hypertrophied hearts from normotensive animals was higher when compared to hypertrophied hearts from age-comparable SHR[21,67]. Based on these and other findings, prevention of LVH by antihypertensive treatment can be expected to normalize capillary density. Indeed, several reports have shown that antihypertensive treatment with different ACE inhibitors increased capillary density when compared to untreated control animals[21,22,68–70] (Figure 1). However, several lines of evidence indicate that the reduction of LVH by chronic ACE inhibitor treatment alone may not account completely for the effect of the drugs on capillary proliferation. First, we recently demonstrated that antihypertensive doses of the ACE inhibitors, ramipril and perindopril, markedly increased cardiac capillary length density following long-term treatment but not in the presence of chronic bradykinin B2 receptor blockade despite an effective prevention of LVH[22] (Figure 1). On the other hand, long-term treatment with the AT1 antagonist, losartan, failed to significantly increase cardiac capillary length density when compared to vehicle-treated SHRSP, although blood pressure and LVH was effectively reduced[22] (Figure 1).

Second, in two separate studies in SHR and SHRSP we demonstrated an increased cardiac capillary length density in hearts from low-dose ramipril treated rats independent

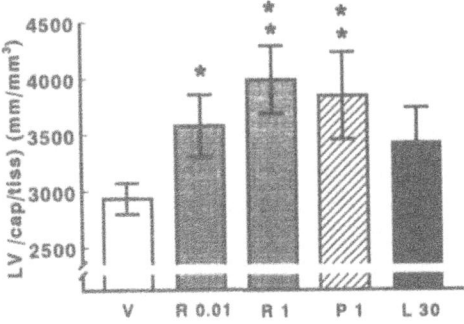

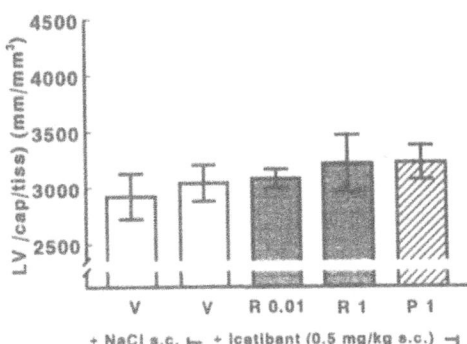

+ NaCl s.c. ⊢ + icatibant (0.5 mg/kg s.c.) ⊣

Figure 1. Upper panel: Effect on cardiac capillary length density (LV [cap/tiss]) of long-term oral treatment of SHRSP with the ACE inhibitors, ramipril (0.01 mg/kg per day; R 0.01 and 1 mg/kg per day; R 1) and perindopril (1 mg/kg per day; P 1) and the AT1 receptor antagonist, losartan (30 mg/kg per day; L 30). Control animals received vehicle (destilled water; V). **Lower panel:** Effect on cardiac capillary length density (LV [cap/tiss]) of chronic oral treatment with ramipril (0.01 mg/kg per day and 1 mg/kg per day) and perindopril (1 mg/kg per day) plus co-treatment with the bradykinin B2-receptor antagonist, icatibant, (0.5 mg/kg per day, s.c.). Values are mean ± S.E.M. *p<0.05; **p<0.01 compared to vehicle-treated animals.

of a reduction in blood pressure and LVH[21,22] (Figure 1). Therefore, these animals may profit from treatment in that their capillary supply and thus, O_2 and nutrient delivery as well as metabolite clearance is increased despite the fact that the hearts had developed hypertrophy to a similar extent as hearts from vehicle-treated controls. Again, the effects of the ACE inhibitor on capillary length density were completely abolished by bradykinin B2 receptor blockade suggesting that bradykinin is a prerequisite for this effect[22] (Figure 1). The potential benefit of a long-term treatment of SHRSP with an ACE inhibitor at subantihypertensive doses has been demonstrated recently by Linz et al.[71] in a survival study. This study showed that low-dose ramipril treatment (0.01 mg/kg per day) can increase survival of SHRSP to about 3 months when compared to vehicle-treated rats. These results also demonstrate the therapeutic importance of blood pressure reduction and prevention of LVH since high dose treated SHRSP lived about one year longer than low dose-treated rats despite similar effect of both doses on capillary density or on cardiac function and metabolism.

The above reported finding that the ACE inhibitors, ramipril and perindopril, but not the AT1 antagonist, losartan, increased cardiac capillary length density at doses which produce similar antihypertensive and antihypertrophic actions needs to be explained (Figure 2). First, the ACE inhibitor effects could be due to the bradykinin potentiating action in addition to inhibition of the renin angiotensin system (RAS) while losartan may act more specifically on the RAS by blocking the AT1 receptors. However, there is also some evidence from studies in isolated rat hearts as well as in cell cultures for an interaction between ANG II and the bradykinin/nitric oxide system possibly mediated by an AT2 receptor stimulation[72,73]. In recent studies we demonstrated that losartan and ramipril show strikingly similar effects with regard to an improvement in myocardial function and myocardial metabolic parameters in ex vivo isolated hearts from SHRSP following long-term

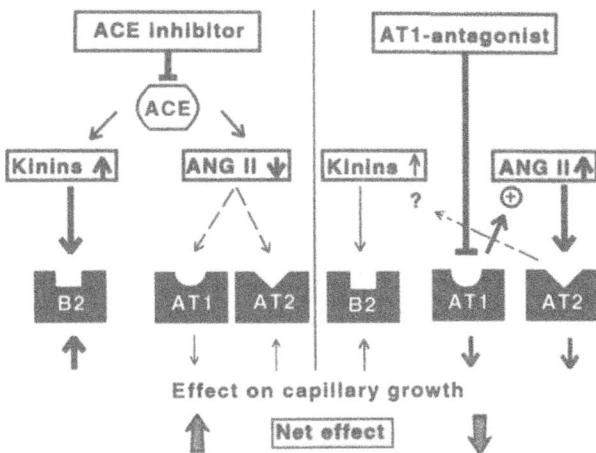

Figure 2. Left panel: Effect of ACE inhibition on capillary growth. Inhibition of ACE causes a decrease in kinin degradation and an inhibition of angiotensin II (ANG II) generation. As a result, the activation of B2 receptors by increased kinins can lead to a stimulation of capillary growth. On the other hand, the AT1 receptor-mediated growth stimulating effects of ANG II as well as the AT2 receptor-mediated growth inhibiting effects of ANG II were both attenuated by a decrease in ANG II levels. The net effect of ACE inhibition is a kinin-mediated stimulation of capillary growth. **Right panel:** Effect of AT1 receptor blockade on capillary growth. The blockade of AT1 receptors inhibits directly the AT1 receptor-mediated growth stimulating effects of ANG II and causes an abolition of the feedback inhibition of renin secretion in the kidney. As a result, plasma ANG II levels increase and can stimulate the AT2 receptor-mediated inhibition of capillary growth. A stimulation of kinin generation by ANG II possibly mediated by activation of AT2 receptors may lead to stimulation of capillary growth. However, the net effect of AT1 receptor blockade is an inhibition of capillary growth.

treatment. In these studies both compounds increased myocardial contractility and coronary flow, reduced the release of the intracellular enzymes LDH and creatine kinase and of lactate, increased myocardial tissue levels of glycogen, and the energy-rich phosphates ATP and creatine phosphate and decreased myocardial lactate concentration[20,74] (Figure 3a). All these effects of the ACE inhibitor were completely abolished by chronic bradykinin B2 receptor blockade[20] (Figure 3b). Thus, the bradykinin-dependent effects of the ACE inhibitor were mimicked by losartan. Moreover, the effects of losartan on coronary flow, an important factor involved in the stimulation of capillary growth, were even more pronounced when compared to ramipril (Figure 3a) and the drug produced a 2.6 fold higher increase in aortic cGMP content which can be regarded as a measure of vascular nitric oxide release[20,30,74]. Therefore, losartan could have been expected to be at least as effective as ramipril in increasing cardiac capillary length density due to its antihypertrophic effect and due to a possible interaction with the bradykinin/nitric oxide system. Therefore, the failure of losartan to increase cardiac capillary length density might involve an additional activation of growth inhibiting mechanisms and may be related to a chronic stimulation of non-AT1 receptors such as the AT2 receptor. A stimulation of AT2 receptors can be expected because: First, the AT2 receptor remains unblocked by losartan at therapeutic doses[75] and second, plasma levels of ANG II increased following AT1 receptor blockade due to an inhibition of the negative feedback regulation of renin secretion by ANG II[76].

Indeed, stimulation with ANG II via AT2 receptors mediates anti-growth effects on coronary endothelial cells[57,77]. Furthermore, there is evidence that ANG II exerts a mito-

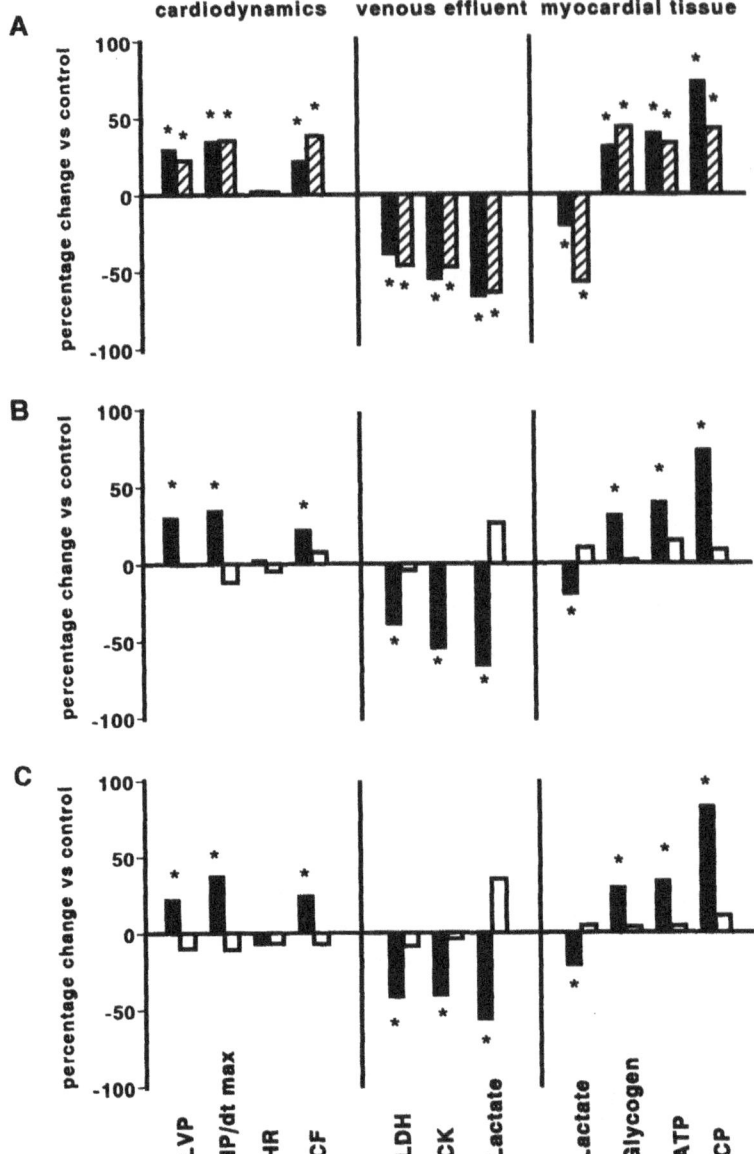

Figure 3. **A:** Effect of oral treatment of SHRSP with the ACE inhibitor, ramipril, at the high dose of 1 mg/kg per day (black bars) and the AT1 antagonist, losartan at an equihypotensive dose of 30 mg/kg per day (hatched bars) on myocardial function and myocardial metabolism. Both substances similarly prevented the development of hypertension and cardiac hypertrophy. **B:** Effect of early-onset long-term oral treatment of SHRSP with the high dose of 1 mg/kg per day ramipril alone (black bars) and following co-treatment with the bradykinin B_2-receptor antagonist, icatibant, (500 μg/kg per day, s.c.) (open bars) on myocardial function and myocardial metabolism. Blockade of bradykinin B2 receptors had no effect on the antihypertensive and antihypertrophic actions of ramipril. **C:** Effect of early-onset long-term oral treatment of SHRSP with the low dose of 0.01 mg/kg per day ramipril alone (black bars) and following co-treatment with the bradykinin B_2-receptor antagonist, icatibant, (500 μg/kg per day, s.c.) (open bars) on myocardial function and myocardial metabolism. The low dose of ramipril did not affect the development of hypertension and cardiac hypertrophy. LVP, left ventricular pressure; dp/dt max, differentiated left ventricular pressure; HR, heart rate; CF, coronary flow; LDH, lactate dehydrogenase; CK, creatine kinase; ATP, adenosine triphosphate; CP, creatine phosphate. *P<0.05 compared with the vehicle control group.

genic effect on coronary endothelial cells by an AT1 receptor mechanism[57]. In vascular smooth muscle cells (VSMC) which only express the AT1 receptor, ANG II exerts a growth-promoting action. However, in the presence of AT2 receptors, that is in VSMC transfected with the AT2 receptor, an anti-growth effect of ANG II could be observed[78].

In a study in rat cremaster muscle, Munzenmaier & Greene[79] demonstrated that in the microcirculation the AT1 receptor mediates angiogenic actions while AT2 receptor stimulation causes inhibition of angiogenesis.

Therefore, losartan treatment might have caused an inhibition of capillary growth by both, the inhibition of the AT1 receptor mediated growth-promoting action of ANG II and by stimulation of the AT2 receptor mediated anti-proliferative action of ANG II (Figure 2). Obviously, the inhibitory effects of losartan on capillary growth could not be compensated by the effects of the drug on LVH and on cardiac function and metabolism[20].

On the other hand, the angiogenic action of ramipril was completely abolished by bradykinin B2 receptor blockade suggesting that endogenous bradykinin is a least a prerequisite of this effect and that ANG II does not contribute to the capillary growth process under these conditions.

However, it is also possible that due to the inhibition of ANG II generation, the ACE inhibitor caused an inhibition of the AT1 receptor-dependent growth promoting actions of ANG II on the one hand, as well as an inhibition of the AT2 receptor-dependent anti-proliferative effects of ANG II, on the other hand. Therefore, growth and anti-growth mechanism may have compensated each other under these conditions leaving as a net effect the bradykinin-mediated angiogenic action of the ACE inhibitor (Figure 2).

Angiogenesis is normally not an isolated event. In the process of angiogenesis, several potential growth-regulating factors have been identified including growth factors, extracellular matrix, cell-cell interactions and mechanical forces. Although physical forces such as changes of intravascular pressure have been postulated as transduction signals for mitosis of vascular endothelial cells[80], recent observations favor a more important role of biochemical transmitters. In addition, vasoactive metabolites produced in hypoxic tissues, e.g. ATP- and NAD breakdown products, have been implicated in the vascular growth process[81]. Peptide growth factors have been intensively studied in recent years, and different peptide mitogens such as fibroblast growth factor (FGF), platelet derived growth factor (PDGF) and transforming growth factor b1 (TGF b1) have been purified from heart tissue[82–84]. Adair et al.[85] incorporated these findings into a hypothesis on growth regulation in the vascular system proposing that changes in the metabolic requirements of the heart could trigger a cascade comprising all of the above mentioned parameters to finally induce capillary proliferation.

There are several pieces of evidence supporting the idea that bradykinin could induce processes leading to neovascularization. Bradykinin can be involved in the angiogenic process either directly or indirectly, e.g. by increasing coronary flow or by alteration of myocardial metabolism[86]. A direct angiogenic action of bradykinin has been suggested in a study in cultured endothelial cells isolated from coronary venules. In this study, bradykinin (10^{-11}–10^{-7} mol/l) dose-dependently increased DNA synthesis as evaluated by [3H] thymidine incorporation[87].

The common denominator of all experimental conditions associated with myocardial capillary proliferation appears to be an enhancement of myocardial capillary blood flow[66]. Therefore, bradykinin may also exert an indirect stimulus for capillary growth by a long-term increase in coronary flow and thus, by increasing the shear stress-induced release of growth factors involved in the angiogenic process[85]. Bradykinin has been shown to improve myocardial blood flow under different experimental conditions even at very low concentrations[9,88]. In a recent study, we demonstrated that low dose ramipril treatment caused an increase in coronary flow and an increase in cardiac contractility independent of its antihypertensive and antihypertrophic action[20] (Figure 3c). In addition, ACE inhibitor treatment caused a marked alteration in cardiac metabolism as demonstrated by decreased tissue levels of lactate and increased levels of glycogen and the energy-rich phosphates ATP and creatine phosphate. In both cases, the effects of the ACE inhibitor were sensitive to bradykinin B2 receptor blockade by icatibant (Figure 3c).

The beneficial effects of bradykinin on cardiac function and metabolism are in accord with the above cited concept of the growth regulation in the vascular system[66]. Assuming that this hypothesis on capillary growth induction is correct, bradykinin could provide two prerequisites for the induction of angiogenesis by improving myocardial blood flow and myocardial metabolism. The potentiation of bradykinin by ACE inhibition could thus trigger a cascade leading to myocardial capillary proliferation.

4. CONCLUSION

There is abundant evidence from animal studies that kinins participate in the cardio-vascular effects of ACE inhibitors under different pathophysiological conditions. For example, some renin-dependent models of hypertension kinin potentiation contributes to the antihypertensive and antihypertrophic actions of ACE inhibitors. However, in genetic hypertension, ANG II reduction appears to be the predominant mechanism of the antihypertensive and antihypertrophic effect of chronic ACE inhibitor treatment. The involvement of kinins in the cardioprotective effects of ACE inhibitors after myocardial infarction appears to be dependent on the time point when treatment is started. Pretreatment or treatment during the acute incident of myocardial infarction with ACE inhibitors appears to limit infarct size rather by potentiation of kinins than by reduction of ANG II. A kinin-induced increase in blood flow to the marginal zone of the ischemic area has been implicated in this respect. It is still controversely discussed, whether inhibition of ANG II generation or blockade of AT_1 receptors, respectively, or the accumulation of kinins is more important for cardioprotection once congestive heat failure has developed after myocardial infarction. Rarefication of myocardial capillaries contributes to cardiac failure and the overall risk of LVH. ACE inhibition can induce myocardial capillary growth by a kinin-dependent mechanism, irresepective of a reduction in blood pressure or LVH. Whether kinins engender capillary growth by a direct effect or indirectly by improving cardiac perfusion and metabolism is still under investigation. Clinical studies will have to show whether or not the compelling evidence in various animal models for cardio- and vasculoprotective actions of kinins under ACE inhibition holds true in human cardiovascular disease.

REFERENCES

1. Bhoola KD, Figuero CD, Worthy K: Bioregulation of kinins: kallikreins, kininogens, and kininases. *Pharmacol Rev* 1992;44 (1):1–80
2. Linz W, Wiemer G, Gohlke P, Unger T, Schölkens BA: Contribution of kinins to the cardiovascular actions of angiotensin-converting enzyme inhibitors. *Pharmacol Rev* 1995;47:25–49
3. Margolius HS: Kallikreins and kinins. Molecular characteristics and cellular and tissue responses. *Diabetes* 1996;45 (Suppl. 1):S14–S19
4. Scicli AG, Mindrooiu T, Scicli G, Carretero OA: Blood kinins their concentrations in normal subjects and in patients with congenital deficiency in plasma prekallikrein and kininogen. *J Lab Clin* 1982;100:81–93

5. Shimamoto K, Ando T, Tanaka S, Nakahashi Y, Nishitani T, Hosoda S, Ishida H, Iimura O: An improved method for the determination of human blood kinin levels by sensitive kinin radioimmunoassay. *Endocrinol Jpn* 1982;29:487–494

6. Ryan JW, Robelero J, Stewart JM: Inactivation of bradykinin in the pulmonary circulation. *Biochem J* 1986;110:795–797

7. Farhy RD, Carretero OA, Ho K-L, Scicli AG: Role of kinins and nitric oxide in the effects of angiotensin converting enzyme inhibitors on neointima formation. *Circ Res* 1993;72:1202–1210

8. Becker RHA, Wiemer G, Linz W: Preservation of endothelial function by ramipril in rabbits on a long-term atherogenic diet. *J Cardiovasc Pharmacol* 1991;18 (suppl. 2):S110–S115

9. Schölkens BA, Linz W, König W: Effects of the angiotensin converting enzyme inhibitor, ramipril, in isolated ischaemic rat heart are abolished by a bradykinin antagonist. *J Hypertens* 1988;(suppl. 4):S25–S28

10. Daniell HB, Carson RR, Ballard KD, Thomas GR, Privitera PJ: Effects of captopril on limiting infarct size in conscious dogs. *J Cardiovasc Pharmacol* 1984;6:1043–1047

11. Ertl G: Angiotensin converting enzyme inhibitors and ischemic heart disease. *Eur Heart J* 1988;9:716–727

12. Kass RW, Kotler MN, Yazdanfar S: Stimulation of coronary collateral growth: current developments in angiogenesis and future clinical applications. *Am Heart J* 1992;123(2):486–496

13. Lefer AM, Peck RC: Cardioprotective effects of enalapril in acute myocardial ischemia. *Pharmacol* 1984; 29:61–69

14. Hock CE, Ribeiro GT, Lefer AM: Preservation of ischemic myocardium by a new converting enzyme inhibitor, enalaprilic acid, in acute myocardial infarction. *Am Heart J* 1985;109:222–228

15. Stauss HM, Zhu YC, Redlich T, Unger T: Early and late treatment of infarction-induced heart failure with a converting enzyme inhibitor: Bradykinin potentiation versus angiotensin II reduction. *Hypertension* 1993;22(3):429(abstract)

16. Stauss HM, Zhu YC, Redlich T, Adamiak D, Mott A, Kregel KC, Unger T: ACE inhibition in infarct-induced heart failure. bradykinin versus angiotensin II. *J Cardiovasc Risk* 1994;1:255–262

17. Stauss HM, Zhu YC, Redlich T, Adamiak D, Moot A, Unger T: Mechanism involved in the reduction of infarct size by ACE inhibition after left coronary ligation in rats. *J Hypertens* 1994;12 (suppl 13):S2 (abstract)

18. Duncan AM, Burell LM, Kladis A, Campbell DJ: Effects of angiotensin-converting enzyme inhibition on angiotensin and bradykinin peptides in rats with myocardial infarction. *J Cardiovasc Phamacol* 1996; 28:746–754

19. Linz W, Schölkens BA: A specific B2-bradykinin receptor antagonist HOE 140 abolishes the antihypertrophic effect of ramipril. *Br J Pharmacol* 1992;105:771–772

20. Gohlke P, Linz W, Schölkens BA, Kuwer I, Bartenbach S, Schnell A, Unger T: Angiotensin converting enzyme inhibition improves cardiac function: role of bradykinin. *Hypertension* 1994;23:411–418

21. Unger T, Mattfeldt T, Lamberty V, Bock P, Mall G, Linz W, Schölkens BA, Gohlke P: Effect of early onset angiotensin converting enzyme inhibition on myocardial capillaries. *Hypertension* 1992;20:478–482

22. Gohlke P, Kuwer I, Schnell A, Amann K, Mall G, Unger T: Bradykinin B2-receptor blockade prevents the increase in capillary growth density induced by chronic ACE inhibitor treatment in SHRSP. *Hypertension* 1997;29:478–482

23. Nolly H, Carbini LA, Scicli G, Carretero OA, Scicli AG: A local kallikrein-kinin system is present in rat hearts. *Hypertension* 1994;23 (2):919–923

24. Campbell DJ, Kladis A, Duncan A-M: Bradykinin peptides in kidney, blood, and other tissues of the rat. *Hypertension* 1993;21:155–165

25. Maeceau F: Kinin B1 receptors: a review. *Immunopharmacol* 1995;30(1):1–26

26. Vavrek RJ, Stewart JM: Competitive antagonists of bradykinin. *Peptides* 1985;6:161–164

27. Bao G, Qadri F, Stauss B, Stauss H, Gohlke P, Unger T: HOE 140, a new highly potent and long-acting bradykinin antagonist in conscious rats. *Eur J Pharmacol* 1992;200:179–182

28. Hock FJ, Wirth K, Linz W, Gerhards HJ, Wiemer G, Henke ST, Breipohl G, König W, Knolle J, Schölkens BA: Hoe 140 a new potent and long acting bradykinin-antagonist: In vitro studies. *Br J Pharmacol* 1991; 102:769–773

29. Wirth K, Hock FJ, Albus U, Linz W, Alpermann HG, Anagnostopoulos H, Henke St, Breipohl G, König W, Knolle J, Schölkens BA: Hoe 140 a new potent and long acting bradykinin-antagonist: in vivo studies. *Br J Pharmacol* 1991;102:774–777

30. Gohlke P, Lamberty V, Kuwer I, Bartenbach S, Schnell A, Linz W, Schölkens BA, Wiemer G, Unger T: Long-term low-dose angiotensin converting enzyme inhibitor treatment increases vascular cyclic guanosine 3′,5′-monophosphate. *Hypertension* 1993;22:682–687

31. Bao G, Gohlke P, Qadri F, Unger T: Chronic kinin receptor blockade attenuates the antihypertensive effect of ramipril. *Hypertension* 1992;20:74–79

32. Fabris B, Jackson B, Kanazawa M, Johnston CI: Increased cardiac ACE in rats with chronic heart failure. *Clin Exp Pharmacol Physiol* 1990;17:309–314

33. Schunkert H, Dzau VJ, Tang SS, Hirsch AT, Apstein AT, Apstein CS, Lorell BH: Increased rat cardiac angiotensin converting enzyme activity and mRNA expression in pressure overload left ventricular hypertrophy. *J Clin Invest* 1990;86:1913–1920

34. Falkenhahn M, Franke F, Bohle RM, Zhu Y, Stauss HM, Bachmann S, Danilov S, Unger T: Cellular distribution of angiotensin-converting enzyme after myocardial infarction. *Hypertension* 1995;25:219–226

35. Liang CS, Gavras H, Black J, Sherman LG, Hood WB: Renin-angiotensin system inhibition in acute myocardial infarction in dogs: effects on systemic hemodynamics, myocardial blood flow, segmental myocardial function and infarct size. *Circulation* 1982;66:1249–1255

36. Brown EJ, Swinfor RD, Shatkin BJ, Honig SC, Cohn PF: Massive reperfusion injury: paradoxical effect of combined angiotensin-converting enzyme inhibition plus myocardial perfusion. *J Am Coll Cardiol* 1988; 11:50A

37. De Lorgeril M, Ovize M, Delaye G, Renaud S: Importance of the flow perfusion deficit in the response to captopril in experimental myocardial infarction. *J Cardiovasc Pharmacol* 1992;19:324–325

38. The Acute Infarction Ramipril Efficacy (AIRE) Study Investigators: Effect of ramipril on mortality and morbidity of survivors of acute myocardial infarction with clinical evidence of heart failure. *Lancet* 1993;342:821–828

39. Trandopril Cardiac Evaluation (TRACE) Study group: A clinical trial of the angiotensin-converting-enzyme inhibitor trandolapril in patients with left ventricular dysfunction after myocardial infarction. *N Engl Med* 1995;333 (25):1670–1676

40. Hashimoto K, Hirose M, Furukawa S, Hayakawa H, Kimura E: Changes in hemodynamics and bradykinin concentration in coronary sinus blood in experimental coronary occlusion. *Jpn Heart J* 1977;18:679–689

41. Baumgarten CR, Linz W, Kunkel G, Schölkens BA, Wiemer G: Ramiprilat increases bradykinin outflow from isolated rat hearts. *Br J Pharmacol* 1993;108:293–295

42. Lamontagne D, Nadeau R, Adam A: Effect of enalaprilat on bradykinin and des-Arg^9-bradykinin release following reperfusion of the ischaemic rat heart. *Br J Pharmacol* 1995;115:476–478

43. Lamontagne D, Nakhostine N, Couture R, Nadeau R: Mechanism of kinin B$_1$-receptor-induced hypotension in the anesthetized dog. *J Cardiovasc Pharmacol* 1996;28:645–650

44. Rosas R, Montague D, Gross M, Bohr DF: Cardiac action of vasoactive polypeptides in the rat. *Circ Res* 1965;16:150–161

45. Groves P, Kurz S, Just H, Drexler H: Role of endogenous bradykinin in human coronary vasomotor control. *Circulation* 1995;92:3424–3430

46. Linz W, Schölkens BA, Han YF: Beneficial effects of the converting enzyme inhibitor, ramipril, in ischemic rat hearts. *J Cardiovasc Pharmacol* 1986;8 (suppl. 10):S91–S99

47. Van Gilst WH, De Graeff PA, Leeuw MJ, Scholtens E, Wesseling H: Converting enzyme inhibitors and the role of their sulfhydryl group in the potentiation of exo- and endogenous nitrovasodialtors. *J Cardiovasc Pharmacol* 1991;18:429–436

48. Ertl G, Kloner RA, Alexander RW, Braunwald E: Limitation of experimental infarct size by an angiotensin-converting enzyme inhibitor. *Circulation* 1982;65:40–48

49. Przyklenk K, Kloner RA: Cardioprotection by ACE-inhibitors in acute myocardial ischemia and infarction?. *Basic Res Cardiol* 1993;88 (Suppl 1):139–154

50. Smits JFM, van Krimpen C, Schoemaker RG, Cleutjens JPM, Daemen MJAP: Angiotensin II receptor blockade after myocardial infarction in rats: effects on hemodynamics, myocardial DNA synthesis, and interstitial collagen content. *J Cardiovasc Pharmacol* 1992;20:772–778

51. Raya TE, Fonken SJ, Lee RW, Daugherty S, Goldman S, Wong PC, Timmermans PB, Morkin E: Hemodynamic effects of direct angiotensin II blockade compared to converting enzyme inhibition in rat model for heart failure. *Am J Hypertens* 1991;4:334S–340S

52. Spitznagel H, Stauss HM, Gohlke P, Zhu YZ, Falkenhahn M, Unger T: Angiotensin II and bradykinin in hypertensive heart disease and myocardial infarction. *High Blood Press* 1996;5:119–123

53. Zhu YC, Stauss HM, Bao G, Gohlke P, Zhu YZ, Redlich T, Unger T: Role of bradykinin in the antihypertensive and cardioprotective actions of converting enzyme inhibitors. *Can J Physiol Pharmacol* 1995;73:827–831

54. Geisterfer AAT, Peach MJ, Owens GK: Angiotensin II induces hypertrophy, not hyperplasia, of cultured rat aortic smooth muscle cells. *Circ Res* 1988;62:749–756

55. Paquet J-L, Baudouin-Legros M, Brunelle G, Meyer P: Angiotensin II-induced proliferation of aortic myocytes in spontaneously hypertensive rats. *J Hypertens* 1990;8:565–572

56. Schelling P, Ganten D, Speck G, Fischer H: Effects of angiotensin II and angiotensin II antagonist saralasin on cell growth and renin in 3T3 and SV3T3 cells. *J Cell Physiol* 1979;98:503–514

57. Stoll M, Steckelings UM, Paul M, Bottari SP, Metzger R, Unger T: The angiotensin AT2-receptor mediates inhibition of cell proliferation in coronary endothelial cells. *J Clin Invest* 1995;95:651–657
58. Freeman GL, Little WC, Haywood JR: Reduction of left ventricular mass in normal rats by captopril. *Cardiovasc Res* 1987;21:323–327
59. Nakashima Y, Fouad FM, Tarazi RC: Regression of left ventricular hypertrophy from systemic hypertension by enalapril. *Am J Cardiol* 1984;53:1044–1049
60. Dahlöf B, Pennert K, Hansson L: Reversal of left ventricular hypertrophy in hypertensive patients. *Am J Hypertens* 1992;5:95–110
61. Lievre M, Guéret P, Gayet C, Roudaut R, Haugh MC, Delair S, Boissel J-P, on behalb of the HYCAR Study Group: Ramipril-induced regression of left ventricular hypertrophy in treated hypertensive individuals. *Hypertension* 1995;25:92–97(abstract)
62. Fernandez PG, Snedden W, Idikio H, Fernandez D, Kin BK, Triggle CR: The reversal of left ventricular hypertrophy with control of blood pressure in experimental hypertension. *Scand J Clin Lab Invest* 1984;44:711–716
63. Clozel J-P, Hefti F: Cilazapril prevents the development of cardiac hypertrophy and the decrease of coronary vascular reserve in spontaneously hypertensive rats. *J Cardiovasc Pharmacol* 1988;11:568–572
64. Linz W, Schölkens BA, Ganten D: Converting enzyme inhibition specifically prevents the development and induces regression of cardiac hypertrophy in rats. *Clin Exper Hypertens* 1989;A11(7):1325–1350
65. Rhaleb N-E, Yang X-P, Scicli AG, Carretero OA: Role of kinins and nitric oxide in the antihypertrophic effect of ramipril. *Hypertension* 1994;23 (part 2):865–868
66. Mall G, Zimmer G, Baden S, Mattfeldt T: Capillary neoformation in the rat heart — Stereological studies on papillary muscles in hypertrophy and physiologic growth. *Basic Res Cardiol* 1990;85:531–540
67. Mattfeldt T, Mall G: Growth of capillaries and myocardial cells in the normal rat heart. *J Mol Cell Cardiol* 1987;19:1237–1246
68. Clozel J-P, Kuhn H, Hefti F: Effects of chronic ACE inhibition on cardiac hypertrophy and coronary vascular reserve in spontaneously hypertensive rats with developed hypertension. *J Hypertens* 1989;7:267–275
69. Olivetti G, Cigola E, Lagrasta C, Ricci R, Quaini F, Monopoli A, Ongini E: Spirapril prevents left ventricular hypertrophy, decreases myocardial damage and promotes angiogenesis in spontaneously hypertensive rats. *J Cardiovasc Pharmacol* 1993;21:362–370
70. Gohlke P, Stoll M, Lamberty V, Mattfeldt T, Mall G, Von Even P, Martorana PA, Unger T: Cardiac and vascular effects of chronic angiotensin converting enzyme inhibition at subantihypertensive doses. *J Hypertens* 1992;10 (suppl. 6):S141–S144
71. Linz W, Wiemer G, Becker RHA, Schölkens BA: Long-term treatment with the ACE-inhibitor ramipril prolongs survival in stroke-prone rats: Interim analysis. *J Hypertens* 1996;14 (suppl. 1):S232 (P1055)
72. Wiemer G, Schölkens BA, Busse R, Wagner A, Heitsch H, Linz W: The functional role of angiotensin II — subtype AT2 — receptors in endothelial cells and isolated ischemic rat hearts. *Pharm Pharmacol Lett* 1993;3:24–27
73. Seyedi N, Xu XB, Nasjiletti A, Hintze TH: Coronary kinin generation mediates nitric oxide release after angiotensin receptor stimulation. *Hypertension* 1995;26:164–170
74. Gohlke P, Linz W, Schölkens BA, Wiemer G, Unger T: Cardiac and vascular effects of long-term losartan treatment in stroke-prone spontaneously hypertensive rats. *Hypertension* 1996;28:397–402
75. Timmermans PBMWM, Wong PC, Chiu AT, Herblin WF, Benfield P, Carini DJ, Lee RJ, Wexler RR, Saye JA, Smith RD: Angiotensin II receptors and angiotensin II receptor antagonists. *Pharmacol Rev* 1993;45:205–251
76. Campbell DJ, Kladis A, Valentijn AJ: Effects of losartan on angiotensin and bradykinin peptides and angiotensin-converting enzyme. *J Cardiovasc Pharmacol* 1995;26:233–240
77. Metsärinne KP, Stoll M, Gohlke P, Paul M, Unger T: Angiotensin II is antiproliferative for coronary endothelial cells in vitro. *Pharm Pharmacol Lett* 1992;2:150–152
78. Nakajima M, Hutchinson HG, Fujinaga M, Hayashida W, Morishita R, Zhang L, Horiuchi M, Pratt RE, Dzau VJ: The angiotensin II type 2 (AT$_2$) receptor antagonizes the growth effects of the AT$_1$ receptor: gain-of-function study using gene transfer. *Proc Natl Acad Sci* 1995;92:10663–10667
79. Munzenmaier DH, Greene AS: Opposing actions of angiotensin II on microvascular growth and arterial blood pressure. *Hypertension* 1996;27 (3):760–765
80. Schaper W, De Brabander M, Lewi P: DNA synthesis and mitosis in coronary collateral vessels of the dog. *Circ Res* 1971;28:671–679
81. Meiniger C, Granger H: Mechanisms leading to adenosine-stimulated proliferation of microvascular endothelial cells. *Am J Physiol* 1990;258:H198–H206
82. Quinkler W, Maasberg M, Bernotat-Danielowski S, Lüthe N, Sharma H.S., Schaper W: Isolation of heparin-binding growth factors from bovine, porcine and canine hearts. *Eur J Biochem* 1989;1989:67–73

83. Roberts AB, Sporn MB, Assoian RK, Smith JM, Roche NS, Wakefield L, Heine V, Liotta L, Falanga V, Kehr JH, Fauci AS: Transforming growth factor type-beta: rapid induction of fibrosis and angiogenesis in vivo and stimulation of collagen formation in vitro. *Proc Natl Acad Sci USA* 1986;83:4167–4171

84. Casscells W, Speir E, Sasse J, Klagsbrun M, Allen P, Lee M, Calvo B, Chiba M, Haggroth L, Folkman J, Epstein S: Isolation, characterization, and localization of heparin-binding growth factors in the heart. *J Clin Invest* 1990;85:433–441

85. Adair TH, Gay WJ, Montani J-P: Growth regulation of the vascular system: evidence for a metabolic hypothesis. *Am J Physiol* 1990;259:R393–R404

86. Tschöpe C, Stoll M, Gohlke P, Unger T: Potential effects of bradykinin on myocardial capillary growth after angiotensin converting enzyme inhibition. *Exp Opin Invest Drugs* 1994;3:501–510

87. Morbidelli L, Parenti A, Granger HJ, Ziche M, Ledda F: Activation of DNA synthesis and inositol-phosphate turnover in coronary venular endothelial cells exposed to bradykinin. *Pharmacol Res* 1992;25 (Suppl. 2): 150–151

88. Linz W, Martorana PA, Schölkens BA: Local inhibition of bradykinin degradation in ischemic hearts. *J Cardiovasc Pharmacol* 1990;15 (suppl. 6):S99–S109

18

LEFT VENTRICULAR HYPERTROPHY AND SYMPATHETIC ACTIVITY

Guido Grassi,[1,2*] Gino Seravalle,[2,3] and Giuseppe Mancia[1,2,3]

[1]Cattedra di Medicina Interna I
Ospedale S.Gerardo
Monza, Italy
[2]Università di Milano
Centro di Fisiologia Clinica e Ipertensione
Ospedale Maggiore, IRCCS
Milano, Italy
[3]Centro Auxologico Italiano, IRCCS
Milano, Italy

1. INTRODUCTION

Pressure and/or volume overload has been regarded in the past as the leading mechanism through which an increase in blood pressure may trigger the development of left ventricular hypertrophy[1]. However, studies performed in recent years both in experimental animals and in man have suggested that not only mechanical but also sympathetic, genetic and hormonal factors (e.g. angiotensin II, insulin, thyroid hormones, etc) may significantly contribute to the development of the cardiac structural alterations frequently detected in the clinical course of the hypertensive state[2,3].

In this paper the complex interactions between sympathetic neural factors and hypertensive left ventricular hypertrophy will be critically reviewed, taking into account three major issues. One, the evidence that sympathetic activation is a common hallmark of essential hypertensive states, even in their earlier clinical stages. Two, the functional relationships between the sympathetic overactivity and the hypertensive left ventricular hypertrophy. Finally, a third issue will be examined, i.e. the possibility that a pathological increase in cardiac wall thickness represents a factor capable to trigger an increase in sympathetic cardiovascular drive.

* Correspondence: Dr. Guido Grassi, Centro di Fisiologia Clinica e Ipertensione, Policlinico, Via Sforza 35, 20122 Milano, Italy. Fax: +39 2 5457666, Phone: +39 2 55184606.

Hypertension and the Heart, edited by Zanchetti et al.
Plenum Press, New York, 1997

2. SYMPATHETIC ACTIVATION IN HYPERTENSION

Biochemical assessment of plasma levels of norepinephrine, i.e. the adrenergic neurotransmitter directly secreted from sympathetic nerve endings into the bloodstream, represents the approach most widely used to evaluate sympathetic function in man. The method, however, encompasses a number of biological and technical limitations, which weaken its ability to faithfully reflect changes in sympathetic neural discharge in physiological and/or pathological conditions[4,5]. This may represent one of the reasons responsible for the discrepancy of the results reported in the published studies, aimed at evaluating by this approach sympathetic activity in normotensive and essential hypertensive subjects. However, when data collected in various studies were pooled together, an increase in plasma concentration of norepinephrine was evident in the hypertensive group as compared to the normotensive one[6]. This result has been recently confirmed by studies employing the norepinephrine radiolabeled technique to directly quantify, via intravenous infusion of tritiated norepinephrine, the amount of the neurotransmitter spilling over from the neuroeffector junctions and entering the circulation[7].

By employing this interesting approach it has been shown that essential hypertensive patients, particularly at young age, display an increased norepinephrine release as compared to age-matched normotensive individuals[8]. To this increase contributes to a large extent sympathetic drive in the heart and the kidney[8], i.e. two organs of fundamental importance in blood pressure and blood volume homeostatic control. In addition recent findings, obtained through the same approach, indicate that hypertensive patients display an increased norepinephrine release also at the level of the cerebral circulation[9]. It can thus be concluded that sympathetic activation characterizing essential hypertension is not peculiar of a single cardiovascular district but widespread to the whole circulation.

Further information on the sympathetic abnormalities occurring in essential hypertension can be derived from the results of electrophysiological studies employing the microneurographic technique to assess efferent postganglionic muscle sympathetic nerve traffic in a peroneal or brachial nerve[10]. The technique, which is at present the only method available in humans which allows sympathetic activity to be directly quantified, has been shown to provide a sensitive and reproducible evaluation of neural adrenergic influences in physiological and pathological conditions[11]. By this approach it has been

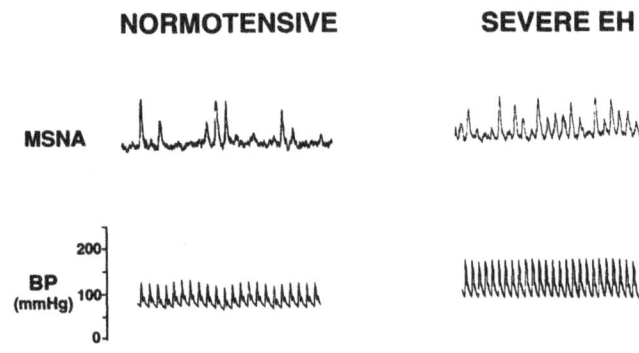

Figure 1. Original recordings of muscle sympathetic nerve traffic (MSNA) and beat-to-beat arterial blood pressure (BP) in a normotensive subject (left panels) and in a patient with severe essential hypertension (EH, right panels). Note that the blood pressure increase observed in hypertension is paralleled by an increased MSNA burst frequency.

shown that an increase in the number of sympathetic bursts (and therefore a sympathetic activation) can be detected in normotensive subjects with a family history of hypertension and in borderline essential hypertensives[12,13]. In addition our group has recently provided evidence[14,15] that 1) severe hypertension displays a further sympathetic nerve traffic increase as compared to mild hypertension (Figure 1), 2) the degree of sympathetic activation characterizing the hypertensive condition parallels the concomitant blood pressure increase and 3) hypertensive states of secondary nature are not characterized by an increased central sympathetic outflow. Taken together these findings support the concept that sympathetic factors play an important role both in the development and in the progression of the essential hypertensive state.

3. SYMPATHETIC ACTIVATION AND LEFT VENTRICULAR HYPERTROPHY

The hypothesis that sympathetic influences may exert cardiotrophic effects and thus favour the development of myocardial hypertrophy has been advanced on the basis of the results provided by animal studies. These experimental evidences can be summarized as follows. First, as shown in Table 1, in almost all experimental models of cardiac hypertrophy, the increase in left and/or right ventricular wall thickness was paralleled by an increase in cardiac sympathetic drive[16,17]. Second, studies performed in dogs have provided evidence that chronic infusion of norepinephrine in the systemic circulation, even when devoid of any pressor effect, was capable to increase left ventricular weight, myocyte cross-sectional area and nucleic acid synthesis from the myocardial tissue[18,19] (Figure 2). Finally, it has been reported that in spontaneously hypertensive rats only antihypertensive drugs which effectively inhibit adrenergic cardiovascular drive are capable to reduce the elevated values of ventricular weight displayed by these animals[20,21]. Taken together these findings appear to support the concept that sympathetic influences play a key role in the pathophysiological process leading to cardiac hypertrophy.

The evidence in favour of a cause-effect relationship between adrenergic factors and cardiac hypertrophy is more controversial in humans. This because 1) plasma and urinary catecholamine levels are not invariably reported to be increased in hypertensive patients

Table 1. Behaviour of cardiac sympathetic activity in experimental conditions leading to adaptive cardiac hypertrophy

Conditions	Cardiac sympathetic activity
Generalized cardiac hypertrophy	
•Physical exercise	Increased
•Cold acclimation	Increased
•Isoprenaline administration	Increased
•Hyperthyroidism	Unchanged
Left ventricular hypertrophy	
•Aortic coarctation	Increased
•Renal hypertension	Increased
•Deoxycorticosterone hypertension	Increased
•Genetic spontaneous hypertension	Unchanged
Right ventricular hypertrophy	
•Hypoxia	Increased
•Experimental pulmonary hypertension	Increased

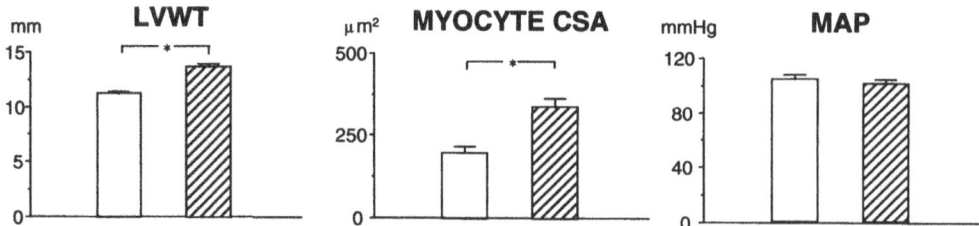

Figure 2. Effects of infusion of subpressor doses of norepinephrine on left ventricular wall thickness (LVWT), myocyte cross-sectional area (myocyte CSA) and mean arterial pressure (MAP) in adult mongrel dogs. Data are shown as means ± SEM. Open histograms: baseline values, hatched histograms: values obtained following a 4 week infusion of norepinephrine. *p<0.05 from baseline values. Modified from reference 19, with permission from the American Heart Association.

with left ventricular hypertrophy[3,22], 2) no relationship has been found between left ventricular mass and cardiac norepinephrine release in essential hypertensives with cardiac hypertrophy[23] and 3) in studies from our own laboratory no significant correlation was found between sympathetic nerve traffic in the muscle circulation and left ventricular mass index in a group of essential hypertensive patients[15]. Whether these negative results depend on a real absence of a cause-effect relationship between sympathetic activity and cardiac hypertrophy or on the limitations in assessing systemic and regional sympathetic cardiovascular drive remains to be clarified.

4. LEFT VENTRICULAR HYPERTROPHY AS A SOURCE OF SYMPATHETIC ACTIVATION

Animal studies have shown that reflex influences stemming from vagally innervated volume sensitive receptors, anatomically located at the level of the cardiac chambers, the lungs and the pulmonary arteries (the so-called "cardiopulmonary receptors"), exert in physiological conditions a tonic restraint on efferent sympathetic outflow to the peripheral circulation, modulating also renin release from the kidney and vasopressin secretion from the hypothalamus[24]. Evidences collected by our group and others[25–29] have shown that this is the case also in man, with the only difference that in the human species cardiac receptors predominate over receptors located in the lungs, because both vascular and neurohumoral reflex responses to cardiopulmonary receptor deactivation and stimulation are markedly blunted in heart transplant recipients, i.e. subjects with a denervated heart.

The effects of hypertension and hypertension-related left ventricular hypertrophy on the cardiopulmonary receptor reflex have been extensively investigated in man. In one of these studies[30], we examined the changes in forearm vascular resistance, plasma norepinephrine and plasma renin activity induced by manoevers capable to alter central venous pressure (i.e. the stimulus determining cardiopulmonary receptor activity[31]) in 3 groups of age-matched subjects, one normotensive and two hypertensive, respectively without and with echocardiographic evidence of left ventricular hypertrophy. In all subjects cardiopulmonary receptor reflex was studied by 1) lower body negative pressure application which, by reducing central venous pressure, deactivated cardiopulmonary receptors and 2) passive leg raising manoeuver which, by increasing central venous pressure, stimulated cardiopulmonary receptors. As shown in Figure 3, similar changes in central venous pressure caused comparable reflex

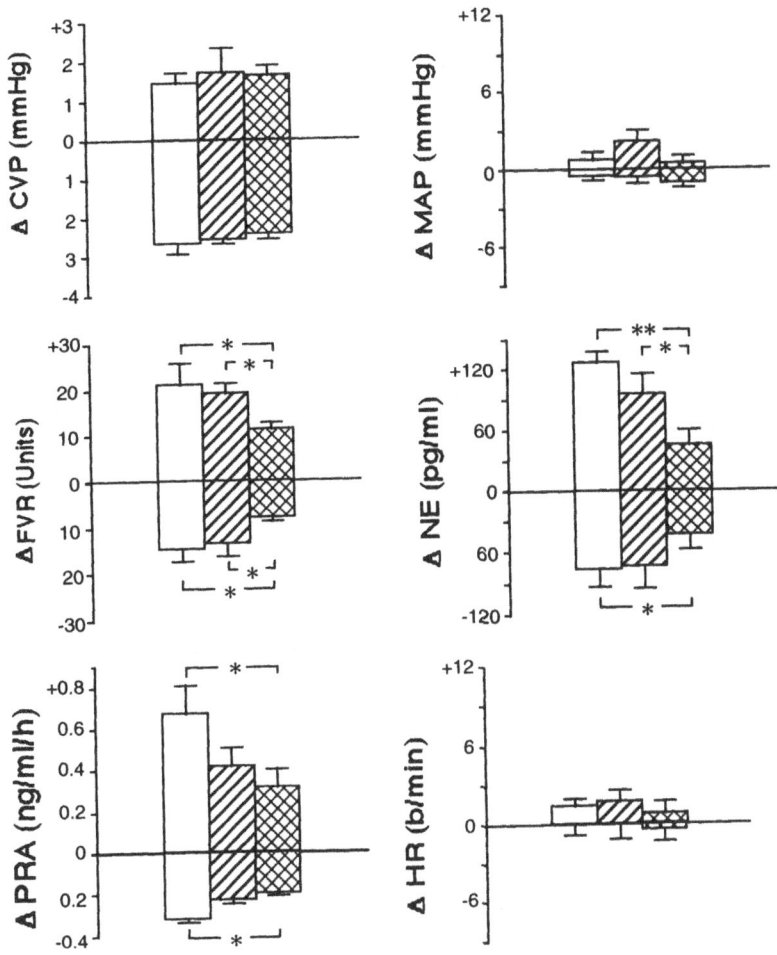

Figure 3. Changes in central venous pressure (ΔCVP), mean arterial pressure (ΔMAP), heart rate (ΔHR), forearm vascular resistance (ΔFVR), plasma norepinephrine (ΔNE) and plasma renin activity (ΔPRA) induced by lower body negative pressure and passive leg raising in normotensive subjects (n=10, open histograms), essential hypertensive patients without (n=10, hatched histograms) and with echocardiographically detected left ventricular hypertrophy (n=10, cross hatched histograms). *p<0.05, **p<0.01 between groups. Data are shown as means ± SEM. Modified from reference 30 with permission from the American Heart Association.

responses in normotensive and hypertensive subjects without cardiac structural alterations. In hypertensives with left ventricular hypertrophy, however, the reflex changes in forearm vascular resistance, plasma norepinephrine and plasma renin activity were all markedly blunted. These data, although in favour of the importance of structural alterations of the heart in determining the cardiopulmonary reflex impairment described in hypertensive patients with cardiac organ damage, did not allow, however, to establish whether high blood pressure "per se" or cardiac hypertrophy "per se" was the major factor responsible for this reflex abnormality. Two experimental evidences collected by our group in subsequent studies are in favour of the last possibility, because 1) an impairment of the cardiopulmonary receptor reflex has been described also in normotensive professional athletes, in which an intense and prolonged

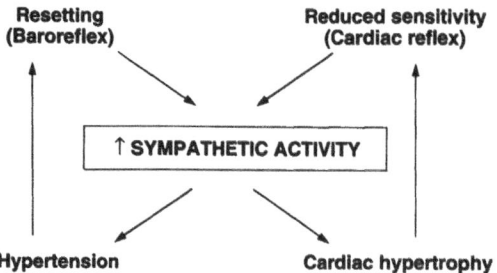

Figure 4. Schematic drawing of the interrelationships between sympathetic activation, left ventricular hypertrophy, essential hypertension and alterations in reflex cardiovascular control occurring in the hypertensive state.

physical training program favoured the development of cardiac hypertrophy[32] and 2) regression of cardiac hypertrophy by long-term antihypertensive treatment or by long-term physical deconditioning has been shown to fully restore the cardiopulmonary reflex function in hypertensive patients and in normotensive athletes respectively[30,33].

Taken together these findings suggest that cardiac hypertrophy, by reducing the inhibitory influences physiologically exerted by cardiopulmonary receptors on sympathetic drive, may represent, together with the resetting of the arterial baroreceptors (i.e. the other major reflexogenic area involved in homeostatic cardiovascular control[34]), a factor which favours the progression of the sympathetic activation characterizing the early hypertensive stages. This activation may in turn promote a further blood pressure rise, thereby establishing a vicious circle further aggravating the hypertensive state (Figure 4).

REFERENCES

1. G.Evans. A contribution to the study of arteriosclerosis, with special reference to its relation to chronic disease. Q.J.Med. 1921;14:215–282.
2. E.D.Frohlich and R.C.Tarazi. Is arterial pressure the sole factor responsible for hypertensive cardiac hypertrophy? Am J Cardiol. 1979;44:959–963.
3. R.B.Devereux and M.J.Roman. Cardiac structure and function in hypertension. In A.Zanchetti, G.Mancia (eds) Handbook of Hypertension: vol.17 Pathophysiology of Hypertension. Elsevier Science, Amsterdam 1997:58–116.
4. G.Mancia, A.Ferrari, L.Gregorini, G.Leonetti, G.Parati, G.B.Picotti, C.Ravazzani and A.Zanchetti. Plasma catecholamines do not invariably reflect sympathetically induced changes in blood pressure in man. Clin Sci 1983;65:227–235.
5. G.Mancia, G.Grassi, G.Parati and A.Daffonchio. Evaluating sympathetic activity in human hypertension. J Hypertens 1993;11 (suppl 5):S13–S19.
6. D.S.Goldstein. Plasma catecholamines and essential hypertension: an analytical review. Hypertension 1983;5:86–99.
7. M.Esler, G.Jackman, A.Bobik, D.Kelleker, G.Jennings, P.Leonard, H.Skews and P.Korner. Determination of norepinephrine apparent release rate and clearance in humans. Life Sci 1979;25:1461–1470.
8. M.Esler, G Lambert and G.Jennings. Regional norepinephrine turnover in human hypertension. Clin Exper Hypertens 1989;11 (suppl 1):75–89.
9. C.Ferrier, M.Esler, G.Eisenhofer, B.G.Wallin, M.Horne, H.Cox, G.Lambert and G.Jennings. Increased norepinephrine spillover into the cerebrovascular circulation in essential hypertension: Evidence of high central nervous system norepinephrine turnover? Hypertension 1992;19:62–69.
10. A.B.Vallbo, K.E.Hagbarth, H.E.Torebjork and B.G.Wallin. Somatosensory, proprioceptive and sympathetic activity from peripheral nerves. Physiol Rev 1979;59:919–957.
11. G.Grassi, G.B.Bolla, G.Seravalle, C.Turri, A.Lanfranchi and G.Mancia. Comparison between reproducibility and sensitivity of muscle sympathetic nerve traffic and plasma noradrenaline in man. Clin Sci 1997; 92: 285–289.
12. Y.Yamada, E.Miyajima, O.Tochikubo, T.Matsukawa, H.Shionoiri, M.Ishii and Y.Kaneko. Impaired baroreflex changes in muscle sympathetic nerve activity in adolescents who have a family history of essential hypertension. J Hypertens 1988;6 (suppl 4):S525–S528.

13. E.A.Anderson, C.A.Sinkey, W.J.Lawton and A.L.Mark. Elevated sympathetic nerve activity in borderline hypertensive humans: evidence from direct intraneural recording. Hypertension 1989;14:177–183.

14. G.Mancia and G.Grassi. Baroreceptor control of the circulation in man. An update. Clin Exper Hypertens 1995;17:387–397.

15. G.Grassi, G.Seravalle, A.Lanfranchi, S.Vailati, C.Turri, G.B.Bolla and G.Mancia. Sympathetic nerve traffic and baroreflex control of circulation in secondary hypertension. J Hypertens 1996;14 (suppl 1):114 (abstract).

16. I.Östman-Smith. Cardiac sympathetic nerves as the final common pathway in the induction of adaptive cardiac hypertrophy. Clin Sci 1981;61:265–272.

17. R.C.Tarazi, S.Sen, M.Saragoca and P.Khairallah. The multifactorial role of catecholamines in hypertensive cardiac hypertrophy. Eur Heart J 1982;3 (suppl A):103–110.

18. M.M.Laks, F.Morady and H.J.C.Swan. Myocardial hypertrophy produced by chronic infusion of subhypertensive doses of norepinephrine in the dog. Chest 1973;64:75–78.

19. M.B.Patel, J.M.Stewart, A.V.Loud, P.Anversa, J.Wang, L.Fiegel and T.H.Hintze. Altered function and structure of the heart in dogs with chronic elevation in plasma norepinephrine. Circulation 1991;84:2091–2100.

20. S.Sen, R.C.Tarazi, P.Khairallah and M.Bumpus. Cardiac hypertrophy in spontaneously hypertensive rats. Circ Res 1974;35:775–781.

21. W.Zierhut and H.G.Zimmer. Significance of myocardial α- and β-adrenoceptors in catecholamine-induced cardiac hypertrophy. Circ Res 1989;65:1417–1425.

22. E.D.Frohlich. Physiologic considerations in left ventricular hypertrophy. In F.H.Messerli (ed) The heart and hypertension. Yorke Medical Books, New York 1987: 43–52.

23. M.Esler, G.Lambert and G.Jennings. Increased regional sympathetic nervous activity in human hypertension: causes and consequences. J Hypertens 1990;8 (suppl 7):S53–S57.

24. G.Mancia, R.R.Lorenz and J.T.Shepherd. Reflex control of circulation by heart and lungs. In: A.C.Guyton and A.W.Cowley (eds) Cardiovascular physiology II, vol 9. Baltimore, University Park Press 1976:111–144.

25. B.M.Egan, S.Julius, C.Cottier, K.J.Osterziel and H.Ibsen. Role of cardiovascular receptors on the neural regulation of renin release in normal man. Hypertension 1983;5:779–786.

26. G.Grassi, C.Giannattasio, A.Saino, E.Sabadini, A.Capozi, L.Sampieri, C.Cuspidi and G.Mancia. Cardiopulmonary receptor modulation of plasma renin activity in normotensive and hypertensive subjects. Hypertension 1988;11:92–99.

27. G.Grassi, C.Giannattasio, C.Cuspidi, G.B.Bolla, J.Cleroux, P.Ferrazzi, R.Fiocchi and G.Mancia. Cardiopulmonary receptor regulation of renin release. Am J Med 1988;84 (suppl 3A):97–104.

28. P.K.Mohanty, M.D.Thames, J.A.Arrowod, J.R.Sowers, C.McNamara and S.Szentpetery. Impairment of cardiopulmonary baroreflex after cardiac transplantation in humans. Circulation 1987;75:914–922.

29. C.Giannattasio, A.Del Bo, B.M.Cattaneo, C.Cuspidi, E.Gronda, M.Frigerio, M.Mangiavacchi, M.Marabini, C.De Vita, G.Grassi, A.Zanchetti and G.Mancia. Reflex vasopressin and renin modulation by cardiac receptors in humans. Hypertension 1993;21:461–469.

30. G.Grassi, C.Giannattasio, J.Cleroux, C.Cuspidi, L.Sampieri, G.B.Bolla and G.Mancia. Cardiopulmonary reflex before and after regression of left ventricular hypertrophy in essential hypertension. Hypertension 1988;12:227–237.

31. A.L.Mark and G.Mancia. Cardiopulmonary baroreflexes in humans. In: J.T.Shepherd and F.M.Abboud (eds) Handbook of Physiology, sect 2, The cardiovascular system, Bethesda, Md, American Physiological Society 1983, vol III:795–813.

32. C.Giannattasio, G.Seravalle, G.B.Bolla, B.M.Cattaneo, J.Cleroux, C.Cuspidi, L.Sampieri, G.Grassi and G.Mancia. Cardiopulmonary receptor reflexes in normotensive athletes with cardiac hypertrophy. Circulation 1990;82:1222–1229.

33. C.Giannattasio, G.Seravalle, B.M.Cattaneo, C.Cuspidi, L.Sampieri, G.B.Bolla, G.Grassi and G.Mancia. Effects of detraining on the cardiopulmonary reflex in professional runners and hammer throwers. Am J Cardiol 1992;69:677–680.

34. G.Grassi and G.Mancia. Arterial baroreflexes and other cardiovascular reflexes in hypertension. In: J.D.Swales (ed): Textbook of Hypertension, Oxford, Blackwell Scientific Publications 1994:394–408.

19

HYPERTENSION, LEFT VENTRICULAR HYPERTROPHY, AND HEART RATE VARIABILITY

Federico Lombardi and Cesare Fiorentini

Cardiologia, Istituto di Scienze Biomediche
Ospedale S. Paolo
Università di Milano
via A. di Rudinì 8
20142 Milano, Italy

The occurrence of left ventricular hypertrophy in hypertensive patients is associated with a greater incidence of cardiovascular fatal and non fatal events despite conventional antihypertensive treatment (1).

The mechanisms by which left ventricular hypertrophy plays such a role remains however largely undefined, although a possible negative effect on autonomic control mechanisms has been proposed to explain the increased cardiac mortality observed in patients with left ventricular hypertrophy.

Several clinical and experimental observations have indicated that alterations in neural regulatory mechanisms play a critical role in the development of the hypertensive state, particularly in the initial phases where signs of sympathetic activation are easily detected, and in the progression of the disease (2,3).

It has been also suggested that (4,5) when left ventricular mass augments in response to a persistent increase in arterial blood pressure, the functional activity of cardiopulmonary vagal and sympathetic afferent fibers may also altered leading to a further impairment of autonomic regulatory mechanisms and to an abnormal control of pulse interval and arterial blood pressure. It remains also to be established whether the beneficial effect of a reduction of left ventricular mass induced by active drug treatment might also be associated with a functional recovery of neural regulatory mechanisms.

The appraisal of alteration in neural regulatory mechanisms has been facilitated by the development and large clinical utilisation of a non invasive approach based on time and frequency domain analysis of heart rate variability (6). In the last decades several studies have indicated that this non invasive methodology can provide relevant information on the changes of neural regulatory mechanisms which characterise different physiopathological conditions such as ischemic heart disease, hypertension and congestive heart failure (6,7).

Hypertension and the Heart, edited by Zanchetti et al.
Plenum Press, New York, 1997

181

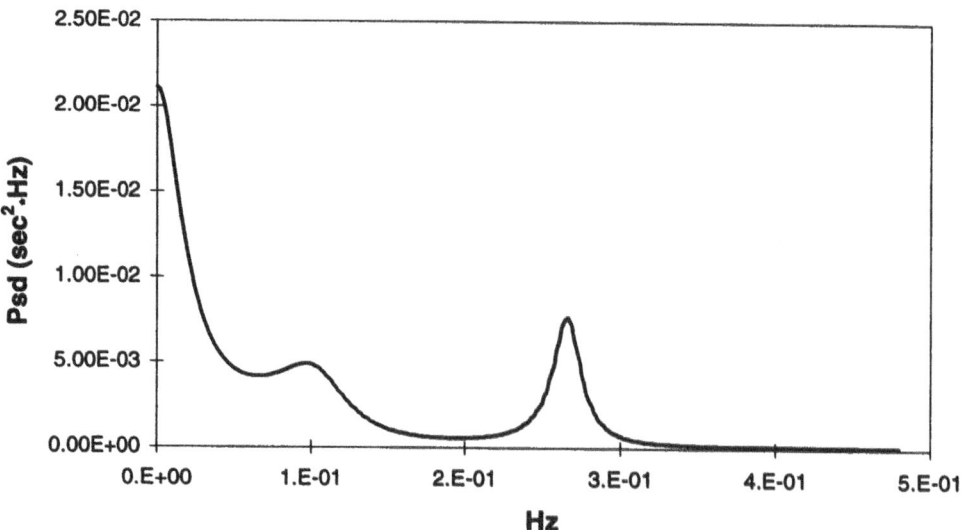

Figure 1. Spectral analysis of heart rate variability of 24-year-old normal subject during resting controlled conditions. Two major components at low (0.10 Hz) and high (0.27 Hz) frequency are clearly detectable.

The hypothesis underlying the analysis of heart rate variability is that beat to beat variations of heart period reflect the continuous interaction between sinus node pacemaker cell activity and vagal and sympathetic efferent activity directed to the heart. Thus, the quantification of the principal rhythmical oscillations detectable in the RR variability signal may provide information on the autonomic modulatory activity responsible of such a rhythmicity. For example, the occurrence of fluctuations in heart rate synchronous with respiration has been known for long time and considered to reflect vagal modulation of sinus node (6–10). On the other hand, the presence of low frequency oscillations, corresponding to the 0.1 Hz frequency oscillations of arterial pressure, has been considered to mainly reflect sympathetic activity (6,7,10). At variance with time domain analysis which provides statistical measures of RR interval distribution or of the differences between intervals, spectral analysis allows the identification and quantification of the oscillatory components present in the variability signal which can be defined in relation to their center frequency and power (6,7,10). As illustrated in Figure 1, spectral analysis of heart rate variability in a normal subject during resting controlled condition is characterised by two major components at low (LF;~0.10 Hz) and high (HF;~0.25 Hz) frequency. In addition a consistent part of the spectral energy is distributed in the 0–0.03 Hz frequency range which corresponds to the very low frequency (VLF) component.

Measurements of power of LF and HF in normalised units as well as of LF/HF ratio have been therefore utilised to detect alterations of sympatho-vagal balance: an increase in LF in nu and in LF/HF ratio was considered to reflect a predominance of sympathetic modulation as well as a reduction of vagal activity, whereas a predominance of HF with a LF/HF ratio <1 was interpreted as a sign of an enhanced vagal modulation (6,7). Despite initial suggestions (5,11), less certain is the physiological interpretation of measures of total 24 hour variability such as the standard deviation or the variance of normal RR intervals whose reduction from normal values was considered to reflect a diminished vagal tone (11).

It is therefore not surprising that time and frequency domain analysis of heart rate variability has been applied by several groups of investigators to evaluate the presence of alterations of neural regulatory mechanisms of hypertensive patients in the different phases of the disease. However, as recently pointed out by the Task Force on heart Rate Variability of the European Society of Cardiology and of the North American Society of Pacing and Electrophysiology (5), in order to make appropriate comparisons of the different results reported in the literature, it is important to pay particular attention for the different methodological characteristics of each study, in relation, for example, to the duration of the recordings, to the expression of power of spectral component in absolute, percent or normalised units and to the experimental setting.

1. METHODOLOGICAL ASPECTS

Whereas time domain analysis of heart rate variability is traditionally performed on the entire 24 hour recording period, spectral analysis is generally performed on short term recordings corresponding to 300–500 RR intervals. When spectral analysis is performed on 24 hour Holter recordings two modalities of analysis may be followed: the first provides an estimation of a single autospectrum of the entire 24 hour period, the second one computes about 200 consecutive autospectra of a five minute duration which can be averaged in order to obtain hourly or preselected interval values (6). The autospectrum of the entire 24hour period provides information on total and fractional power which are essentially similar to those derived from time domain analysis, whereas only by considering hourly spectral values it is possible to trace the circadian pattern of variation of sympathetic and parasympathetic modulatory mechanisms and to detect its alteration (6,7).

In our opinion, however, the most rewarding application of the spectral approach is the possibility of obtaining information on autonomic modulation of heart period during controlled conditions in relation to the presence or absence of a disease, in response to physiological stimuli capable of modifying sympatho-vagal balance, or before and after pharmacological and non pharmacological interventions.

A second aspect to take into consideration is the type of units (absolute versus normalised) used to measure the power of spectral components (6,7,10).

It is evident that the absolute power of LF and HF is correlated with total power and that a reduction in total power is generally accompanied by a reduction of the relative power of spectral components, whereas an increase in total power, as the one occurring in almost all subjects during night time, is associated with a proportional increase in the power of each spectral component. This mathematical relationship makes the interpretation of the physiological meaning of LF and HF (in absolute units) very difficult and has prevented a large clinical utilisation of this methodology. To overcome these limitations, Malliani and coll. (6,8,10,12) proposed to express the power of spectral components in normalised units. The normalisation procedure has been proven to facilitate the appraisal of changes in LF and HF independently of the concomitant variations in total power and to reflect the reciprocal interaction which characterise sympathetic and vagal outflows in most physiological and pathological conditions. A similar evaluation of sympatho-vagal balance can be derived by computing the LF/HF ratio (10).

A final point to be considered is the recording environment. It is evident that controlled conditions can be obtained only during short term recordings. However, also in this condition the modality of respiration my exert profound influences on heart rate variability. It has been reported (9,10) that controlled breathing at a fixed rate markedly alters the autospectrum, by determining a significant increase in HF and a reduction in LF and LF/HF ratio in respect to a free breathing condition. Moreover, the increase in LF component observed in response to tilt is markedly blunted if this stimulus is applied during controlled respiration.

For the above reasons, it is sometimes difficult to compare results obtained by applying different methodologies or derived from recordings performed in different experimental conditions.

2. TIME AND FREQUENCY DOMAIN ANALYSIS OF HEART RATE VARIABILITY

2.1 In Hypertensive Patients

For the purpose of this article only the first or most relevant reports will be considered.

In a study (13) comparing short term heart rate variability of hypertensive patients with that of an age matched normotensive control group, it was found that LF was greater (68±3 versus 54±3 nu) and HF was smaller (24±3 versus 33±2 nu) in mild hypertensive patients. The overall spectral profile of these patients was consistent with an enhanced sympathetic modulation and a reduced vagal activity. Of interest was the finding that in hypertensive patients with signs of sympathetic excitation at rest, the LF response to a sympathetic stimulus such as 90° head up tilt, was blunted in respect to controls.

A predominance of LF in normalised units over HF was also reported by Pagani and coll. (14) who studied the adaptive effects of physical training on cardiovascular control mechanisms in a small group of mild hypertensive subjects. After a six month training period, these Authors were able to observe a normalisation of the spectral pattern with a reduction of LF and an increase in HF. These changes were also associated with an increase of the gain of the relationship between heart period and systolic arterial pressure.

A reduced response of LF component to tilt was also reported by Radaelli and coll. (15) who analysed heart rate variability in a group of hypertensive subjects. At variance with previous studies, recordings were performed during controlled respiration: i.e. an experimental condition in which the power of HF component is increased and is often predominant over LF. This may explain why these Authors were unable to observe a clear predominance of LF component in both absolute and normalised units at rest.

Of particular interest were the results reported by Piccirillo and coll. (16) who studied a group of patients at the time of the first diagnosis of mild hypertension and observed that during high sodium intake, salt-sensitive hypertensive patients had a significant higher (59±2.4 nu) LF component than salt-resistant subjects (55±3.2 nu) and normotensive control subjects (41.6±2.9 nu). A finding which confirmed the multifactorial origin of the mechanisms leading to an abnormal autonomic regulation in the initial phases of hypertension.

When RR variability was analysed along the 24 hours, different results were reported. Furlan and coll. (17) studied 18 hospitalised patients with a history of border line hypertension and found a circadian pattern of variation of spectral indices of sympathetic and vagal modulation similar to that observed in controls: signs of sympathetic activation were predominant during day time whereas signs of a sympathetic withdrawal and of a vagal predominance were detectable during night time. Guzzetti and coll. (18) reported that patients with mild hypertension were characterised by a loss of the circadian variation of spectral indexes of sympathetic and parasympathetic modulation. In comparison to normal control subjects, patients did not present a significant reduction of LF during nighttime whereas a small increase in HF was still detectable. Thus, in patients with mild to moderate hypertension, the analysis of heart rate variability suggested not only the presence of signs of sympathetic activation at rest but also a blunted response of sinus node to sympathetic and vagal stimulation.

2.2 In Hypertensive Patients with Left Ventricular Hypertrophy

In a small group of hypertensive patients with left ventricular hypertrophy spectral analysis of short term recordings obtained during controlled respiration did not reveal any significant difference from that of patients without evidence of left ventricular hypertrophy (15). In particular the Authors observed a blunted increase of LF component during tilt.

By analysing 24 hour recording, Chakko and coll. (19) reported the alterations in heart rate variability and its circadian rhythm in hypertensive patients with left ventricular hypertrophy and normal coronary arteries. They observed that the difference between mean RR interval of day and night time period was significantly smaller in hypertensives in comparison to controls. The latter group also presented a greater standard deviation of normal 24 hour RR intervals. Moreover they reported (19) that the nocturnal increase of PNN50 (i.e. the percentage of difference of RR intervals exceeding 50 msec) was not detectable in patients with left ventricular hypertrophy. When considering spectral components in absolute units, they noticed that the power of HF was smaller among the hypertensive patients who did not exhibit a physiological pattern of variations of LF component. These findings led the Authors to conclude that in hypertensive patients with left ventricular hypertrophy a partial withdrawal of parasympathetic activity and an altered day-night interaction of sympathetic and vagal regulatory mechanisms were present.

Similar findings were reported subsequently by Kohara and coll. (20) who analysed the relationship between heart rate variability and left ventricular mass in essential hypertension. These Authors reported that left ventricular mass index had a significant negative correlation with the absolute power of LF and HF spectral components. Of particular interest was the finding that LF/HF ratio of hypertensive patients was not significantly different from that of normotensive subjects and that LF/HF ratio did not correlate with left ventricular mass index. These findings were interpreted as an evidence that the level of end-organ damage could correlate with the neuronal alteration in essential hypertension. However, despite the reduction in total power, the absence of a correlation between LF/HF ratio and left ventricular mass suggested the persistence of a physiological balance between the two neural regulatory outputs which could have been more easily appreciated by considering the power of spectral components in normalised rather than absolute units.

Two recent studies (21,22) have focused the attention on a relevant physiopathological problem: the effect of left ventricular mass reduction on heart rate variability in hypertensive patients.

Petretta and coll. (22) studied the effects of drug induced left ventricular hypertrophy regression on autonomic control mechanisms, by means of 24 hour heart rate variability analysis. Recordings were obtained at baseline, after one year of lisinopril treatment and after one month of drug withdrawal. In patients with left ventricular mass normalisation, the Authors observed a significant increase in the absolute power of HF component which was interpreted as an indirect evidence of an improvement of neural cardiac control.

More recently, Muiesan and coll. (22) reported the result of a study carried out in three groups of subjects: controls and hypertensives with and without left ventricular hypertrophy. Fourteen patients were studied for a second time during a wash-out period after a six month therapy which determined a regression of left ventricular hypertrophy in eight patients. The most interesting finding of the study was the reappearance, in patients with regression of left ventricular hypertrophy, of a circadian pattern of variation of LF component which was not detectable at the time of the first recording and remained absent in patients in whom treatment was not associated with a normalisation of left ventricular mass.

3. FINAL CONSIDERATIONS

All the above studies indicate that time and frequency domain analysis of heart rate variability can be effectively utilised to study the alterations of neural regulatory mechanisms that characterise patients with essential hypertension.

Signs of sympathetic activation are mainly evident in the initial phases of the disease, whereas a reduction in heart rate variability and in particular a marked attenuation of the circadian variation of spectral indices of sympathetic and vagal modulation of heart period seem to characterise the most advanced phases of the disease.

Regarding this point, it is important to recall that a similar pattern of change in heart rate variability has been also observed in patients after myocardial infarction (5,23–25). In post myocardial infarction patients with an uncomplicated outcome we observed signs of sympathetic activation and of a reduced vagal tone that were indicated by a predominant LF and by a smaller HF at rest and by an attenuation of the circadian pattern of variations of spectral indices of sympathetic and vagal modulation. In patients with signs of left ventricular dysfunction and with a complicated outcome there was a significant reduction in heart rate variability and a less detectable LF component, i.e. a spectral pattern which seemed to suggest a diminished responsiveness of sinus node to neural modulation (25).

For an appropriate interpretation of these findings it is important to recall (6,7) that spectral methodology cannot provide information on the specific neural circuits whose activation or inhibition is responsible for the alteration of neural regulatory mechanisms reflected by a change in total power or in the power of LF and HF or in LF/HF ratio; rather the analysis of heart rate variability may provide an indirect evaluation of what can be defined as sympatho-vagal balance and of its alterations in several physiopathological conditions such as hypertension. Moreover, the interpretation of the results obtained with spectral methodology is often based on the assumption of a linear relationship between neural regulatory outflows and sinus node responsiveness which is unlikely to be true in all physiopathological conditions (6,26).

The above results indicate that the presence of left ventricular hypertrophy might further altered time and frequency domain parameters of heart rate variability. Available data are limited, however suggest that hypertensive patients with left ventricular hypertrophy present a greater reduction in heart rate variability in comparison to patients without left ventricular hypertrophy. It is possible that in these patients, the structural abnormality of the heart might alter the mechanical sensitivity of cardiac vagal and sympathetic afferent fibres (4,5) and their reflex function, thus contributing to the abnormal autonomic modulation of sinus node which is detected by time and frequency domain analysis of heart rate variability.

REFERENCES

1. Levy D, Garrison RJ, Savage DD, Kannel WB, Castelli WP. Prognostic implications of echocardiographically determined left ventricular mass in the Framingham heart study. N Engl J Med 1990;322:1561–1666.
2. Malliani A, Pagani M, Lombardi F: Positive feedback reflexes. In Zanchetti A, Tarazi RC (eds): Handbook of Hypertension: Volume 8. Pathophysiology of Hypertension. Amsterdam, Elsevier Science Pubblishing Co, Inc,1986,pp 69–81.
3. Goldstein DS. Plasma catecholamines and essential hypertension: An analytical review Hypertension 1983,5:86–89.

4. Bishop VS, Malliani A, Thoret P: Cardiac mechanoreceptor. In Shepherd JT, Abboud FM, Geiger SR (eds) Handbook of Physiology, section 2: The Cardiovascular System: Vol 3, peripheral circulation and organ blood flow. Bethesda, Md, Am Phys Soc 1983:497–555.

5. Giannattasio C, Cattaneo BM, Serravalle G, Grassi G, Mancia G: Left ventricular hypertrophy and the "cardiogenic reflex" in man. J of Hypertension 1991;9:S43–S50.

6. Task Force of the European Society of Cardiology and the North American Society of Pacing and Electrophysiology. Heart Rate Variability. Standards of measurement, physiological interpretation, and clinical use. Circulation 1996;93:1043–1065.

7. Malliani A, Pagani M, Lombardi F, Cerutti S. Cardiovascular neural regulation explored in the frequency domain. Circulation 1991;84:482–492.

8. Akselrod S, Gordon D, Ubel FA, Shannon DC, Barger AC, Cohen RJ: Power spectrum analysis of heart rate fluctuation: a quantitative probe of beat-to-beat cardiovascular control. Science 1981;213:220–222.

9. Pomeranz B, Macaulay RJB, Caudill MA, Kutz I, Adam D, Gordon D, Killborn KM, Barger AC, Shannon DC, Cohen RJ, Benson H. Assessment of autonomic function in humans by heart rate spectral analysis. Am J Physiol 1985;248:H151–H153.

10. Pagani M, Lombardi F, Guzzetti S, Rimoldi O. Furlan R, Pizzinelli P, Sandrone G, Malfatto G, Dell'Orto S, Piccaluga E, Turiel M, Baselli G, Cerutti S, Malliani A: Power spectral analysis of heart rate and arterial pressure variabilities as a marker of sympathovagal interaction in man and conscious dog. Cir Res 1986; 59:178–193.

11. Kleiger RE, Miller JP, Bigger JT, Moss AR, Multicenter Post-Infarction Research Group: Decreased heart rate variability and its association with increased mortality after acute myocardial infarction. Am J Cardiol 1987;59:256–262.

12. Malliani A, Lombardi F, Pagani M. Power spectrum analysis of heart rate variability: a tool to explore neural regulatory mechanisms. Br Heart J 1994;71:1–2.

13. Guzzetti S, Piccaluga E, Casati R, Cerutti S, Lombardi F, Pagani M and Malliani A: Sympathetic predominance in essential hypertension: a study employing spectral analysis of heart rate variability. J Hypert 1988,6:711–717.

14. Pagani M, Somers V, Furlan R, Dell'Orto S, Conway J, Baselli G, Cerutti S, Slight P, Malliani A: Changes in autonomic regulation induced by physical training in mild hypertension. Hypertension 1988,12:600–610.

15. Radaelli A, Bernardi L, Valle F, Leuzzi S, Salvucci F, Pedrotti L, Marchesi E, Finardi G, Sleight P. Cardiovascular autonomic modulation in essential hypertension. Effect of tilting. Hypertension 1994;24:556–563.

16. Piccirillo G, Bucca C, Durante M, Santagada E, Munizzi MR, Cacciafesta M, Marigliano V. Heart rate and blood pressure variabilities in salt-sensitive hypertension. Hypertension 1996;28:994–952.

17. Furlan R, Guzzetti S, Crivellaro W, Dassi S, Tinelli M, Baselli G, Cerutti S, Lombardi F, Pagani M, Malliani A: Continous 24 hours assessment of the neural regulation of systemic arterial pressure and R-R variabilities in ambulant subjects. Circulation 1990, 81:537–547.

18. Guzzetti S, Dassi S, Pecis M, Casati R, Masu AM, Longoni P, Tinelli M, Pagani M, Malliani A: Altered pattern of circadian neural control of heart rate period in mild hypertension. J of Hypertension 1991;9:831–838.

19. Chakko S, Mulingtapang RF, Huikuri HV, Kessler KM, Materson BJ, Myerburg RJ: Alterations in heart rate variability and its circadian rhythm in hypertensive patients with left ventricular hypertrophy free of coronary artery disease. Am Heart J 1993;126:1364–1372.

20. Kohara K, Hara-Nakamura N, Hiwada K. Left ventricular mass index negatively correlates with heart rate variability in essential hypertension. Am Journal of Hypertension 1995;8:183–188.

21. Petretta M, Bonaduce D, Marciano F, Bianchi V, Valva G, Apicella C, de Luca N, Gisonni P. Effect of 1 year lisinopril treatment on cardiac autonomic control in hypertensive patients with left ventricular hypertrophy. Hypertension 1996;27:330–338.

22. Muiesan ML, Rizzoni D, Zulli R, Castellano M, Bettoni G, Porteri E, Agabiti-Rosei E. Power spectral analysis of heart rate in hypertensive patients with and without left ventricular hypertrophy. The effect of left ventricular mass reduction. Am Journal of Cardiology, submitted for publication.

23. Lombardi F, Sandrone G, Perpruner S, Sala R, Garimoldi M, Cerutti S, Baselli G, Pagani M, Malliani A: Heart rate variability as a an index of sympathovagal interaction after acute myocardial infarction. Am J Cardiol 1987,60:1239–1245.

24. Lombardi F, Sandrone G, Mortara A, La Rovere MT, Colombo E, Guzzetti S, Malliani A: Circadian variation of spectral indices of heart rate variability after myocardial infarction. Am Heart J 1992;123: 1521–1529.

25. Lombardi F, Malliani A, Pagani M, Cerutti S. Heart rate variability and its sympatho-vagal modulation. Cardiovasc Res 1996;32:208–216.

26. Parati G, Saul JP, Di Rienzo M, Mancia G. Spectral analysis of blood pressure and heart rate variability in evaluating cardiovascular regulation. A critical appraisal. Hypertension 1995;25:1276–1286.

COMPARISON OF META-ANALYSES OF THERAPEUTIC STUDIES ON REGRESSION OF LEFT VENTRICULAR HYPERTROPHY

Lennart Hansson[*]

Division of Clinical Hypertension Research
Department of Geriatrics
University of Uppsala
P.O. Box 609
751 25 Uppsala, Sweden

ABSTRACT

In recent years several meta-analyses have been performed of studies in which the effect of various antihypertensive therapies on left ventricular hypertrophy (LVH) has been assessed. It is the purpose of this review to briefly discuss three of these meta-analyses. All data in the reviewed studies have been obtained with the echocardiographic technique.

INTRODUCTION

Left ventricular hypertrophy (LVH) has been recognized as a very potent risk indicator of cardiovascular morbidity, both when the diagnosis of LVH has been based on electrocardiographic criteria (EKG) (1) and echocardiographic studies (2). In fact, a report from the Framingham Heart Study described echocardiographically determined left ventricular (LV) mass as a more powerful risk indicator than established risk factors such as blood pressure and serum-cholesterol (2).

Against this background reversal of LVH through the use of antihypertensive therapy assumes great interest. It is logical to expect, but remains to be shown, that a reduction in LV mass would be associated with a decrease in risk. Numerous studies have shown that most antihypertensive therapies reduce LV mass, and many of these studies have been analyzed together in meta-analyses (3–5).

---

[*] Fax: +46-18-17 79 73.

Hypertension and the Heart, edited by Zanchetti et al.
Plenum Press, New York, 1997

METHODS

Studies dealing with the reversal of LVH in hypertensive patients treated with various antihypertensive compounds, using echocardiography as the technique, were included in the three meta-analyses (3–5). Strict selection criteria were applied for inclusion, e.g. that the studies were published in the established scientific literature in peer-reviewed journals (3). Papers in which only EKG criteria had been used for the evaluation of LV mass (LVM) were excluded (3–5). The first meta-analysis included papers published in 1990 or earlier (3) whereas the other two meta-analyses included more recent papers (4,5).

RESULTS

All three meta-analyses showed that the various antihypertensive regimens reduced LVM. The reduction in LVM was significantly correlated to the fall in mean arterial pressure (3).

A better than expected reversal of LVH, in relation to the obtained reduction in blood pressure, was found for the angiotensin converting enzyme (ACE) inhibitors in the meta-analysis including studies published before 1990 (3). However, the latest meta-analysis on this topic, which included more recent studies, showed that calcium antagonists are at least equally effective as ACE inhibitors in this regard (5).

DISCUSSION

The three meta-analyses are similar in many ways; they all show that antihypertensive therapies can reduce LVM. They also show that all therapies are not alike in this regard. Some of the more novel classes of agents, in particular ACE inhibitors and calcium antagonists are obviously more effective than the older therapies such as diuretics and beta-blockers. What this means in terms of affecting cardiovascular morbidity and mortality remains to be shown in prospective randomized intervention trials. It is logical to assume, however, that a greater reduction of LVH will be associated with a better protective effect against cardiovascular disease, in view of the powerful prediction of cardiovascular complications that can be obtained by assessing LVM.

It should be stressed that the quality of a meta-analysis is never better than the data used in the analysis. Unfortunately, many studies included in these meta-analyses have methodological flaws that limit the possibilities of making useful conclusions.

REFERENCES

1. Levy D. Left ventricular hypertrophy. Epidemiological insights from the Framingham Heart Study. *Drugs* 1998; *35* (suppl 5):1–5.
2. Levy D, Garrison RJ, Sagae DD et al. Prognostic implications of echocardiographically determined left ventricular mass in the Framingham Heart Study. *N Engl J Med* 1990; *322*:1561–1566.
3. Dahlöf B, Pennert K, Hansson L. Reversal of left ventricular hypertrophy in hypertensive patients. A metaanalysis of 109 treatment studies. *Am J Hypertens* 1992; *5*:95–110.
4. Schmieder RE, Martus P, Klingbeil A. Reversal of left ventricular hypertrophy in essential hypertension. A meta-analysis of randomized double-blind studies. *JAMA* 1996; *275*:1507–1513.
5. Jennings GL, Wong J. Reversibility of left ventricular hypertrophy and malfunction by antihypertensive treatment. In: *Handbook of Hypertension, Vol 18, Assessment of Hypertensive Organ Damage.* Eds: Hansson L, Birkenhäger WH. Elsevier, Rotterdam 1997; 184–223.

COMPARISON OF THERAPEUTIC STUDIES ON REGRESSION OF LEFT VENTRICULAR HYPERTROPHY

Roland E. Schmieder[*] and Markus P. Schlaich

Dept. of Medicine IV
University of Erlangen-Nürnberg
Germany

SUMMARY

In numerous studies left ventricular hypertrophy has been clearly established to be a strong, blood-pressure independent risk factor for cardiovascular morbidity and mortality. In fact, increased echocardiographic left ventricular mass has been shown to predict cardiovascular complications not only in patients with hypertension, but also in the general population. Preliminary data revealed that regression of left ventricular hypertrophy indeed reduces cardiovascular complications. As a consequence, regression of left ventricular hypertrophy by drug treatment has emerged as a desirable goal in patients with echocardiographically determined left ventricular hypertrophy. These findings raised the question, whether certain antihypertensive drugs differ in their ability to reduce left ventricular mass. To resolve this issue several comparative studies and some meta-analyses have been carried out.

In a meta-analysis by Dahlöf et al., comprising 109 treatment studies published until december 1990 with a total of 2357 patients, ACE-inhibitors (−15%) were most effective in reducing left ventricular mass followed by diuretics (−11.3%), calcium channel blockers (−8.5%) and β-blockers (−8%). Reduction in left ventricular mass was mainly due to a decrease in wall thickness except for diuretics which predominantly reduced ventricular diameter. Although reduction in blood pressure was similar for all antihypertensive agents, the correlation between changes in mean arterial pressure and effect on left ventricular mass was only significant for β-blockers with a modest correlation for ACE-inhibitors and no clearcut relation for diuretics and calcium channel blockers.

---

[*] Correspondence and requests for reprints to: Prof. Dr. Roland E. Schmieder, Medizinische Klinik IV/Nephrology, Universität Erlangen-Nürnberg, Breslauer Str. 201, D-90471 Nürnberg, Germany. Tel: 0049-911-398 3119, Fax: 0049-911-398 3183.

Hypertension and the Heart, edited by Zanchetti et al.
Plenum Press, New York, 1997

191

Another meta-analysis by Cruickshank et al., screening articles for the same publication period and comprising 104 studies with a total of 2107 patients also showed best results in reducing left ventricular mass for ACE-inhibitors as single antihypertensive therapy. Calcium channel blockers were more effective than β-blockers with diuretics in the intermediate range.

In a meta-analysis of Schmieder et al, only double-blind, randomized, controlled clinical studies with parallel group design were considered.Out of a large sample size of 471 studies identified by extensive literature search, only 39 studies of presumably high scientific quality, published until July 1995 fulfilled inclusion criteria. After adjustment for different durations of treatment, left ventricular mass decreased with ACE-inhibitors by 13% (95% CI: 9.9–16.8%), with calcium channel blockers by 9% (95% CI: 5.5–13.1%), with β-blockers by 6% (95% CI: 2.3–8.6%) and with diuretics by 7% (95% CI: 3.0–10.7%) at similar fallen blood pressure. An update of this meta-analysis including all available data until the end of 1996, comprising a total of 1715 patients found a reduction of left ventricular mass by 12% (95% CI: 9.0–14.5%) for ACE-inhibitors, by 11% (95% CI: 7.8–13.7%) for calcium channel blockers, by 5% (95% CI: 1.2–7.3%) for β-blockers and by 8% (95% CI: 3.9–11.1%) for diuretics.

Regarding the available data, blockade of angiotensin II by ACE-inhibitors emerged as the most potent approach for the treatment of left ventricular hypertrophy. The most recent updated meta-analysis revealed that calcium channel blockers emerged to be similarly potent or according to other studies to be at least the second choice of drug class.

THERAPEUTICAL APPROACHES FOR REDUCTION OF LEFT VENTRICULAR HYPERTROPHY

As shown in numerous studies, left ventricular hypertrophy has been clearly established to be a strong, blood pressure independent risk factor for cardiovascular morbidity and mortality[1,2]. Therefore, regression of left ventricular hypertrophy has emerged as a desirable therapeutical goal. Preliminary data have indeed been found that cardiovascular complications are reduced after regression of left ventricular hypertrophy[3,4]. This issue raises the question, how regression of left ventricular hypertrophy can be ideally achieved. Numerous hemodynamic and non-hemodynamic factors seem to be involved in the process of cardiac adaptation in essential hypertension. Thus, the ability of different therapeutical approaches for the reduction of left ventricular hypertrophy need to be adressed thoroughly.

NON-PHARMACOLOGICAL INTERVENTION

Several risk factors for the development of left ventricular hypertrophy have been identified, some of which can be treated by non-pharmacological intervention. Weight reduction for example has been shown to lower blood pressure in obese patients[5,6]. Additionally, MacMahon et al[7] found that weight reduction was directly associated with reduced left ventricular mass in overweight hypertensive patients, independently of changes in blood pressure. MacMahon et al[6] also demonstrated a greater decrease in left ventricular mass by weight loss opposed to treatment with β-blockers in mildly obese and hypertensive subjects. In accordance, intensive nutritional hygienic intervention, accomplishing the important role of sustained weight reduction was shown to decrease left ventricular mass[8]. Strict salt depletion has been shown by Ferrara et al[9] to reduce left ventricular mass in hypertension. Even salt restriction seems to be capable to reduce left ventricular mass in mild to moderate essential hypertensive patients[9,10]. According to the large-scale TOMHS study, salt reduction emerged as most effective measure to reduce left ventricular mass independent of blood pressure changes[11].

The role of alcohol consumption has been assessed by Manolio et al[12], who found that in addition to a blood pressure rising effect alcohol increases left ventricular mass. Although there is a lack of prospective studies adressing the ability of alcohol moderation to reduce left ventricular mass, alcohol should be avoided in patients with left ventricular hypertrophy, since alcohol consumption beyond certain limits (approximately 40 g/day) increases blood pressure and increases the risk of ventricular arrhythmias in patients with left ventricular hypertrophy (F.H. Messerli, personal communication), prone to have 3 to 5 fold elevated risk for cardiac sudden death.

Several studies revealed, that regular exercise can result in satisfactory blood pressure control[13]. However, although no reduction in left ventricular mass was observed under regular exercise, the pattern of left ventricular hypertrophy may change from concentric towards eccentric left ventricular hypertrophy in echocardiographic terms and from fetal abnormal myosin isoform pattern to the physiological adult composition in the myocardium. Hence, non-pharmacological intervention, especially when adjusted to an individual´s risk profile and possibly combined with other forms of pharmacological therapy seem to be beneficial not only in reducing blood presssure, but also in decreasing left ventricular hypertrophy.

ANTIHYPERTENSIVE TREATMENT

Since regression of left ventricular hypertrophy by drug treatment has emerged as a desirable goal in patients with echocardiographically determined left ventricular hypertrophy, several comparative studies and so far three meta-analyses have been carried out to analyze, whether certain antihypertensive drugs differ in their ability to reduce left ventricular mass.

COMPARATIVE STUDIES

Far more than 500 trials in patients with arterial hypertension have been undertaken to test the effects of different antihypertensive drugs on the regression of left ventricular hypertrophy. Although results from these studies are inconsistent and vary in a large extent, it has been shown that left ventricular mass decreased by almost all classes of antihypertensive drugs, if blood pressure was reduced substantially. Therefore, sustained blood pressure control seems to be of crucial importance to achieve reduction of left ventricular hypertrophy in hypertensive patients.

In the Treatment of Mild Hypertension Study (TOMHS)[11], 844 mildly hypertensive patients were randomly allocated to one of 5 antihypertensive therapies or placebo in a double blind fashion. Echocardiographically determined left ventricular mass decreased to a similar extent in the placebo group as well as in the active treatment group. In other words, the non-pharmacologic intervention treatment was most effective in reducing left ventricular mass. This lack of an additional effect on the active treatment groups may be related to the fact that mild hypertensive patients were included with only few characterized by echocardiographic left ventricular hypertrophy. Within the active compound groups regression of left ventricular mass was most pronounced in the chlortalidon group and least in the β-blocker group. Therefore, data of TOMHS provide only limited information concerning direct effects of antihypertensive drugs on left ventricular hypertrophy.

In a comparative study by Senior et al[14], including 151 hypertensive patients, the effect of 6 months of treatment with indapamide on regression of left ventricular hypertrophy was compared to the effect of the calcium antagonist nifedipine, the ACE inhibitor enalapril and the diuretic hydrochlorothiazide in four parallel, double blind studies. An 8–17% reduction in left ventricular mass index was found, with no significant differences between antihypertensive therapies used in this trial with the exception of hydrochlorothiazide, that did not decrease left ventricular mass. The results of Senior et al are in contrast to the findings of the Veterans Administration Study[15], in which more than 400 patients were randomly assigned to various antihypertensive treatment with a mean follow-up of two years. In this trial a reduction of left ventricular mass occured only in patients treated with hydrochlorothiazide, whereas no significant decrease occured with atenolol, clonidine or diltiazem. These results are divergent from several other comparative studies and may be associated to the large portion of black patients that was observed. Black patients are well known and were also found in the Veterans Administration Study to have a better response to diuretics than to ACE-inhibitors. This finding stresses the importance of further separate investigations in black and white hypertensive patients, known to have a different systemic hemodynamic profile and might be clarified by subsequent analysis of Gottdiener et al comparing various active drug treatments in 452 black and white men separately (J.S. Gottdiener, personal communication).

META-ANALYSES

Although one may critisize that pooling of results from the literature as done in meta-analysis is less satisfactory than adequately sized single studies, meta-analyses are helpful in increasing statistical power, resolving uncertainty when results differ between studies and improving accurate estimation of the magnitude of effect. Since reliability of resulting conclusions of meta-analyses depend on the methods used in the original studies, the methodologic and scientific quality of the studies to be combined is the most critical issue[16].

In a meta-analysis by Dahlöf et al[17], comprising 109 treatment studies published until december 1990 and including a total of 2357 patients with an average age of 49 years it was analyzed, whether the four classes of antihypertensive first-line treatment (ACE-inhibitors, calcium channel blockers, β-blockers and diuretics) induce different degrees of regression of left ventricular mass, whether reduction in left ventricular mass was equally linked to the fall in blood pressure and whether therapies differently affected wall thickness and left ventricular diameter. The average follow up of patients was 10.1 months, but 56% of studies had a follow up shorter than 6 months.

According to this meta-analysis, antihypertensive drug treatment is effective in reducing left ventricular mass. Overall, there was a reduction in MAP of 14.9% (95% CI: 14.0–15.8%) in parallel with a reduction in left ventricular mass of 11.9% (95% CI: 10.1–13.7%). ACE-inhibitors (−15%) were most effective in reducing left ventricular mass followed by diuretics (−11.3%), calcium channel blockers (−8.5%) and β-blockers (−8%). Although reduction in blood pressure was similar for all antihypertensive agents, the correlation between changes in mean arterial pressure and effect on left ventricular mass was only significant for β-blockers. The correlation for ACE-inhibitors was only modest and no clearcut relation was observed for diuretics and calcium channel blockers. Reduction in left ventricular mass was mainly due to a decrease in wall thickness except for diuretics which predominantly reduced ventricular diameter.

The data of Dahlöf et al need to be interpreted with caution, since of the 109 studies fulfilling the inclusion criteria for analysis, only 17% (n = 18) were randomized, double blind, parallel group comparisons, 10% (n = 11) were single blind comparative trials and the remaining 79% (n = 80) were open and uncontrolled.

Another meta-analysis[18] published in parallel screened articles for the same publication period and included 104 studies with a total of 2107 patients. Of the 104 studies evaluated, only 8% were randomized placebo-controlled, 21% were randomized active comparisons and 71% were uncontrolled studies. Besides the four major drug classes (ACE-inhibitors, calcium channel blockers, β-blockers and diuretics), alpha-blockers, alpha-methyldopa, vasodilators and combination therapy were analyzed with respect to reduced left ventricular mass. The combined results of all active treatments differed significantly from placebo, suggesting an overall effect of antihypertensive treatment on reduction of left ventricular mass. In between comparisons revealed significant differences for the different drug classes. ACE-inhibitors as single antihypertensive therapy also emerged as the most potent drug class in reducing left ventricular mass, followed by alpha-methyldopa and alpha-blockers. Calcium channel blockers (non-dihydropyridines) were more effective than β-blockers, and diuretics were in the intermediate range. Drug effects on posterior wall thickness and interventricular septal wall thickness were not significantly different between drug classes but showed similar trends to those observed for left ventricular mass. There were only small differences in MAP reduction between the examined drug classes, that according to the authors did not account for the effects on left ventricular mass. The average duration of treatment was rather short for dihydropyridine calcium channel blockers (4.1 months) compared to the other treatment arms (9.2 months). Therefore, decrease in left ventricular mass for the dihydropyridines was directly compared with the ACE inhibitor studies lasting 6 months or less. Nevertheless, ACE-inhibitors were still found to be significantly more effective in reducing left ventricular mass than dihydropyridine calcium channel blockers.

Conclusions of these two meta-analyses need to be interpreted with caution, since non-randomized, open, non-comparative studies were included. This situation was improved by a meta-analysis of Schmieder et al[19], that only considered double-blind, randomized, controlled clinical studies with parallel group design in order to minimize any observer bias due to non-blinded evaluation of echocardiograms or treatment of patients, conflict of interest with potential sponsors, and the so called effect of a self-fulfilling hypothesis.

Out of a large sample size of 471 studies identified by extensive literature search, only 39 studies of presumably high scientific quality, published until July 1995 fulfilled the preset inclusion criteria. Final analysis of studies included 1394 patients, with 189 (age: 51 ± 3 years) in the placebo arm and 1205 (age: 54 ± 8 years) in the active treatment arm. Overall, significant differences were observed in reduction of both systolic and diastolic blood pressure in parallel to those of left ventricular mass index between placebo and active antihypertensive treatment groups.

Independent determinants for the reduction of left ventricular mass were decline in blood pressure, pretreatment left ventricular mass, duration of antihypertensive pharmacologic therapy, and antihypertensive drug class. After adjustment for different durations of treatment, left ventricular mass decreased with ACE-inhibitors by 13% (95% CI: 9.9–

16.8%), with calcium channel blockers by 9% (95% CI: 5.5–13.1%), with β-blockers by 6% (95% CI: 2.3–8.6%) and with diuretics by 7% (95% CI: 3.0–10.7%) at similar control of blood pressure. Overall, there existed a significant difference for drug classes in reduction of left ventricular mass and posterior wall thickness, but not for septal wall thickness. Direct comparisons revealed that ACE-inhibitors effected a greater decrease in left ventricular mass index than diuretics and β-blockers. No significant difference was found between ACE-inhibitors and calcium channel blockers.

An update of the meta-analysis by Schmieder et al, comprising studies until december 1996 confirms the data discussed above. Thirteen recently published controlled clinical studies, in particular studies with calcium channel blockers of long duration with a double-blind, randomized, parallel group design were additionally evaluated. The results of all 50 studies comprised a total of 1715 essential hypertensive patients with 165 (age: 50 ± 3 years) in the placebo arm and 1550 (age: 56 ± 10 years) in the active treatment arm.

The update version found a reduction of left ventricular mass by 12% (95% CI: 9.0–14.5%) for ACE-inhibitors, by 11% (95% CI: 7.8–13.7%) for calcium channel blockers, by 5% (95% CI: 1.2–7.3%) for β-blockers and by 8% (95% CI: 3.9–11.1%) for diuretics (Figure 1).

In comparison to our first meta-analysis, one study was reevaluated due to concomitant treatment with an exercise program[13]. Between July 1995 and December 1996, thirteen double blind, randomized, controlled clinical trials have been carried out. Of note, nine treatment arms were with calcium channel blockers with five studies lasting for one year. This explains, that there was no need to adjust for different duration of treatment, as done in our first meta-analysis. The new update of our meta-analysis with clearly more treatment groups randomized to calcium channel blockers revealed an almost similar decrease of left ventricular mass for ACE-inhibitors and calcium channel blockers. Two studies analyzing dihydropyridine-calcium channel blockers to non-dihydropyridine-calcium channel blockers observed no difference between these two subclasses of calcium channel blockers.

CONCLUSIONS

Both ACE-inhibitors and calcium channel blockers were more effective in reducing left ventricular mass than β-blockers, with diuretics in the intermediate range. Blockade of the renin-angiotensin-aldosterone system as an effective measure to reduce left ventricular hypertrophy is supported by numerous experimental data that documented growth stimulating effects of angiotensin II on the myocardium. Although intracellular accumulation of calcium has been reported to exert growth stimulating properties, the experimental evidence that blockade of calcium channels exerts reduction of left ventricular mass in addition to its blood pressure lowering properties is less profound, but supported by a most recent double blind, randomized clinical trial (Schmieder 1997, unpublished data).

Regarding the available data, blockade of angiotensin II by ACE-inhibitors emerged as the most potent approach for the treatment of left ventricular hypertrophy. According to our updated meta-analysis calcium channel blockers emerged to be similarly potent or according to other studies to be at least the second choice of drug class. Despite early expressed scepticism by some researchers, diuretics are able to reduce left ventricular mass, whereas β-blockers are the least effective drug class. The latter was nearly uniformly found.

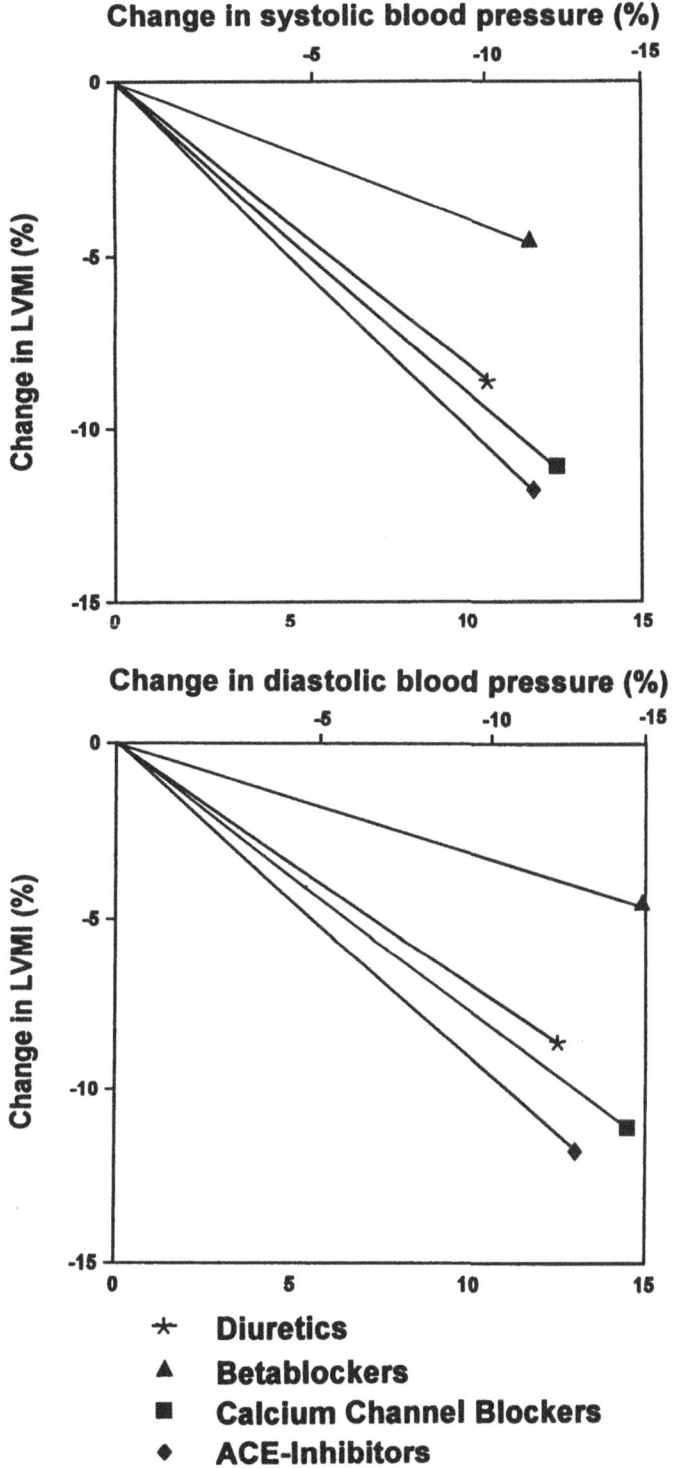

Figure 1. Meta-analysis: antihypertensive therapy and LVH-regression.

REFERENCES

1. Levy D, Garrison RJ, Savage DD, Kannel WB, Castelli WP. Prognostic implications of echocardiographically determined left ventricular mass in the Framingham Heart Study. *N Engl J Med 1990; 322: 1561–66*
2. Kannel WB. Left ventricular hypertrophy as a risk factor: the Framingham experience. *J Hypertens 1991; 9 (Suppl): S3–S9*
3. Koren MJ, Savage DD, Casale PN, Laragh JH, Devereux RB. Changes in left ventricular mass predict risk in essential hypertension [abstract]. *Ciculation 1990; 82 (suppl III): 20*
4. Muiesan ML, Salvetti M, Rizzoni D, et al. Association of change in left ventricular mass with prognosis during long-term antihypertensive treatment. *J Hypertens 1996; 13: 1091–95*
5. Jennings, G, Dart A, Meredith I, Korner P, Laufer E, Dewar E. Effects of exercise and other non-pharmacologic measures on blood pressure and cardiac hypertrophy. *J Cardiovasc Pharmacol 1991; 17 (suppl 2): S70–S74*
6. MacMahon SW, McDonald GJ, Bernstein L, et al. Comparison of weight reduction with metoprolol and treatment of hypertension in young overweight patients. *Lancet 1986; 1: 1233–1236*
7. MacMahon SW, Wilcken DEL, McDonald GJ. The effect of weight reduction on left ventricular mass: a randomized controlled trial in young, overweight hypertensive patients. *N Engl J Med 1986; 314: 334–339*
8. Liebson PR, Grandits TA, Dianzumba S, et al. Comparison of five antihypertensive monotherapies and placebo for change in left ventricular mass in patients receiving nutritional hygienic therapy in the Treatment of Mild Hypertension Study (TOMHS). *Circulation 1995; 91: 698–706*
9. Ferrara LA, DeSimone G, Pasanisi F, et al. Left ventricular mass reduction during salt depletion in arterial hypertension. *Hypertension 1984; 6: 755–759*
10. Jula AM, Karanko HM. Effects on left ventricular hypertrophy of long-term non-pharmacological treatment with sodium restriction in mild to moderate hypertension. *Circulation 1994; 89: 1023–1031*
11. Neaton JD, Grimm RH, Prieas RJ, et al. Treatment of Mild Hypertension Study. Final results. *JAMA 1993; 270: 713–724*
12. Manolio TA, Levy D, Garrison RJ et al. Relation of alcohol intake to left ventricular mass: The Framingham Study. *J Am Coll Cardiol 1991; 17: 717–721*
13. Kelemen MH, Effron MB, Valenti SA, Stewart KJ. Exercise training combined with antihypertensive drug therapy. Effects on lipids, blood pressure and left ventricular mass *JAMA 1990; 263: 2766–2771*
14. Senior R, Imbs JL, Bory M, et al. Indapamide reduces hypertensive left ventricular hypertrophy: an international multicenter study. *J Cardiovasc Pharmacol 1993; 22 (suppl 6): S106–S110*
15. Gottdiener JS. Hypertensive heart disease in blacks. *Cardiovasc Clin 1991; 21: 133–134*
16. Sacks HS, Berrier J, Reitman D, Ancona-Berc VA, Chalmers TC. Meta-analyses of randomized controlled trials. *N Engl J Med 1987; 316: 450–455*
17. Dahlöf B, Pennert K, Hansson L. Reversal of left ventricular hypertrophy in hypertensive patients: a meta-analysis of 109 treatment studies. *Am J Hypertens 1992; 5: 95–110*
18. Cruickshank J, Lewis J, Moore EV, Dodd C. Reversibility of left ventricular hypertrophy by differing types of antihypertensive thearpy. *J Hum Hypertens 1992; 6: 85–90*
19. Schmieder RE, Martus P, Klingbeil A. Reversal of left ventricular hypertrophy in essential hypertension: a meta-analysis of randomized double-blind studies. *JAMA 1996; 275: 1507–1513*

PROGNOSTIC SIGNIFICANCE OF LEFT VENTRICULAR HYPERTROPHY REGRESSION

Enrico Agabiti-Rosei[*] and Maria Lorenza Muiesan

Cattedra Semeiotica e Metodologia Medica
Universita' di Brescia

INTRODUCTION

In hypertension, left ventricular hypertrophy (LVH) is initially a useful compensatory process, that represents an adaptation to increased ventricular wall stress; however, it is also the first step toward the development of overt clinical disease, such as congestive heart failure, cardiac dysrrhythmias, and ischemic heart disease. In fact, the Framingham Study has shown that once LVH is recognized clinically it constitutes a powerful independent risk factor for future cardiovascular morbid events whether assessed by ECG or echocardiography, the latter being a specific, repeatable and far more sensitive measure of LVH[1,2]. The echocardiographic technique has demonstrated that the geometric adaptation of the left ventricle to increased cardiac load may be different among patients. Concentric hypertrophy is characterized by increased mass and increased relative wall thickness, whereas eccentric hypertrophy is characterized by increased mass and relative wall thickness < 0.45; on the other hand, concentric remodeling occurs when there is increased thickness with respect to radius, without increased LV mass. Concentric hypertrophy appears to carry the highest risk and eccentric hypertrophy an intermediate risk, whereas concentric remodeling is probably associated with a smaller, albeit still consistent risk[3].

Several pathophysiological changes and clinical alterations consequent to the development of myocite growth and fibrosis that characterize hypertensive LVH have been invoked to explain the association with increased risk: these include an impairment of diastolic function, and, probably, also of systolic performance during exercise; a reduced coronary reserve and a predisposition to ventricular arrhythmias. Autonomic nervous system activity dysfunction, and reduced cardiac responsiveness to β-adrenergic stimulation have also been reported. In addition, LVH may be an indicator of vascular structural

* Address for correspondence: Prof Enrico Agabiti-Rosei, Cattedra Semeiotica e Metodologia Medica, UOP Scienze Mediche, Universita' di Brescia, c/o Spedali Civili, 1a Medicina, Brescia 25100, Italy. Telephone and fax: 39-30-3384348, e-mail: Agabiti@master cci.unibs.it

Hypertension and the Heart, edited by Zanchetti et al.
Plenum Press, New York, 1997

199

changes in both large and small arteries. Since LVH in hypertension represents an independent risk factor for cardiovascular morbidity and mortality, the possibility of reversing or even preventing LVH through a decrease of elevated BP values and modification of some other pathogenetic factors is likely to represent a major therapeutic goal for the treatment of hypertensive patients[4].

REVERSIBILITY OF LVH BY ANTIHYPERTENSIVE TREATMENT

Several hundred human or experimental studies have established that blood pressure reduction may reverse hypertensive LVH. It has been observed that different classes of antihypertensive drugs do not have the same effect in reducing LV mass, probably because, beyond the control of blood pressure, they may differently interfere with several non hemodynamic factors, including the renin-angiotensin and adrenergic nervous system activity and other growth factors, may contribute to the development and the reversal of LVH. This was suggested for the first time by the elegant studies of Sen and Tarazi[5] in spontaneously hypertensive rats (SHR); they observed that, although methyldopa, hydralazine and minoxidil resulted in an equivalent reduction of BP, ventricular mass was reduced by methyldopa but actually increased by minoxidil. They suggested that the failure of LVH regression by direct vasodilators may be a result of adrenergic stimulation. In man, few studies with sympatholytics, including methyldopa, clonidine and reserpine have been found to be associated with significant regression of LVH; in addition, one study reported that methyldopa led to a significant reduction of LV mass despite only small changes of BP[6]. On the other hand, vasodilators such as minoxidil and hydralazine did not induce a significant regression of LVH despite a satisfactory control of BP[7]. Converting enzyme inhibitors which reduce BP through peripheral vasodilatation but, in contrast to other vasodilators, do not induce a reflex adrenergic stimulations, were consistently found able to reduce LV mass. Some conflicting results have been reported with the use of diuretics and β-blockers, although most studies with these agents have reported that their antihypertensive effect is associated to a reduction of LV mass. The different pharmacological classes of calcium antagonists were all found able to reduce significantly LV mass, despite the fact that dihydropyridine compounds are sometimes associated with a measurable, albeit small, adrenergic stimulation[8].

In order to extract the maximal amount of information from such studies, Dahlof et al.[9] performed a meta-analysis of all relevant published studies on echocardiographically demonstrable reversal of LVH obtained through the use of antihypertensive drugs. A total of 109 studies comprising more than 2.300 patients were considered.

They concluded that ACE inhibitors, β-blockers and calcium antagonists all reduced LVH by reversing wall hypertrophy, whereas diuretics reduced LVM mainly through a decrease in LV volume. The authors calculated in their meta-analysis that the reduction of LVM was most pronounced with ACE inhibitors. Similar conclusions were reached by Cruickshank et al.[10] in their meta-analysis of 104 published studies. They observed that significant LV mass reduction was never obtained in studies using direct-acting vasodilators and only in a minority of trials using diuretic therapy, as compared to virtually all trials using ACE inhibitors, and a majority of those using calcium antagonists, beta- and/or alpha adrenoceptor blockers. However, these data cannot be considered definitive because of serious limitations of most available studies. In fact, most of the studies considered in meta-analysis were of a small size (average 10 to 15 subjects/study), open, non randomized, non comparative. Further problems include short study duration (less than six months), poor characterizations of patients, lack of blinding of echocardiographic measurements[11]. Schmieder[12] found only 39 out of 471 (or 8%) of available studies that were randomized, double-blind, parallel group comparisons, performed in patients with WHO class I or II hypertension without concomitant cardiac disease. His analysis indicated that 1) the fall in BP and the initial LV mass determines the reduction of LVH, and that 2) both ACE inhibitors and calcium antagonists do better than the β-blockers or diuretics in this respect. In addition, it should be considered that the efficacy of different classes of drugs on specific populations may modify the final effect on LVH. Thus Dahlof et al.[13] observed a greater effect on LV mass of ACE inhibitors in comparison with diuretics in a group of 28 caucasian men, while Shulman et al.[14] found that a calcium antagonists induced greater reduction of LV mass than did a β-blocker in a group of 42 elderly patients, predominantly African Americans. These results are in keeping with the expected differences in efficacy of different classes of antihypertensive drugs between black and white, young and elderly patients.

In order to add useful information to the existing knowledge what we really need are large, randomized, double-blinded studies able to compare the effect of a drug vs placebo, or of two different antihypertensive drugs.

In the large multicenter trial TOMHS (Treatment of Mild Hypertension Study)[15] a total of 819 mildly hypertensive subjects underwent an echocardiographic study at baseline and subsequently at least once during the four year treatment period. All participants received a highly effective nutritional-hygienic intervention. Approximately seventy per cent (668/819) of patients were randomized to additional active therapy with low doses of either a representative diuretic, β-blocker, alpha blocker, ACE-inhibitor or calcium antagonist. In TOMHS, the nutritional-hygienic therapy was very effective, and reduced BP and LV mass so successfully that only limited information about the effects of antihypertensive drugs on the heart could be obtained. In fact, only chlortalidone slightly reduced further LV mass (minus 7 grams in respect to placebo) and did so mainly by decrease of LV volume.

We have carried out a study designed to compare the effect of BP lowering by the ACE-inhibitor Ramipril with that of a similar BP reduction by the β-blocker Atenolol on LV hypertrophy[16]. The study was multicentric, with central blind readings of the echocardiograms, in accordance with the PROBE (Perspective Randomized Open Blinded Endpoint) design. From 193 patients enrolled in 16 centers, 111 had echocardiograms that could be quantitatively evaluated. The study demonstrated that for the same reduction of BP, LVM was significantly reduced by Ramipril only. Thus, the conclusion of this study is in keeping with the results of the metaanalyses performed by both Dahlof et al. and Cruickshank et al.

Gottdiener et al.[17] have recently published the results of the Veterans Affairs Cooperative Study on Single-drug therapy in Mild–Moderate Hypertension that was designed in order to compare the effects on echocardiographic LV mass of antihypertensive monotherapy with six different agents in a group of 584 male hypertensive patients (58% black race). After one year of treatment, the greatest reduction of LV mass were obtained by captopril (-15g, $p = .05$), and hydrochlorothiazide(-14 g, $p = .08$), while no significant changes were observed with atenolol, diltiazem, clonidine and prazosin. However, the lack of women and the high drop-out rate that left less than 40 patients in each treatment arm, seem to limit the consistency of the conclusions of this study.

In order to add useful information to the existing knowledge what we really need are large, randomized, blinded studies, able to compare the effect of two different antihypertensive drugs. At present several such trials have begun in hypertensive patients.

PROGNOSTIC SIGNIFICANCE OF LVH REGRESSION

The pathophysiological consequences of the increased LV mass reduction could explain the potential reduction of cardiovascular events associated with LVH regression. In fact, it has been shown that reduction of LV mass does not impair systolic function, as assessed by the usual echocardiographic indices of LV performance[18-20]. Controversial results have been obtained regarding the changes of diastolic filling after reversal of LVH, probably related to the use of different methodologies; in several studies an improvement of the diastolic filling pattern has been demonstrated with the reduction of cardiac hypertrophy. A change toward normalization of autonomic nervous system activity[21], and in particular of cardiopulmonary reflexes[22], and a possible reduction of arrhythmias[23,24] have also been described in association with the reversal of LVH. In addition, a possible improvement of coronary flow reserve has been found associated with LVH regression as well[25].

To date only four studies have examined the potential clinical prognostic benefit from regression of LVH. Levy et al.[26] analyzed the data from 524 participants to the Framingham study in which the diagnosis of LVH was based on ECG criteria. They observed that the decrease of ECG LVH toward normal, assessed by biannual serial examination, over a mean follow-up period of 5 years, was associated with a reduction of cardiovascular risk. Two other studies have measured LV mass changes by echocardiography. The initial study, by Koren et al.[27], presently available only in abstract form, has shown that in 166 hypertensive patients studied by echocardiography and followed up for 5.5 years, cardiovascular events occurred in 16% of patients whose LV mass increased from baseline and in only 6% of patients whose LV mass decreased. In a second relevant study by Yurenev et al.[28], 304 patients, all with LVH or high normal LV mass at baseline echocardiographic examination, were followed for 4 years and retrospectively divided in two groups, according to the presence or absence of cardiovascular complications; LVH regression or progression was strongly associated with the likelihood of morbid events; in fact LVH resulted significantly reduced only in the group without complications. However, in this study there was no central blind reading of echocardiograms.

In a more recent study[29], a total of 151 uncomplicated hypertensive patients were followed and recalled after 7–13 years (on average 10 years follow-up). A blind reading of all echocardiographic baseline and follow-up tracings was performed and echocardiograms that had been performed for clinical purposes during the follow up were also assessed.

All patients were not taking therapy when examined at baseline and received antihypertensive medication as prescribed by their general practitioner during all the follow up period. In the 151 patients who completed the follow up with final echocardiogram and clinical evaluation, 23 had a documented non fatal cardiovascular event. LVH was present at baseline in 49% of males and 36% of females (44% of total patients). Patients were grouped according to the presence or absence of LVH at baseline and at follow-up: with normal LVMI at both examinations (n = 78), with LVH at baseline and regression of hypertrophy (n = 32), with LVH at baseline and at follow up (n = 34), and with normal LV mass at baseline who developed cardiac hypertrophy (n = 7).

At baseline and at follow up no significant differences were observed between groups for other traditional risk factors (lipid and glucose plasma concentration, smoking habits, clinic systolic and diastolic blood pressure values).

Life-table analyses showed significant differences in event-free survival between patients of the three groups (Fig 1).

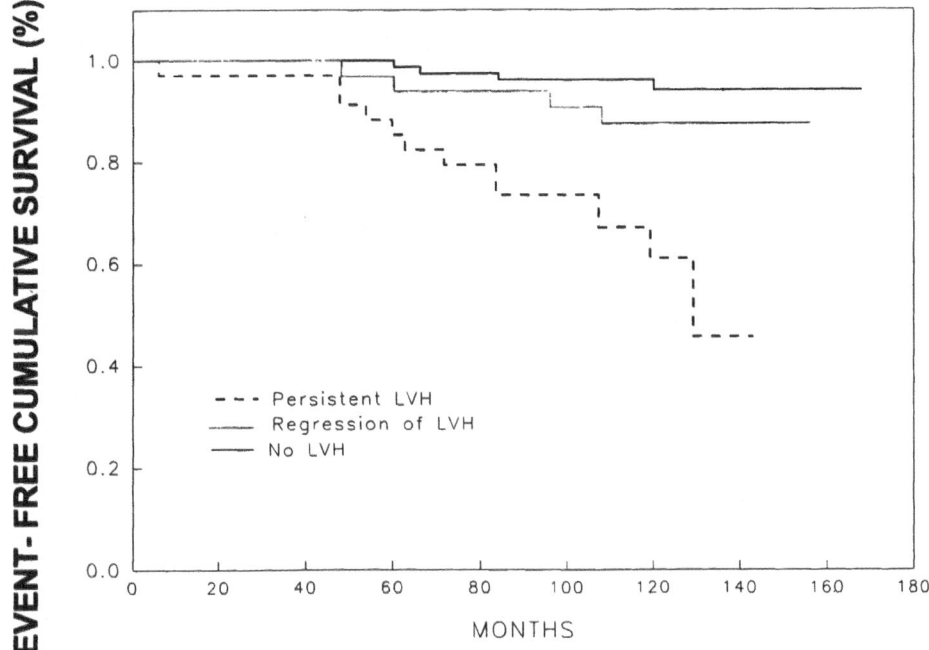

Figure 1. Cardiovascular event-free survival curve in patients with LVH persistence (dotted line), in patients with regression of LVH (continuous gray line) and in patients with normal LV mass at baseline and at follow-up (continuous black line). (Reference 29.)

In patients with regression or persistence of LVH the incidence of cardiovascular events was also examined according to percent changes of LV mass index (taking into account our laboratory variability), despite or not a normalization of LV mass index was obtained at follow up: 13 events were observed in patients with a decrease of less than 10% or an increase of LV mass index (n = 22), while 4 events occurred in those with a decrease greater than 10% in respect to baseline (n = 44).

The relative importance of prognostic factors such as age, sex, clinic systolic or diastolic blood pressure, presence of LVH, dyslipidemia, presence of diabetes, smoking status at baseline and/or at follow up was evaluated and the association of these variables to cardiovascular risk was assessed by univariate analyses. Only age and LVH status resulted significantly associated to the occurrence of non fatal cardiovascular events, while male sex was of borderline significance. No significant interaction between sex, age and LVH status was detected. The relative risk for cardiovascular events, adjusted for age, sex and systolic blood pressure, was significantly greater only in patients with persistence of LVH, in respect to the other two groups.

After adjustment for traditional cardiovascular risk factors the cumulative incidence of morbid cardiovascular events was significantly higher in the group of patients without regression of LVH; in addition, the presence of LVH at the end of follow-up study resulted the most important factor related to cardiovascular events.

In conclusion, the available data, on more than 1100 patients strongly suggest that the lack of decrease or the increase of LV mass after antihypertensive treatment is associated with a higher risk of CV events; in addition, the increased risk is significantly reduced and seems to be almost normalized by complete regression of LVH.

Future studies will provide definitive information whether differences in reversal of LVH exist among various antihypertensive drugs, including the new class of Angiotensin II receptor antagonists. At present time, ACE inhibitors and calcium antagonists seem to be more effective than other antihypertensive classes of drugs for the reduction of LV mass.

Ongoing treatment trials and epidemiological studies will adequately assess the relationship between changes of LV mass and subsequent prognosis, in different populations, taking into account changes of blood pressure, measured in the clinic and by ambulatory monitoring, treatment type and other variables that may influence the results, such as race or gender. These studies will provide additional and definitive information in order to solve the question as whether or not LVH changes can be considered an established intermediate end-point for the development of cardiovascular events in hypertensive patients.

REFERENCES

1. Kannel WB, Gordon T, Offut T. Left ventricular hypertrophy by electrocardiogram. Prevalence, incidence and mortality in the Framingham study. Ann. Int. Med., 71: 89 (1969).
2. Levy D, Garrison RJ, Savage DD, Kannel WB, Castelli WP. Prognostic implications of echocardiographically determined left ventricular mass in the Framingham Heart Study. N. Engl. J Med, 322: 1561–1566 (1990).
3. Koren MJ Devereux RB, Casale PN et al. Relation of left ventricular mass and geometry to morbidity and mortality in uncomplicated essential hypertension Ann Intern Med, 114: 345–352 (1991).
4. Zanchetti A. Goals of antihypertensive treatment: prevention of cardiovascular events and prevention of organ damage. Blood Pressure, 1: 201–211 (1992).
5. Sen S, Tarazi RC. Reversal of myocardial hypertrophy and influence of the adrenergic system. Am J Physiol, 244: H97–H101 (1983).
6. Fouad FM, Nakashima Y, Tarazi RC, Salcedo EE. Reversal of left ventricular hypertrophy in hypertensive patients treated with methyldopa. lack of association to blood pressure control. Am J Cardiol, 49: 759–801 (1982).
7. Drayer JIM, Gardin JM, Weber MA, Aronow WS. Cadiac muscle mass during vasodilation therapy in hypertension. Clin Pharmacol Ther, 33: 727–732 (1983).
8. Agabiti-Rosei E, Muiesan ML, Romanelli G, et al. Reversal of cardiac hypertrophy by long term treatment with calcium antagonists in hypertensive patients. J Cardiovasc Pharmacol, 12(suppl 6): 75–77 (1988).
9. Dahlöf B, Pennert K, Hansson L. Reversal of Left Ventricular Hypertrophy in Hypertensive Patients. A Metaanalysis of 109 Treatment Studies. Am J Hypertens, 5: 95–110 (1992).
10. Cruickshank J.M. Lewis J, Moore V, Dodd A. Reversibility of left ventricular hypertrophy by differing types of antihypertensive therapy. J. Human Hypertens,6: 85–90 (1992).
11. Agabiti-Rosei E, Muiesan ML, Castellano M. Methodology of studies on reversal of left ventricular hypertrophy. High Blood Press, 2 (suppl 1):11–13 (1993).
12. Schmieder AM. Reversal of left ventricular hypertrophy in essential hypertension: a meta-analysis of randomized double blind studies. JAMA, 275: 1507–1513 (1996).
13. Dahlöf B, Hansson L: The influence of antihypertensive therapy on the structural vascular amplifying mechanism in essential hypertension. Different effects of Enalapril and Hydrochlorothiazide. J Hypertens, 10: 1513–1524 (1992).
14. Schulman S, Weiss J Becker L et al. The effects of antihypertensive therapy on left ventricular mass in elderly patients. New Eng J Med, 322, 19: 1350–1356 (1990).
15. Neaton JD, Grimm RH, Prineas RJ, Stamler J, Grandits GA, Emler P, Cutler JA, Flack JM, Schoenberger JA, McDonald R, Lewis CE, Liebson PR, on behalf of Treatment of Mild Hypertension Study Research Group. Treatment of Mild Hypertension Study. Final results. JAMA, 270: 713–724 (1993).
16. Agabiti-Rosei E, Ambrosioni E, DalPalu' C, Muiesan ML, Zanchetti A on behalf of the RACE Study group. Ace-inhibitor ramipril is more effective than β-blocker atenolol in reducing left ventricular mass in hypertension. Results of the RACE (ramipril cardioprotective evaluation) study. J Hypertens, 13: 1325–1335 (1995).
17. Gottdiener JS, Reda DJ, Massie BM, Materson BJ, Williams DW, Anderson RJ, for the VA Cooperative Study group on antihypertensive Agents. Effect of single-drug therapy on reduction of left ventricular mass in mild to moderate hypertension Comparison of six antihypertensive agents. The Departement of Veterans Affairs Cooperative Study Group on Antihypertensive Agents. Circulation, 95: 2007–2014 (1997).

18. Trimarco B, De Luca N, Ricciardelli B, Rosiello G, Volpe M, Condorelli G, Lembo G, Condorelli M. Cardiac function in systemic hypertension before and after reversal of left ventricular hypertrophy. Am J Cardiol, 62: 745–750 (1988).

19. Schmieder RE, Messerli FH, Sturgill D, Garavaglia GE, Nunez BD. Cardiac performance after reduction of myocardial hypertrophy. Am J Med, 87: 22–27 (1989).

20. Muiesan ML, Agabiti-Rosei E, Romanelli G, et al. Improved left ventricular systolic and diastolic function after regression of cardiac hypertrophy, treatment withdrawal and revedelopment of hypertension. J. Cardiovasc. Pharmacol, 17: 179s–181s (1991).

21. Agabiti Rosei E. Romanelli G, Muiesan ML et al. Impaired response of the hypertrophied left ventricle to beta adrenergic stimulation in hypertensive patients. Circulation, 70 (Suppl. II): 61 (1984).

22. Grassi G Gianattasio C, Cleroux J, Cuspidi C, Sampieri L, Mancia G Cardiopulmonary reflex before and after regression of left ventricular hypertrophy in essential hypertension. Hypertension, 12: 227–231 (1988).

23. Messerli FH Ventura HO, Elizardi DJ, Dunn FG, Frolich ED. Hypertension and sudden death: disparate effects of calcium entry blocker and diuretic therapy on cardiac disrrhythmias. Arch. Intern. Med, 149: 1263–1267 (1989).

24. Muiesan ML Rizzoni D, Rulli R, Calebich S, Malerba M, Porteri E, Agabiti-Rosei E. Effect of changes in blood pressure and left ventricular mass induced by antihypertensive treatment on ventricular arrhythmias in essential hypertension. J Hypertens, 11 (suppl 5): s300–301 (1993).

25. Magrini F, Reggiani P, Roberts N, Meazza R, Ciulla M, Zanchetti A. Effects of angiotensin blockade on coronary circulation and coronary reserve. Am J Med, 84: 55–60 (1988).

26. Levy D, Salomon M, D'Agostino R, Belanger A, Kannel WB. Prognostic implications of baseline electro-cardiographic features and their serial changes in subjects with left ventricular hypertrophy. Circulation, 90: 1786–93 (1994).

27. Koren MJ, Savage DD, Casale PN, Laragh JH, Devereux RB. Changes in left ventricular mass predict risk in essential hypertension. Circulation, 82 (suppl III): III29 (Abstract) (1990).

28. Yurenev AP, Dyakonova HG, Novikov ID, Vitols A, Pahl L, Haynemann G et al. Management of essential hypertension in patients with different degrees of left ventricular hypertrophy multicenter trial Am J Hypertens, 5 (suppl): 182s–189s (1992).

29. Muiesan ML, Salvetti M, Rizzoni D, Castellano M, Donato F, Agabiti-Rosei E. Association of change in LV mass with prognosis during long-term antihypertensive treatment. J Hypertens 13: 1091–1105 (1995).

HYPERTENSION AND CORONARY MICROVASCULAR DISEASE[*]

B. E. Strauer and B. Schwartzkopff

Med. Klinik and Policlinic B
Heinrich Heine University
Moorenstr. 5
40225 Düsseldorf, Germany

INTRODUCTION

Arterial hypertension represents the most frequent kind of left ventricular pressure overload in man. As former studies in our clinic have shown, three distinct types of left ventricular hypertrophy may occur: concentric — irregular — eccentric (1). The main functional features of these different types of hypertrophy imply: (I) Left ventricular systolic ejection fraction is normal, despite of significant or excessive increase in left ventricular muscle mass as long as ventricular volume is not increased. Diastolic function is impaired at all stages of LV hypertrophy. (II) There is an inverse relationship between systolic wall stress, i.e. left ventricular afterload, and left ventricular function. (III) Systolic wall stress is directly correlated with LV myocardial oxygen consumption. (IV) In hypertensive hypertrophy there is, even at normal coronary arteriogram, significant reduction in coronary reserve (2) (Fig. 1). Both, reduction in coronary reserve and diastolic dysfunction already may occur in the prehypertrophic state of hypertensive heart disease.

MYOCARDIAL STRUCTURE IN HYPERTENSIVE HEART DISEASE

In order to further analyze the structural hypertrophic characteristics, morphometric studies from human transvenous septal biopsies were examined in more than 50 hypertensive patients. It could be demonstrated that the morphological consequences of chronic pressure overload refer to myocardial, to interstitial and to changes of the intramural coronary arterioles.

---

[*] With support of SFB 242 "Koronare Herzkrankheit — Prävention und Therapie akuter Komplikationen."

Hypertension and the Heart, edited by Zanchetti et al.
Plenum Press, New York, 1997

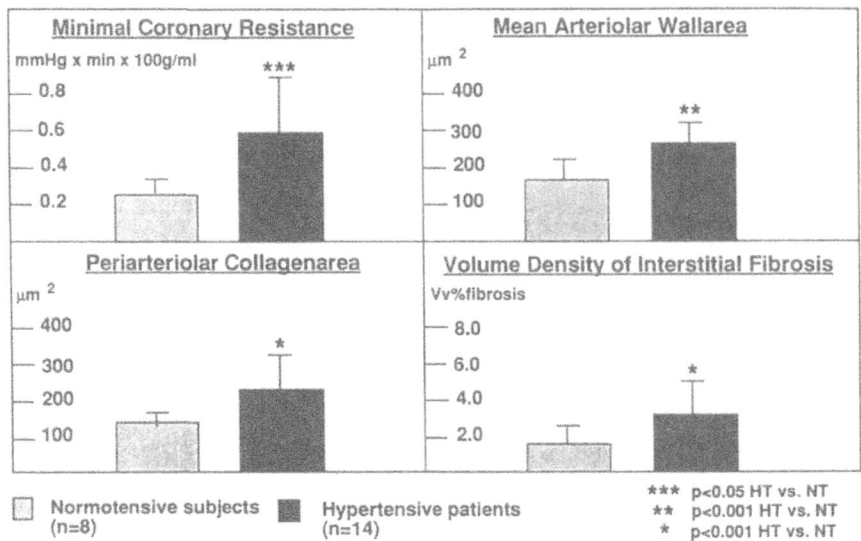

Figure 1. In hypertensive heart disease even without coronary artery disease, there is an inappropriate decrease in coronary resistance, a reduced coronary blood flow after dipyridamole (0.5 mg/kg body weight) resulting in a reduced coronary reserve (1,2).

Myocytes represent the main compartment building 70% of the myocardial mass, but it has to be taken into consideration that myocytes only account for 25% of the cells in the myocardium (3). Increase in wall tension is followed by an augmentation in myocyte cross-section area leading to ventricular wall thickening and reduced wall tension in the initial state (1,2). Thus, myocytic hypertrophy represents an adaptive, appropriate response to increased left ventricular pressure from the standpoint of wall stress regulation. On the other hand, during myocardial hypertrophy, isoforms of fetal contractile proteins, such as β-myosin heavy chain, β-troponin, and skeletal actin, are expressed (4,5). Myocardial hypertrophy therefore is not merely a quantitative augmentation of normal contractile protein production; it reflects reexpression of an early developmental stage of myocardium; the ability of the myocardium to generate new contractile proteins is therefore eventually exhausted, terminating cardiac function (4). Additionally, the increase in myocytic size may reduce oxygen diffusion and substrate supply, reducing intracellular energy generation. A loss of cardiomyocytes, mainly in the subendocardium, and the appearance of scars were reported in the late stage of left ventricular hypertrophy due to experimental arterial hypertension (6).

Structural alterations of the interstitium may be precursors of myocardial remodeling in hypertensive heart disease. The interstitium of the myocardium contains fibrillar connective tissue, which consists mainly of type I and III collagen (7). The fibrillar collagen network is an essential element for maintaining the structural integrity and architecture of the myocardium during systole and diastole, delivering the stress developed by sarcomeres to the ventricular cavity, and distributing diastolic filling stress throughout the ventricle so at least adjacent myocytes are at equivalent levels of stretch. An abnormal increase of collagen (e.g., fibrosis) and its inelastic properties are responsible for increased myocardial stiffness (7).

An increase in interstitial collagen is one of the earliest structural changes in the course of the development of hypertensive heart disease. In established hypertensive hypertrophy, the collagen content, i.e. the amount of interstitial fibrosis, is significantly increased. However, it is important to emphasize that even in hypertensive patients without LV hypertrophy, i.e. in hypertensive left ventricles in the pre-hypertrophic state, there is an increase in collagen content (8). This predisposes to diastolic dysfunction, regarded to be an early indicator of hypertensive heart disease.

The further and clinically important early indicator of alterations in hypertensive heart refers to coronary arteries and arterioles.

Intramural coronary vessels with a luminal diameter of less than 100 μm mainly control coronary blood flow and are regarded as resistance vessels (9). These vessels constitute more than 70 percent of the intramural arterial tree, and a loss in branches (rarefaction) or inadequate growth in relation to hypertrophy of myocytes may diminish oxygen and substrate delivery. Furthermore, structural alterations of the vessel wall have been discussed for years in regard to increase vascular resistance (10,11). In right septal endomyocardial biopsies of 30 patients with arterial hypertension and angina pectoris in the absence of coronary macroangiopathy, we observed wall thickening of intramyocardial arterioles, compared to that of 10 heart donors with no evidence of heart disease. Even in hypertensive individuals without LVH, thickening of the intramyocardial arteriolar wall was observed (8). Therefore it has been assumed that vascular hypertophy is controlled independently from ventricular hypertrophy (8,12) and be an early manifestation of hypertensive heart disease. The arteriolar wall consists mainly of smooth muscle cells and, to a small extent, extracellular matrix. Medial hypertrophy can be caused by hypertrophy or hyperplasia of smooth muscle cell, edema, and increased contents of collagens and other matrix components (i.e., elastin) (8,12,13–16). Other features include intimal hyalinization and endothelial hyperplasia (14). Vascular growth may be induced by many factors. Shear stress and mechanical stretch are reported to induce vascular growth (10). Furthermore hormonal stimulation and growth fac-

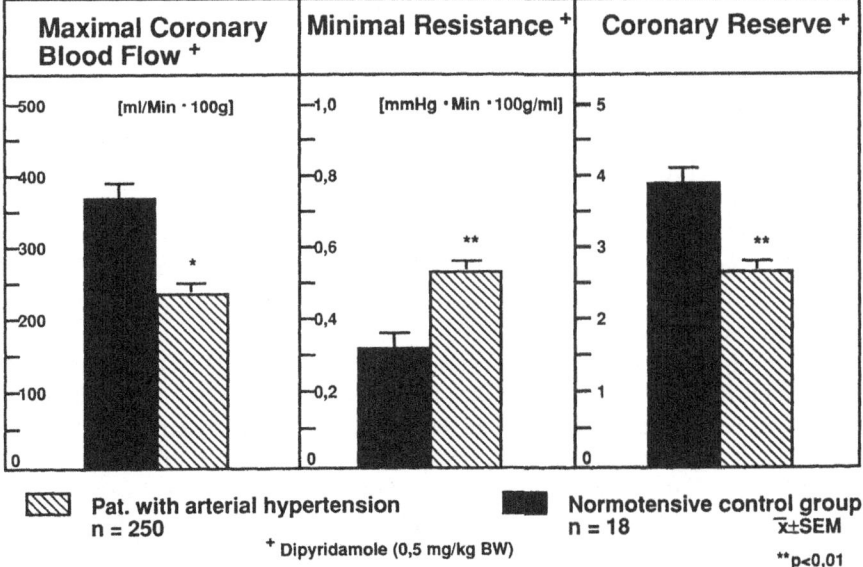

Figure 2. Structural analysis of right septal endomyocardial biopsies reveals in hypertensive heart disease an increase in arteriolar media area, in perivascular fibrosis and in total interstitial collagen content as compared with control subjects. This is associated with higher coronary resistance that is not explained by left ventricular end-diastolic pressure or left ventricular muscle mass (12).

tors are involved (13,15) that may act in endocrine, paracrine, and autocrine ways. The renin-angiotensin system, in particular, modulates the growth of vascular smooth muscle cells and reinforces the process of hypertensive cardiac remodeling via angiotensin II-mediated induction of proto-oncogenes and growth factors (15). Other growth factors, such as plateled-derived growth factor, have been found to modulate medial hypertrophy or hyperplasia.(16) Structural alterations of the intramural arteriolar tree may dispose or even induce myocardial ischemia. Wall hypertrophy at a small lumen is associated with reduced distensibilty and consecutively impairs vascular conductance. Furthermore, an increased wall/lumen ratio may predispose to vessel closures, as every contraction of the thickened vessel wall leads to ever-greater lumen reduction (17). Thus, limited coronary reserve and microvascular spasms could be the consequence of vascular hypertrophy. Furthermore in hypertensive heart disease, perivascular fibroblasts are activated generating collagen (7). In a quantitative morphometric study of autopsied hearts and in biopsy speciments from hypertensives, we observed a marked increase of periarteriolar fibrosis (12,18). This perivascular fibrosis was found in the left hypertensive ventricle as well as in the right, non-pressure-overloaded ventricle. In contrast, no perivascular fibrosis was observed with valvular aortic stenosis (18). Thus, in hypertensive heart disease, the medial wall of intramural arterial vessels as well as the adjacent interstitium are remodelled. These findings predispose to a limited vasodilator-capacity (Fig. 2).

FUNCTIONAL CONSEQUENCES OF MICROVASCULAR REMODELING

It has been reported by our group 20 years ago (1,2) that the coronary reserve in hypertensive heart disease is considerable reduced while coronary arteriogram is normal. Normal coronary reserve amounts 400–500 per cent, i.e. a normal heart may, following maximum coronary vasodilatation, e.g. by dipyridamole, reduce its minimum coronary resistance to 0,2–0,25 (mmHg×min×100g/ml). In coronary artery disease due to epicardial coronary stenosis, coronary reserve is impaired to approximately 200 per cent, i.e. reduced to around 50 per cent of the control value. This refers to both, normotensive and hypertensive coronary artery disease. In contrast, in hypertensives even with normal coronary arteriogram, coronary reserve is already reduced by 30–50 per cent compared with controls. This occurs even in young hypertensive patients between 20–30 years of age (Fig. 1). Accordingly, a significantly increased ischemic risk can be derived for hypertensive heart disease, and this even in young hypertensives. Myocardial ischemia might be one important factor for reported depressed relaxation in diastolic function regarded as an early indicator of hypertensive heart disease.

The reasons for the fundamental decrease in coronary reserve in hypertension are most probably multifactoral. However, as has been shown by human biopsy studies (8,12), one of the crucial reasons refer to vascular, especially to media hypertrophy of coronary resistance vessels in hypertension. In hypertension, various degree of vascular hypertrophy were bioptically found. The comparison of both, normal and excessively hypertrophied coronary arteries encourages the assumption, that coronary reserve is more reduced in the presence of vascular hypertrophy than in the absence of vascular structural changes. We could demonstrate, that, on contrast to normal vessel wall hypertensive patients with thickened walls of arterioles had considerable lower coronary reserve and marked elevation of the minimum coronary resistance following maximum coronary vasodilatation with dipyridamole (12). Thus, media hypertrophy of coronary arteries and arterioles plays an important role for the reduction in coronary reserve and hence, for the increased ischemic risk in hypertensive heart disease with normal coronary arteriogram. It has been demonstrated that both, reduced coronary reserve and diastolic dysfunction already occur in the pre-hypertrophic state, i.e. in hypertensive heart disease in which LV hypertrophy, as detected by echocardiography or by left ventriculography, is absent. However, in the pre-hypertrophic state, both, media hypertrophy of the coronary arterioles and increase in interstitial fibrosis are already present. Accordingly, these results emphasize the importance of these structural changes for the disturbances in coronary reserve that may induce diastolic dysfunction in terms of abnormal relaxation via ischemia or by collagen accumulation. They furthermore demonstrate, that collagen increase and vascular hypertrophy may precede the pressure-induced hypertrophic process and they finally indicate that there exist at least two early structural changes in hypertensive heart disease which are associated with two important clinical correlates, that may be considered manifestations of early cardiac involvement in arterial hypertension.

THERAPEUTIC INTERVENTIONS

Under preventive and therapeutic aspects the questions have to be raised, whether these structural changes are prone to antihypertensive therapy, i.e. whether they are potentially reversible by antihypertensive treatment and whether improvements of coronary reserve and of LV diastolic dysfunction occur. Accordingly, 122 patients were treated over a period of 9–12 months, 64 of them have been analyzed after long-term treatment at that moment. Invasive diagnostics included determinations of LV mass and of coronary reserve. Pharmacotherapeutic regimen consisted of bisoprolol (n = 15), of diltiazem (n = 16), of isradipine (n = 15) and of enalapril (n = 18). Dosages were titrated and maintained until normal blood pressure values were obtained. In a pilote study in hypertensive patients, we showed that after long-term antihypertensive therapy with the ACE inhibitor enalapril, regression of interstitial reactive fibrosis, including collagen type I and collagen type III, was achieved (19). Diez et al. (20), who administered antihypertensive therapy with lisinopril, reported reversal of LVH, decreased serum procollagen types I and III, and an improvement in Doppler echocardiographically determined diastolic function in hypertensive patients.

In a previous study we determined diastolic function of the left ventricle before and after 9–12 months after ACE-inhibitor therapy. Before therapy, relaxation time index was prolonged and the velocity of LV diameter increase was slowed down, so that depressed relaxation performance was present. Following long-term therapy with ACE-inhibitors, relaxation time index almost normalized to values as in normotensive patients and the maximum velocity of LV diastolic diameter increase also improved. Accordingly, the early structural abnormalities of collagen increase and of LV diastolic dysfunction could be reversed following long-term therapy with ACE-inhibitors.

The first evidence for restoration of the coronary microcirculation was reported in an open therapy study comparing the effect of calcium antagonists, ACE inhibition, and β-blockers on the coronary reserve, determined by the argon method (21,22,23,24). In hypertensive patients with microvascular angina pectoris, evidence of myocardial ischemia during the exercise tolerance test or thallium scan, but normal epicardial arteries, long-term therapy (9–12 months) with the ACE-inhibitor enalapril, the calcium antagonist diltiazem and isradipin, and the β-blocker bisoprolol was investigated. During antihypertensive therapy systolic and diastolic blood pressure was in the normotensive range in all three treatment groups. The left ventricular muscle mass decreased in all four groups simi-

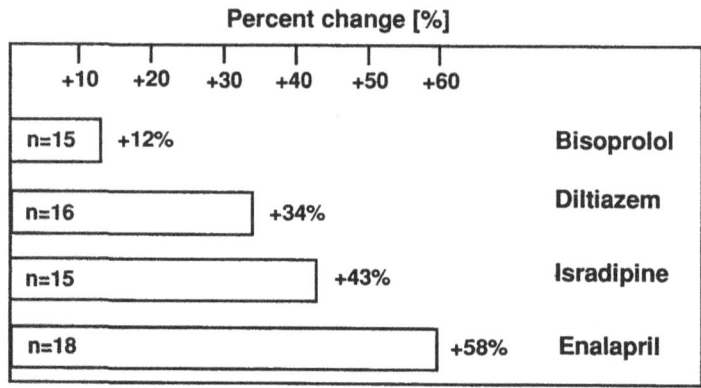

Figure 3. Improvement of coronary reserve after antihypertensive therapy with bisoprolol, diltiazem, isradipine and enalapril in an open study (21–24).

larly, by about 8–10 percent. Coronary reserve increased significantly in the bisoprolol group by 22%, diltiazem group by 34%, isradipin 45%, enalapril by 58%. (Fig. 3)

Possible structural mechanisms that lead to improvement in coronary reserve are regression of myocardial hypertrophy and fibrosis, a decrease in media wall thickening, an increase in capillary densitiy, and a decrease in perivascular fibrosis. Concomitant with reversal of hypertrophy are blood pressure reduction and a decrease in the myocardial component of coronary resistance. Consequently, it is difficult to differentiate between the influence of the myocardial factors (e.g., hypertrophy and fibrosis) and the vascular factors (e.g., medial wall thickness and capillary density) on the coronary flow reserve. An antiproliferative effect of ACE-inhibitors on the vessel wall has been found in experimental studies (25,26), that could explain the favorable disproportionate increase of coronary reserve compared with regression in LVH.

In our opinion the structural vascular changes in hypertensive heart disease may play an important role for the progression of left ventricular dysfunction and especially for the transition of the hypertrophic heart to the dilatative and eccentric state. In hypertensive hypertrophy, vascular structural changes follow pressure overload, resulting in an increase of the wall thickness/radius ration, in a reduction of coronary reserve and consequently in an impairment of the oxygen supply to the heart. Myocardial ischemia, however, leads to myocardial fibrosis, to micro- and macro necroses, to diastolic dysfunction, to an abnormally increased extravascular component of coronary resistance and hence to a further deterioration of myocardial oxygen supply and to worsening of LV systolic function by a self-perpetuating process or a vicious circle. Therefore, coronary small vessel disease in the hypertensive heart exhibits a central and crucial role for the induction of cardiac failure by means of the chronic and progressive impairment of myocardial oxygen supply. Conversely, the regression of the vascular structural changes may initiate the fundamental therapeutical step in preventing hypertensive failure.

REFERENCES

1. Strauer BE: Ventricular function and coronary hemodynamics in hypertensive heart disease. Am J Cardiol 1979; 44: 999–1006
2. Strauer BE: Coronary hemodynamics in hypertensive heart disease. Am J Med 1988; 84: 45–54

3. Anversa P, Ricci R, Olivetti G: Quantitative structural analysis of the myocardium during physiologic growth and induced cardiac hypertrophy. A review. J Am Coll Cardiol 1986; 7: 1140–1149

4. Katz A: cardiomyopathy of overload. A major determinant of prognosis in congestive heart failure. N Engl J Med 1990; 322: 100–110

5. Nadal-Ginard B, Mahdavi V: Molecular mechanisms of cardiac gene expression. pp 65–80. In: Strauer BE (ed): The heart in Hypertension. Springer-Verlag, New York 1993

6. Capasso JM, Palackal T, Olivetti G, Anversa P: Left ventricular failure — induced by long-term hypertension in rats. Circ Res 1990; 66: 1400–1412

7. Weber KT, Sun Y, Guarda E: Structural remodeling in hypertensive heart disease and the role of hormones. Hypertension 1994; 23: 869–877

8. Schwartzkopff B, Motz W, Knauer S, Frenzel H, Strauer BE: Morphometric investigations of intramyocardial arterioles in right septal endomyocardial biopsy of patients with arterial hypertension and left ventricular hypertrophy. J cardiovasc Pharmacol, Suppl 1 1992; 20: 12–17

9. Tillmanns H, Steinhausen M, Leinberger H, Thederau H, Kübler W: Pressure measurement in the terminal vascular bed of the epicardium of rats and cats. Cir Res 1981; 49: 1202–1211

10. Mulvany MJ: Vascular growth in hypertension. J Cardiovasc Pharmacol 1992; 22: 7–11

11. Opherk D, Mall G, Zebe H et al: Reduction of coronary reserve. A mechanism for angina pectoris in patients with arterial hypertension and normal arteries. Circulation 1984; 69: 1–7

12. Schwartzkopff B, Motz W, Frenzel H et al.: Structural and functional alterations of the intramyocardial coronary arterioles in patients with arterial hypertension. Circulation 1993; 88: 993–1003

13. Hudlicka O, Brown M, Egginton S: Angiogenesis in skeletal and cardiac muscle. Physiol Rev 1992; 72: 369–417

14. Moritz AR, Oldt MR: Arteriolar sclerosis in hypertensive and non-hypertensive individuals. Am J Pathol 1937; 13: 679–728

15. Dzau VJ, Gibbons GH, Cooke JP, Omoigui N: Vascular biology and medicine in the 1990's. Scope, concepts, potentials and perspectives. Circulation 1993; 87: 705–719

16. Scott-Burden T, Resink TJ, Baur U, Bürgin M, Bühler FR: Epidermal growth factor responsiveness in smooth muscle cells from hypertensive and normotensive rats. Hypertension 1989; 13: 295–304

17. James JN: Morphologic characteristics and functional significance of focal fibromuscular dysplasia of small coronary arteries. Am J Cardiol 1990; 65: 12G–22G

18. Schwartzkopff B, Frenzel H, Dieckerhoff J et al.: Morphometric investigation of humen myocardium in arterial hypertension and valvular aortic stenosis. Eur Heart J, Suppl D 1992; 13: 17–20

19. Schwartzkopff B, Motz W, Strauer BE: Repair of human myocardial structure by chronic treatment with ACE-inhibitors in hypertensive heart disease. Circulation Suppl. I 1994; 90: 343

20. Diez J, Laviades C, Mayor G, Gil MJ, Monreal I: Increased serum concentrations of procollagen peptides in essential hypertension. Relation to cardiac alterations. Circulation 1995; 91: 1450–1456

21. Motz W, Vogt M, Scheler S et al.: Prophylaxe mit gefäßaktiven Substanzen. Z Kardiol, Suppl. 4 1992; 81: 199–204

22. Motz W, Strauer BE: Improvement of coronary flow reserve after long-term therapy with Enalapril. Hypertension 1996; 27: 1031–1058

23. Vogt M, Motz W, Strauer BE: Antihypertensive Langzeittherapie mit Isradipin. Arzneimittel Forschung; 44: 1321–1318

24. Motz W, Vogt M, Scheler S, Schwartzkopff B, Strauer BE: Verbesserung der Koronarreserve nach Hypertrophieregression durch antihypertensive Therapie mit einem Beta-Rezeptorenblocker. Dtsch Med Wochenschr 1993; 118: 540–553

25. Brilla CG, Janicki JS, Weber KT: Cardioreparative effects of lisinopril in rats with genetic hypertension and left ventricular hypertrophy. Circulation 1991; 83: 1771–1779

26. Schiffrin EL, Deng LY, Larochelle P: Effects of a β-blocker or a converting enzyme inhibitor on resistance arteries in essential hypertension. Hypertension 1994; 23: 83–91

24

MYOCARDIAL PERFUSION IN HYPERTENSIVE PATIENTS WITH NORMAL CORONARY ARTERIES

Carlo Palombo[*], Michaela Kozàkovà, Giovanni Bigalli, Danilo Neglia, Alessandro Distante, Oberdan Parodi, and Antonio L'Abbate

CNR Institute of Clinical Physiology,
  and University of Pisa,
Pisa, Italy

1. INTRODUCTION

Arterial hypertension represents a major risk factor for cardiovascular morbidity and mortality: increasing experimental and clinical evidence suggest that a major role can be played by myocardial ischemia. A reduction of coronary vasodilator reserve, i.e. the capability of coronary system to increase flow in response to an increased metabolic demand, has been reported in several models of animal and human hypertension even in absence of angiographically detectable coronary atherosclerosis (1–4).

Theoretically, in patients with arterial hypertension and without significant atherosclerotic narrowing of coronary epicardial vessels several mechanisms, coronary and myocardial, functional or structural, can be responsible for this reduction of coronary reserve, possibly preventing an adequate increase in myocardial blood flow in response to increments in metabolic demand, and precipitating chest pain and myocardial ischemia (Fig.1):

1. increased myocardial blood flow at rest, due to an increased myocardial oxygen consumption (related to increased left ventricular wall stress, inotropism or heart rate), determining an upward shift of the autoregulated flow (5–6);
2. increased intrinsic coronary vascular resistance, due to functional and/or structural abnormalities of coronary microcirculation (increased coronary vasoconstrictor tone, vascular hypertrophy, decreased vascular density), responsible for a reduced vasodilator capacity (1, 7–9); consequently, the maximal flow attainable at any given perfusion pressure is also reduced, resulting in a decreased slope of the corresponding pressure-flow relation;

* Address for correspondence: Carlo Palombo, MD, CNR Institute of Clinical Physiology, Via Savi, 8-56126 PISA (Italy); Phone: 39-50-583111; Fax: 39-50-553461; E-mail: palombo@po.ifc.pi.cnr.it.

Hypertension and the Heart, edited by Zanchetti et al.
Plenum Press, New York, 1997

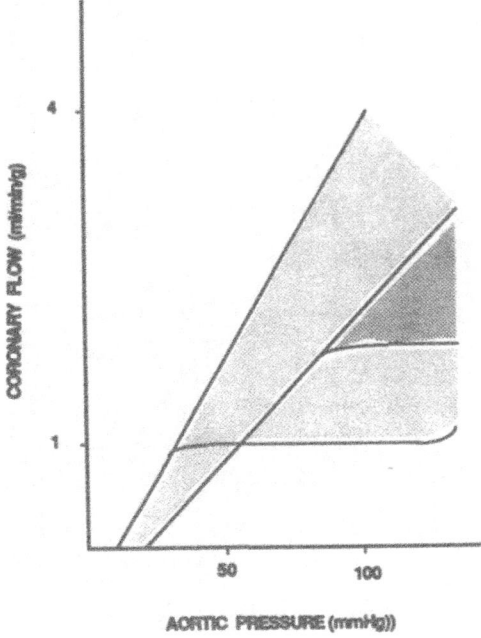

Figure 1. Schematic representation of the different mechanisms contributing to the coronary reserve impairment in hypertensive patients without significant coronary atherosclerosis.

3. increased extravascular component of total coronary resistance, due to increased extravascular compression and myocardial stiffness, shifting the coronary pressure-flow relation to the right on the x-axis (1, 10–11).

A variable combination of these myocardial and vascular mechanisms can be expected to contribute to an extremely wide range of abnormalities of myocardial perfusion in hypertensive patients without significant coronary artery disease. Some of them are associated with the presence of left ventricular hypertrophy, but most may operate even in absence of echocardiographically detectable myocardial hypertrophy.

2. ASSESSMENT OF CORONARY RESERVE AND MYOCARDIAL PERFUSION IN PATIENTS WITH ARTERIAL HYPERTENSION AND ANGIOGRAPHICALLY NORMAL CORONARY ARTERIES

In presence of a significant stenosis of an epicardial coronary artery, the impairment of coronary flow reserve and the occurrence of myocardial ischemia can be qualitatively detected by several noninvasive methods, mostly based on the combination of a physiologic or pharmacological stress with either echocardiographic monitoring of left ventricular wall motion or myocardial perfusion.

Of course, this diagnostic approach is effective in patients with arterial hypertension as well as in normotensive patients, provided a coronary artery disease coexists. However, in patients with high blood pressure and without significant coronary atherosclerosis, the impairment of myocardial perfusion, if present, is related to a variable combination of the myocardial and vascular mechanisms already mentioned and tends to be diffuse and strictly subendocardial (prevalent "horizontal" distribution) instead of regional and transmural (prevalent "vertical" distribution). In these conditions, sensitivity and specificity of stress imaging techniques effective for the assessment of coronary artery disease slow down, and different and more sophisticate techniques are needed to evaluate the mechanisms responsible for an impairment of coronary reserve and myocardial perfusion, as well as to assess the effects of antihypertensive treatment. However, most of the techniques so far utilized, like thermodilution in coronary sinus, intracoronary Doppler, quantitative angiography, are invasive and hardly allow follow-up measurements (12–13).

A significant contribution to solve this problem may be provided by noninvasive, or at least minimally invasive, techniques, such as Transesophageal Echo-Doppler (TEE) and Positron Emission Tomography (PET).

This article summarizes, mainly throughout a review of results collected by our group, the main advantages and limitations of TEE and PET to evaluate the regulation of coronary flow and myocardial perfusion in patients with arterial hypertension and without significant stenosis of epicardial vessels, their relations with myocardial oxygen demand and left ventricular hypertrophy (LVH), as well as the effect of antihypertensive therapy.

2.1. Transesophageal Echo-Doppler of Coronary Arteries

TEE-Doppler allows beat-to-beat monitoring of coronary flow velocity in the left anterior descending artery (LAD) (14–17) in basal conditions and during pharmacologically induced coronary vasodilatation (Fig. 2). The continuous monitoring guarantees that the peak flow response, corresponding to maximal vasodilatation, is actually recorded and coronary flow reserve, assessed as ratio of maximum to basal flow velocity, is not underestimated. This issue is particularly relevant due to the wide interindividual variability of

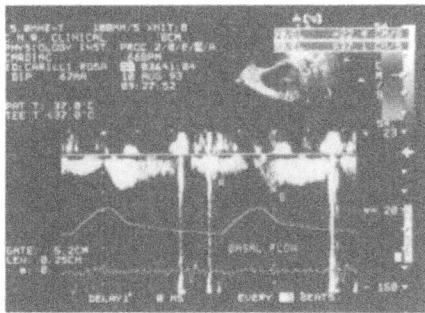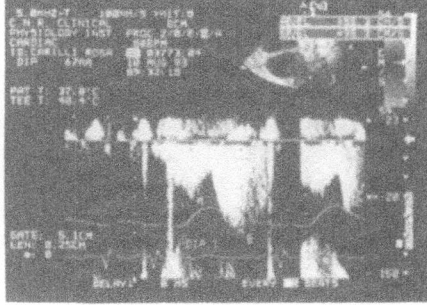
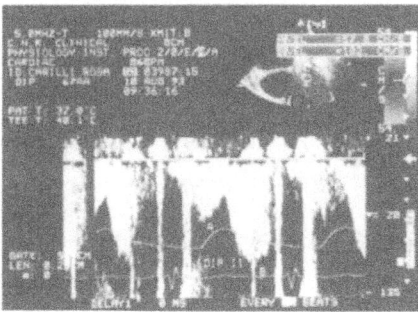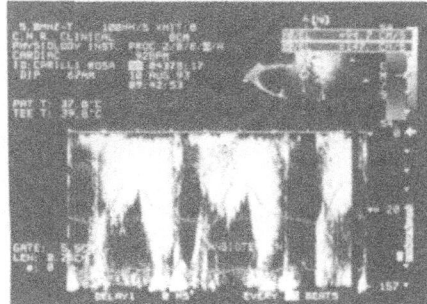

Figure 2. TEE-Doppler monitoring of coronary flow velocity in the left anterior descending artery (LAD) in basal conditions (top, left) and during stepwise pharmacologically induced coronary vasodilation.

the time response to arteriolar vasodilators as dipyridamole (18–19). Furthermore, so far TEE represents the only technique allowing the determine, simultaneously with coronary vasodilator capacity, autoregulatory coronary flow and left ventricular inotropic function and wall stress, i.e. the major determinants of myocardial oxygen consumption together with heart rate and rate-pressure product.

On the other side, the measurement of coronary flow velocity at epicardial level during arteriolar vasodilatation reflects only indirectly the microcirculatory abnormalities reported in hypertensive patients (18, 20), and flow velocity values are not normalized for LV mass. Finally, being the measurements limited to the left main and to the proximal part of left anterior descending artery, the assumption has to be accepted that they are representative of the response of the overall coronary system.

2.2. Positron Emission Tomography

PET provides measurements of myocardial blood flow (MBF) directly at microcirculatory level, which are specific (per gram of myocardial tissue) and regional (rMBF): both these features, together with the possibility to identify and quantify regional perfusion defects (Fig. 3), have crucial relevance when hypertrophy-related abnormalities of MBF and their response to medications are investigated (19).

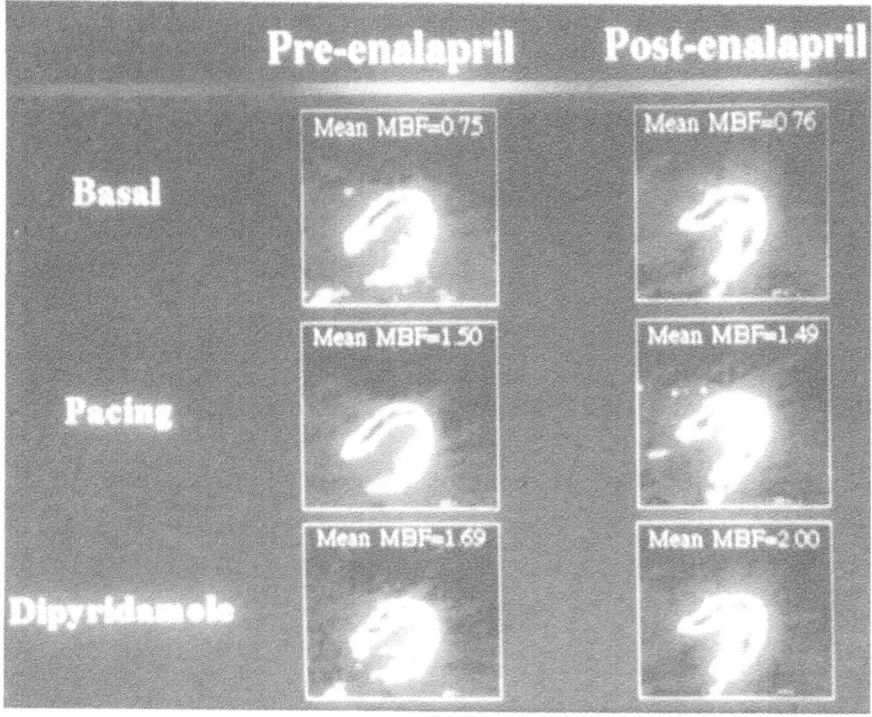

Figure 3.   Regional myocardial blood flow (rMBF) assessed by PET in a hypertensive patient before and after therapy with enalapril. Studies in basal conditions, during pacing and after dipyridamole infusion in one transaxial axis are represented. The map shows relative underperfusion of the anterior and posterolateral wall, reversed after therapy.

Major shortcomings of PET are represented not only by the high cost and limited availability, but also by the low number of physiological steps which can be acquired during one study, always at fixed times; consequently, peak flow response to stimuli can be missed (21).

3. STUDY OF CORONARY FUNCTION BY TEE DOPPLER

3.1. Coronary Flow Reserve in Hypertension and in Physiologic Hypertrophy

The different mechanisms responsible for an impairment of coronary vasodilator capacity in hypertensive patients were investigated by an integrated echocardiographic approach, including TEE Doppler, which allows noninvasive monitoring of coronary flow velocity in the left anterior descending artery during pharmacological vasodilatation, and transthoracic echo for evaluation of LV mass and systolic function (22).

The study population included 17 healthy controls and 33 hypertensive patients. A group of 16 age-matched endurance athletes (marathon runners and triatlonists) with physiologic 23) was also investigated.

Significant coronary artery disease and valvular or myocardial diseases other than LVH were ruled-out by clinical history and noninvasive testing including basal and effort ECG and basal and high-dose dipyridamole-atropine echocardiography.

In hypertensive patients where the suspicion of coronary artery disease, based on anginal symptoms and/or a positive exercise ECG, could not be ruled out on the basis of the noninvasive diagnostic work-up (14/33 patients), coronary angiography was performed. In all subjects, basal echocardiogram did not show regional left ventricular asynergy, and was negative for regional wall motion abnormalities. Coronary angiography, when performed, was negative for coronary artery stenosis.

Left ventricular mass was determined by transthoracic echocardiography (24–25). Hypertensive patients with LVH were further subdivided in mild-moderate and severe LVH according to the diastolic thickness of interventricular septum (>11 and <15 mm and ≥15 mm, respectively), i.e. the region mainly perfused by LAD artery. Within hypertensive patients, 10 did not have LVH (LVMI = 99.4±17.3 g/sqm), 16 showed mild to moderate LVH (LVMI = 157.3±50.3 g/sqm), and 7 severe LVH (LVMI = 230.2±53 g/sqm). When present, LVH was always concentric (26–27).

Left ventricular contractile function was assessed as midwall fractional shortening (MFS; %) (28); left ventricular peak systolic wall stress (PSWS; Pa) and end-systolic wall stress (ESWS; Pa) were calculated (29–30).

Coronary flow velocity in LAD artery was monitored basally and during i.v. peripheral infusion of high-dose dipyridamole (0.84 mg/kg/9min).

Coronary reserve was assessed as ratio of mean diastolic velocity after high-dose dipyridamole and basal diastolic velocity, and minimum coronary resistance as ratio of diastolic blood pressure and diastolic velocity after high-dose dipyridamole.

As compared to controls, in all hypertensive subgroups coronary reserve was similarly decreased (3.54±0.84 vs 2.59±0.42 in patients without LVH, 2.29±0.46 in patients with mild LVH, 2.43±0.71 in patients with severe LVH, p<0.01 vs controls) and minimum resistance increased (0.56±0.15 vs 0.75±0.31, 0.75±0.19, 0.78±0.21 mmHg·s·cm^{-1}, N.S.). By contrast, athletes with physiologic LVH had coronary reserve and minimum resistance

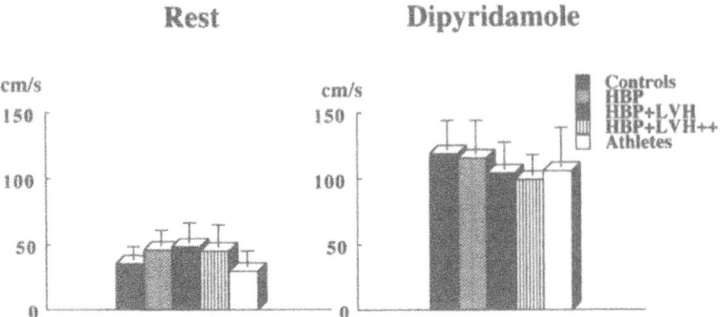

Figure 4. Coronary flow velocity assessed by TEE at rest and after dipyridamole in controls, hypertensive subjects and athletes. HBP+LVH = hypertension plus moderate LVH; HBP+LVH++ = hypertension plus severe LVH.

values comparable to normals (3.9 ± 1.0 and 0.65 ± 0.18 mmHg·s·cm^{-1}, respectively), despite markedly increased LVMI (184 ± 6 g/sqm vs 96.1 ± 25.1 g/sqm in controls, p< .05).

A reduced coronary reserve value can be dependent on both an increase in resting coronary flow and an impairment in the maximal vasodilator capacity. Resting coronary flow velocity was increased in the overall hypertensive group as compared to controls, while flow velocity after dipyridamole was relatively decreased, although not significantly, only in patients with severe LVH (Fig. 4). The increased resting flow was associated to higher heart rate, rate pressure-product and wall stress in patients without LVH, and mainly to increased myocardial mass in patients with LVH (Fig. 5). Athletes showed resting flow velocity slightly decreased compared to controls, with no differences in velocity after dipyridamole.

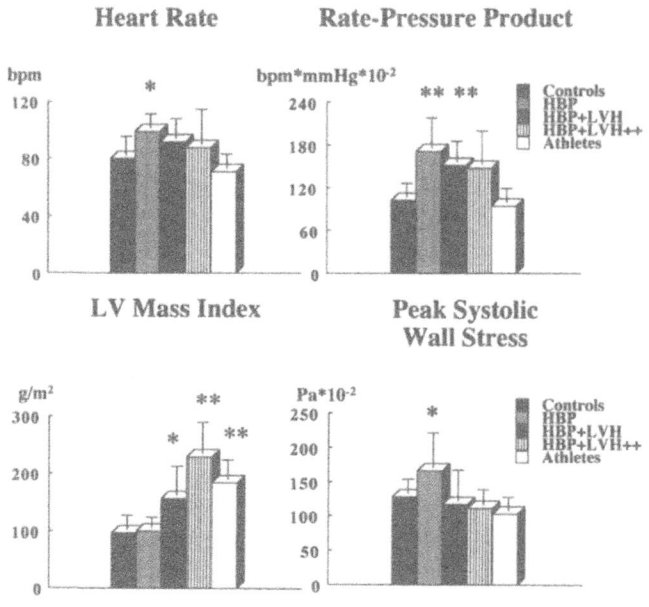

Figure 5. LV geometry and determinants of baseline coronary flow velocity in controls, hypertensive subjects and athletes studied by TEE.

Coronary flow velocity after dipyridamole, which can be assumed to correspond to flow in maximal arteriolar vasodilation, was not significantly different in all hypertensive subgroups as compared to controls. However, in hypertensive patients the flow velocity values were obtained at higher perfusion pressure; due to the pressure-dependence of maximally vasodilated flow (Fig. 1), this approach underestimates the abnormality of coronary vasodilator capacity in hypertensive patients. Using coronary resistance instead of flow can overcome this limitation: by this approach, hypertensive patients were shown to have minimum coronary resistance increased by about 35% as compared to controls, without differences between patients with or without LVH.

3.2. Coronary Flow Velocity in Autoregulation and Determinants of Myocardial Oxygen Demand in Patients with Hypertension and Athletes with Physiologic Hypertrophy

In controls, coronary flow velocity before dipyridamole infusion, i.e. in autoregulation, correlated directly with RPP (r = 0.716, p<0.001) and heart rate (r = 0.634, p<0.01), and non-significantly also with PSWS (r=0.440, p=0.07). Similar relations were found in athletes (for RPP, r = 0.69, p<0.01; for PSWS, r = 0.52, p<0.05), but not in hypertensive patients. Only in athletes basal, autoregulatory, flow velocity was directly related also with ESWS (r=0.65, p<0.01). These data suggest that in hypertensive patients the simple relation between flow in autoregulation and heart rate or RPP is altered by the interplay of other factors like LVH, wall stress or LV inotropic function, all of which may contribute to variable extent to changes in resting oxygen demand. Actually, midwall fractional shortening of LV was comparable in the controls, athletes and hypertensive patients without LVH (18.0±1.7%, 16.5±1.8%, and 17.4± 1.8%, respectively), but significantly reduced in presence of moderate and severe LVH (14.7± 2.4% and 13.8±1.0%, p<0.01 versus controls). On the other side, peak systolic and end-systolic wall stress were significantly increased (p<0.05) in hypertensive patients without LVH (165±51 and 74 ±23 × 10^2 Pa) as compared to controls (128±20 and 55±11 × 10^2 Pa), athletes (103±27 and 51±10 × 10^2 Pa), and hypertensive patients with LVH, either moderate (117±44 and 59±23 × 10^2 Pa) or severe (112±21 and 67±14 × 10^2 Pa).

3.3. Remodeling of Epicardial Coronary Vessels

The diameter of left main artery (LMA) can be measured in 2-D zoomed images in most of patients undergoing a TEE examination (Fig. 6). By this approach, LMA diameter was measured before and after dipyridamole infusion in 47 subjects (71% of the overall population), and the corresponding values of cross-sectional area were calculated. Compared to controls, athletes but not hypertensive patients showed a significantly increased area of LMA (15.2±2.7 sq.mm vs 12.6±3.9 in hypertensives and 12.0±3.1 sq.mm in controls) and an enhanced dilator response of the epicardial vessel to dipyridamole administration (30.4±13.9 vs 7.7±11.2 and 17.4±15.0%) (31); in the same group, the increment in LMA area after dipyridamole was directly related to coronary reserve value (r=0.56, p<0.05).

4. EVALUATION OF MYOCARDIAL PERFUSION BY PET

Together with noninvasiveness, the unique features of PET underlying the increasing role of this technique for investigating the function of coronary microcirculation and

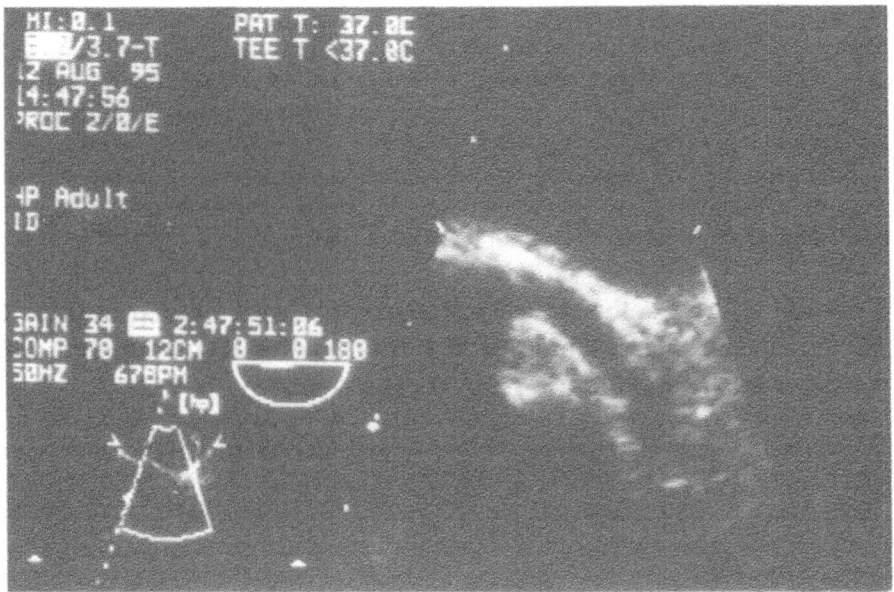

Figure 6. Two-dimensional image of the left main coronary artery and left anterior descending artery visualized by TEE.

nutritive tissue perfusion in various cardiac diseases with normal epicardial arteries are represented by the possibility of quantitative regional measurements normalized for LV mass (19). Thus, a key role of PET in understanding coronary circulation in hypertensive heart disease is obvious.

4.1. Specific Myocardial Blood Flow and Its Response to Pacing Stress and Dipyridamole

Due to the very short half-life of positron-labelled tracers, serial determinations of rMBF can be performed in the same session. Sequential stress including atrial pacing tachycardia and dipyridamole infusion represent a clinical model suitable to explore respectively the capability of coronary bed to reduce the arteriolar tone in response to an increased metabolic demand, still within the autoregulatory range, and to estimate the maximal vasodilator capacity (Fig. 3).

Regional MBF was assessed by dynamic PET and ^{13}N-Ammonia in 20 patients with essential hypertension, ten with and ten without LVH, and in 14 normotensive subjects of comparable age and gender, with chest pain syndrome and angiographically normal coronary arteries, at baseline, during maximal atrial pacing tachycardia and after i.v. dipyridamole infusion (0.56 mg/kg/4 min) (32). Estimation of rMBF was performed by means of a previously reported approach (33). For each study, two postero-lateral, two anterior and two septal wall regions of interest were selected, and regional MBF expressed as ml·min^{-1}·g^{-1}. Flow values in the 6 left ventricular myocardial regions were averaged to obtain a mean MBF value for the whole left ventricle. Regional MBF was highest in the septum and lowest in the postero-lateral wall in both control and hypertensive populations.

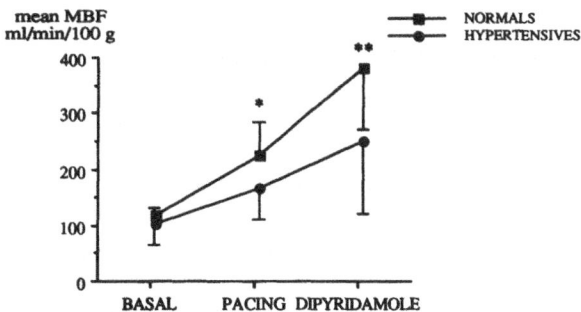

Figure 7. Average mean myocardial blood flow (MBF) assessed by PET in normal subjects and in hypertensive patients before therapy in basal conditions, during pacing and after dipyridamole.

The homogeneity of MBF distribution throughout the left ventricle was evaluated by the coefficient of variation of the flow measurements in the 6 myocardial regions of interest (calculated as the ratio of the standard deviation to the mean). Mean MBF did not differ between hypertensive and normotensive groups at rest. During atrial pacing tachycardia MBF significantly increased in both groups but was significantly lower in hypertensive than in normotensive subjects. After dipyridamole infusion, mean MBF significantly increased compared to baseline values in both groups but was significantly lower in hypertensives (Fig. 7). No differences were found according to the presence or absence of LVH (Fig. 8). Coronary flow reserve was significantly depressed in patients compared with normotensive subjects (2.6 ± 0.8 vs 3.4 ± 1.0, $p<0.01$).

4.2. Effect of Antihypertensive Treatment on Myocardial Perfusion

Hypertensive patients underwent a follow-up PET study according to the same protocol after six months of therapy with an ACE-inhibitor (Enalapril, up to 40 mg per day) or a calcium-antagonist (sustained-release Verapamil, up to 480 mg per day). A comparable blood pressure reduction, by at least 10% of the baseline systo-diastolic values, was

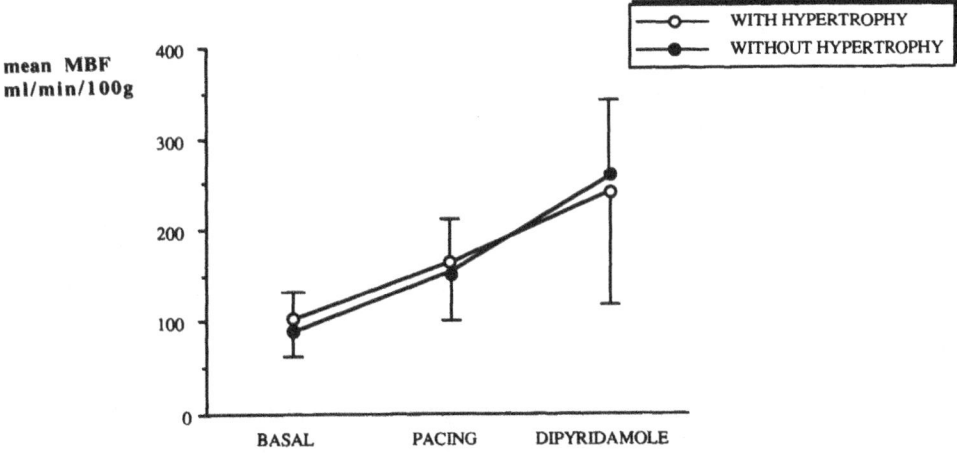

Figure 8. Basal and stress mean MBF in hypertensive patients with or without LVH.

attained with both medications. However, the post-therapy PET study was performed one week after the discontinuation of treatment, when blood pressure had returned to pre-treatment levels, in order to exclude either the acute pharmacological effects of the drugs or the possible interference of different blood pressure levels with the coronary circulatory function.

Mean MBF at rest did not change after therapy as compared to pre-treatment values in both Enalapril (0.96 ± 0.22 vs 0.91 ± 0.27 ml·min^{-1}·g^{-1}, ns) and Verapamil (0.95 ± 0.23 vs 0.96 ± 0.27 ml·min^{-1}·g^{-1}, ns) groups. Mean MBF during pacing tachycardia did not change after enalapril (1.68 ± 0.45 vs 1.50 ± 0.29 ml·min^{-1}·g^{-1}, ns) but significantly increased after verapamil (2.34 ± 0.65 vs 1.71 ± 0.42 ml·min^{-1}·g^{-1}, p<0.01). Similarly, mean MBF after dipyridamole did not change in the enalapril group (2.29 ± 0.80 vs 2.17 ± 0.77 ml·min^{-1}·g^{-1}, ns) but significantly increased in the verapamil group (3.47 ± 1.65 vs 2.69 ± 1.35 ml·min^{-1}·g^{-1}, p<0.05). Coronary reserve did not change in the enalapril-treated patients (2.37 ± 0.59 vs 2.42 ± 0.72, ns) and increased in the verapamil-treated patients (3.73 ± 1.79 vs 2.74 ± 0.80, p<0.05). After therapy, coronary resistance was comparable at rest in the two groups, while during pacing stress and dipyridamole infusion it was significantly reduced compared with the pre-treatment values in the verapamil group (pacing: 63 ± 23 vs 82 ± 28 mmHg/ml·min^{-1}·g^{-1}, p<0.01; dipyridamole: 43 ± 19 vs 52 ± 19 mmHg/ml·min^{-1}·g^{-1}, p<0.05), but not in the enalapril group (77 ± 17 vs 86 ± 20 mmHg/ml·min^{-1}·g^{-1}; 57 ± 22 vs 60 ± 17 mmHg/ml·min^{-1}·g^{-1}, respectively, ns).

A tendency to lesser inhomogeneity of flow distribution was observed at rest after both treatments and also during pacing tachycardia in the enalapril-treated patients (Fig. 3, 9). Within the 10 patients with LVH at the pre-treatment evaluation, six had a not statistically significant reduction of LV mass, with no correlation between percent change in LV mass index after treatment and percent change in resting MBF (r=0.28, ns), pacing MBF (r=0.54, ns) and dipyridamole MBF (r=0.49, ns).

4.3. Inhomogeneity in Myocardial Perfusion: Relation with Myocardial Hypertrophy

In order to specifically address the issue of inhomogeneity of rMBF and its relation with LVH and coronary flow reserve, 30 more untreated hypertensive subjects with low probability of coronary artery disease — estimated on the basis of absent symptoms and negative ECG on effort and dipyridamole-echo test — underwent a PET study at rest and after i.v. infusion of Dipyridamole (0.56 mg/kg/4min) (34). In the overall series of 50 patients, including 22 non hypertrophic and 28 hypertrophic subjects, mean coronary flow after Dipyridamole and coronary flow reserve were confirmed to be lower than in our normal control group (2.18 ± 0.75 vs 3.57 ± 1.0 ml·min^{-1}·g^{-1}, and 2.51 ± 0.88 vs 3.35 ± 1.03, respectively, p<0.05), without differences between hypertrophic and non hypertrophic patients. Coronary vasodilator response to Dipyridamole was impaired in all the considered regions. However, in 18 out 50 patients, a flow heterogeneity responsible for a clear-cut regional perfusion defect was observed in the postero-lateral or in the anterior wall after dipyridamole (Fig. 3), with vasodilated flow within the normal range in the scintigraphically normal territories. Age, gender distribution, mean resting and Dipyridamole MBF were comparable in the group displaying an inhomogeneous distribution of perfusion and in the population with a homogeneous flow pattern. By contrast, patients with regional perfusion heterogeneity had significantly higher LVMI values than those with homogeneously reduced perfusion after Dipyridamole (156 ± 38 vs 141 ± 27 g/m^2, p<0.05).

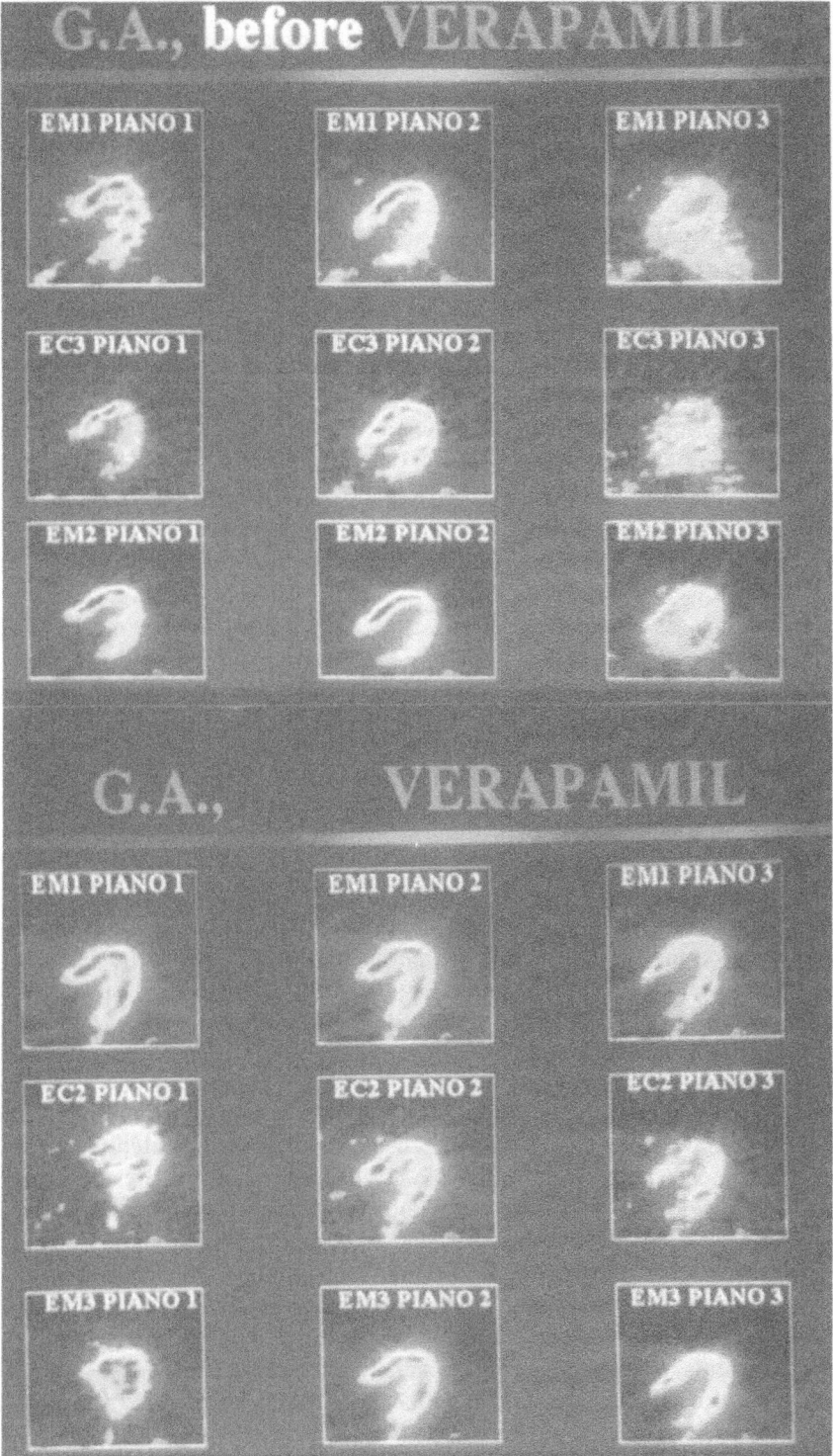

Figure 9. Regional MBF assessed by PET in a hypertensive patient before and after therapy with verapamil, in basal conditions (EM1), during pacing (EC3) and after dipyridamole (EM2) in three transaxial sections. The color maps show regional perfusion defects of the anterior and posterolateral wall before therapy. After treatment, a significant increase of flow is evident, with a reduction of flow inhomogeneity.

5. CFR, CHEST PAIN, AND STRESS ECG (TEE AND PET)

Whether or not chest pain and transient changes of the repolarization phase at ECG during stress correspond to myocardial ischemia or underperfusion in patients with angiographically normal coronary arteries represents a still controversial issue. In our TEE study, sixteen hypertensive patients had history of angina pectoris, while 17 were asymptomatic; those with angina pectoris tended to show higher, although not significantly, basal coronary flow velocity than those without angina (51.2 ± 14.2 vs 41.8 ± 14.7 cm/s, p=0.07). Exercise ECG was positive in 10 out of 33 hypertensive patients, nondiagnostic in 11 and negative in 12. The hypertensive patients with positive exercise ECG had non-significantly higher basal coronary flow velocity as compared to those with negative exercise ECG (52.4 ± 16.8 vs 41.0 ± 10.6 cm/s, p=0.07). Hypertensives with and without angina pectoris as well as those with positive and negative exercise ECG did not differ in coronary flow velocity values after high-dose dipyridamole, LVMI, basal RPP, midwall fractional shortening and wall stress. A similar association between relatively higher resting myocardial flow values and transient ECG abnormalities during stress (pacing and dipyridamole) was observed in the PET study (35).

6. DISCUSSION

6.1. Impairment of Coronary Vasodilator Capacity in Hypertensive Patients

As shown by our TEE and PET studies, hypertensive patients without significant coronary artery disease show a mosaic of changes in coronary function and myocardial perfusion accompanying high blood pressure and LVH.

In the past the reduction of coronary flow reserve in hypertensive patients has been mainly ascribed to a myocardial factor, i.e. the hemodynamic, metabolic and anatomical effects of LVH (1–2, 36–37), as in patients with aortic stenosis (38) and hypertrophic cardiomyopathy (39). However, more recent studies reported a reduced coronary flow reserve also in hypertensives without LVH (2).

Taken together, our data obtained with two different techniques in distinct series of patients show a substantial agreement about the impairment of maximal vasodilator capacity of the coronary microvasculature in hypertensive patients as compared to normotensive controls. Such a global impairment is not merely dependent on the presence of LVH as assessed by echocardiography, being clearly detectable even in non hypertrophied hearts, and without significant correlation between LV mass and minimum coronary resistansce. These finding are in agreement with those obtained by Vogt with the argon technique (40), and by our group with PET (32). These findings suggest a major role of vascular factors in restricting coronary flow reserve and its utilization in hypertensive patients.

Various vascular mechanisms can be theoretically responsible for a reduced maximal vasodilator capacity in hypertensive patients, including inadequate neoangiogenesis (41–42), structural remodeling of the intramyocardial coronary arterioles (43–44), and functional factors as an increase in the tone of coronary resistance vessels (2) and an impairment in endothelium-dependent vasodilation of resistance vessels (45). The coronary vasodilation induced by such stressors as dipyridamole or adenosine is primarily endothelium-independent; however, the increment in coronary blood flow may trigger further vasodilation, which is flow-induced and endothelium-dependent (46–48), and is reported to be impaired in hypertension (45, 49–50).

Our clinical models do not allow any inference on the site of the microcirculatory abnormality along the coronary tree: according to Chilian, 40–50% of the total coronary vascular resistance is reported to be located in vessels less than 100 μm in diameter, which are also those responsible for autoregulation of myocardial blood flow (51–52). Due to the fact that the large conduit vessels, which are unaffected by coronary atherosclerosis in our patients, are responsible for a negligible part of the overall coronary resistance, this model is consistent with the remaining 40–50% resistance being located in prearterioles greater than 100 μm. These vessels receive autonomic innervation and their diameter may be altered by stimulation of these nerves (53).

6.2. Elusive Link between Left Ventricular Hypertrophy and Coronary Reserve Impairment

The elusive link between coronary flow reserve impairment and myocardial hypertrophy, observed in both TEE and PET studies in hypertensive patients (22, 32), is also supported by our TEE study on endurance athletes (23), demonstrating a preserved coronary flow reserve despite LV mass values even higher than those of hypertensive patients with LVH, and by the observation of Camici et al who reported, using PET, an impaired vasodilator response to dipyridamole also in the non-hypertrophied walls of patients with hypertrophic cardiomyopathy (54).

As shown with PET during increased metabolic demand by pacing tachycardia, also the recruitment of coronary vasodilator capacity within the autoregulatory range, i.e. below the limit of maximal vasodilation, can be blunted in hypertensive patients independently of LVH.

On the basis of experimental studies, also this abnormal response to increased metabolic demand may depend on multiple vascular mechanisms such as structural changes of the intramyocardial coronary arterioles (55–57), endothelial dysfunction (58), and myogenic regulation of coronary resistance in response to elevated pressure (59–60).

Myocardial factors like interstitial fibrosis (61) and diastolic dysfunction (57, 62–63) can contribute to the development of subendocardial ischemia during stress in presence as well in absence of myocyte hypertrophy, (64–66).

6.3. Left Ventricular Hypertrophy and Myocardial Flow Inhomogeneity

While LVH seems to play a minor role in determining the impairment of the overall coronary vasodilator capacity, a significant association between increased LV mass and myocardial flow inhomogeneity during stress has been observed by PET, confirming previous results obtained by Houghton using 201-Tl scintigraphy (67). In patients with heterogeneous regional MBF, the flow impairment seems to affect only few districts, whereas others appear to be unaffected. In contrast, in patients with homogeneously impaired perfusion, the whole myocardium displays a reduced vasodilating capacity. Whether these differences stem from variable degrees of capillary neoangiogenesis associated with the development of LVH, regionally different myocardial extravascular forces or other mechanisms remain to be elucidated, as well as the possible clinical relevance of regional relative hypoperfusion.

The role of an increased resting myocardial oxygen demand in decreasing coronary flow reserve through higher basal coronary flow has been already mentioned (68–70). However, technical limitations restricted so far the possibility to investigate by noninvasive means the relations between autoregulatory flow and factors affecting metabolic demand in man.

6.4. Assessment of Coronary Autoregulation by Echocardiographic Techniques

By transthoracic and transesophageal echo, the relative role of decreased vasodilator capacity and increased resting myocardial metabolic demand in the different hypertensive subsets has been explored: a progressively increasing impairment in maximal isobaric coronary flow is observed throughout increasing LV mass in hypertensive patients. As far as autoregulatory flow is concerned, compared to controls all hypertensive patients show an elevated resting coronary flow velocity, which is related to higher rate-pressure product in patients without LVH or in presence of moderate LVH, to the increased wall stress in absence of LVH, and to increased myocardial mass in presence of moderate to severe LVH. Our finding that hypertensive patients with angina pectoris or positive exercise ECG had higher basal coronary flow velocity as compared to asymptomatic patients, suggests a possible clinical relevance of the increased basal coronary flow in hypertensive patients, and may be of interest for the choice of therapeutic approach.

6.5. Effect of Chronic Antihypertensive Treatment on Coronary Function

Evidence that the coronary reserve impairment can be reversed by long-term antihypertensive treatment with calcium-antagonists and ACE-inhibitors has been provided by our group using PET, and by Motz and Strauer using argon (71).

In our PET study, effective long-term therapy with verapamil reduced coronary resistance and increased MBF during both metabolic and pharmacological vasodilation. These favorable changes were unrelated to changes in LV mass, indicating that the improved coronary vasodilating capacity after verapamil is mainly due to a regression of coronary microcirculatory dysfunction. Both treatments, and in particular enalapril, were associated with a more homogeneous MBF distribution (72), compared with the pre-treatment study, suggesting an improved matching between myocardial mass and perfusion after therapy.

The capability shown for calcium-antagonists and ACE-inhibitors to reverse after long-term treatment medial thickening of coronary resistance vessels (73–75) myocardial fibrosis (69, 76) and diastolic dysfunction (77), or endothelial dysfunction and coronary vasomotion disorders (78) may be responsible for the improvement of coronary vascular reserve. In summary, the effect of treatment in reducing total coronary resistance and increasing MBF during vasodilating stimuli can only be explained by a partial regression of structural and/or functional abnormalities of the coronary microcirculation either at the level of the arteriolar segments responsive to metabolic stimula (i.e., less than 100 μm diameter) and/or at the level of the small vessel segment larger than 100 μm, more dependent on endothelial function and NO synthesis (58).

6.6. Coronary and Myocardial Remodeling in Physiologic Left Ventricular Hypertrophy

Endurance athletes show preserved coronary flow reserve, left ventricular function and coronary autoregulatory function. These findings are clearly in keeping with a physiologic integrated remodeling process, possibly including adequate neoangiogenesis and a well regulated growth process involving myocites and intramyocardial vessels. A direct demonstration of structural and functional adaptation involving also epicardial vessels has been provided with our TEE studies (23, 31): in fact, the basal cross-sectional area of left main was higher in endurance athletes, as compared to controls and especially to hypertensive subjects. This finding is in agreement with previous studies (79–84), and suggests an adaptation in conduit vessel to frequent high-flow stimuli caused by the increase in myocardial oxygen demand during frequent submaximal-maximal exercises (79, 85). The enhanced response of left main artery to arteriolar dilation induced by the endothelium-independent vasodilator dipyridamole in our athletes may reflect augmented flow-mediated dilation, already reported in other muscular districts in athletes and in the coronary bed of exercising animals (80, 86–90).

7. CONCLUSIONS

The regulation of myocardial blood flow in subjects with arterial hypertension and or left ventricular hypertrophy with significant epicardial artery stenosis depends on a number of factors such as coronary perfusion pressure, function of coronary microcirculation, extravascular forces, particularly intramyocardial pressure, and vasomotor changes in epicardial conduit vessels. Consequently, interaction between hypertension, hypertrophy and regional myocardial perfusion may lead to variable results in different patients. The comparison of hypertensive patients with or without LVH, sedentary controls, and athletes with physiologic hypertrophy, even when made by using different techniques, indicate a multifaced structural and functional adaptation which is appropriate in athletes and defective in hypertension. In hypertension, a primary abnormality in vascular structure and function and in myocardial oxygen demand appears to be followed by a progressively increasing role of myocardial factors (not only LVH, but even fibrosis, diastolic stiffness and extravascular compressive forces) with the increasing duration and severity of the disease, which may have an additional role in limiting myocardial perfusion. Such abnormalities seem to be at least partly amenable to be reversed with calcium-antagonists and ACE-inhibitors.

REFERENCES

1. Opherk D, Mall G, Zebe H, Schwarz F, Weihe E, Manthey J, Kubler W. Reduction of coronary reserve: a mechanism for angina pectoris in patients with arterial hypertension and normal coronary arteries. Circulation 1984; 69:1–7.
2. Brush JE, Cannon RO, Schenke WH. Angina due to coronary microvascular disease in hypertensive patients without left ventricular hypertrophy. N Engl J Med 1988; 319:1302–1307.
3. Strauer BE. The significance of coronary reserve in clinical heart disease. JACC 1990; 15:775–783.
4. Marcus ML, Harrison DG. Alterations in the coronary circulation in hypertrophied ventricles. Circulation 1987; 75 (Suppl I):119–I25.
5. Harrison DG, Florentine MS, Brooks LA, Cooper SM, Marcus ML. The effect of hypertension and left ventricular hypertrophy on the lower range of coronary autoregulation. Circulation 1988; 77:1108–1115.
6. Polese A, De Cesare N, Montorsi P, Fabbiocchi F, Guazzi M, Loaldi A, Guazzi MD. Upward shift of the lower range of coronary flow autoregulation in hypertensive patients with hypertrophy of the left ventricle. Circulation 1991; 83:845–853.
7. Schwartzkopff B, Motz W, Frenzel H, Vogt M, Knauer S, Strauer BE. Structural and functional alterations of the intramyocardial coronary arterioles in patients with arterial hypertension. Circulation 1993; 88:993–1003.

8. Treasure CB, Klein JL, Vita JA, Manoukian SV, Renwick GH, Selwyn AP, Ganz P, Alexander RW. Hypertension and left ventricular hypertrophy are associated with impaired endothelium-mediated relaxation in human coronary resistance vessels. Circulation 1993; 87:86–93.

9. Cannon RO III, Epstein SE. "Microvascular angina" as a cause of chest pain with angiographically normal coronary arteries. Am J Cardiol 1988; 61:1338–1343.

10. Tomanek RJ, Palmer PJ, Pfeiffer GL, Schreiber KL, Eastham CL, Marcus ML. Morphometry of canine coronary arteries, arterioles, and capillaries during hypertension and left ventricular hypertrophy. Circ Res 1986; 58:38–46.

11. Duncker DJ, Zhang J, Bache RJ. Coronary pressure-flow relation in left ventricular hypertrophy. Importance in changes in back pressure versus changes in minimum resistance. Circ Res 1993; 72:579–587.

12. L'Abbate A. Methodology of coronary blood flow measurements in humans: present status and future advancement. Cardiovasc. Pharmacol. 1987; 10 (Suppl. 5):S120–S122.

13. Wolters-Geldof, Manger Cats V, Bruschke AVG. Clinical methods to determine coronary flow and myocardial perfusion. Int J Card Imag 1997; 13:79–94.

14. Iliceto S, Marangelli V, Memmola C, Rizzon P. Transesophageal Doppler echocardiography evaluation of coronary blood flow velocity in baseline conditions and during dipyridamole-induced coronary vasodilation. Circulation 1991; 83:61–69.

15. Kozàkovà M, Palombo C., Pratali L., Bigalli G., Marzilli M., Distante A., L'Abbate A. Assessment of coronary reserve by transesophageal Doppler echocardiography. Direct comparison beetiween different modalities of dypiridamole and adenosine administation. Eur Heart J1997; 18:514–523.

16. Redberg RF, Sobol Y, Chou TM, Malloy M, Kumar S, Botvinick E, Kane J. Adenosine-induced coronary vasodilation during transesophageal Doppler echocardiography. Rapid and safe measurement of coronary flow reserve ratio can predict significant left anterior descending coronary stenosis. Circulation. 1995; 92:190–196.

17. Palombo C, Kozàkovà M, Pratali L, Bigalli G, Galetta F, L'Abbate A. Transesophageal Echo-Doppler for Study of Coronary Flow Reserve: Feasibility and Normalcy Criteria. J Am Coll Cardiol 1997; 2 (supplement A):364A.

18. Wilson RF, Laughlin DE, Ackel PH, Chilian WM, Holida CJ. Transluminal, subselective measurement of coronary artery blood flow velocity and vasodilator reserve in man. Circulation 1985; 72:82–92.

19. Camici PG, Gropler RJ, Jones T, L'Abbate A, Maseri A, Melin JA, Merlet P, Parodi O, Schelbert HR, Schwaiger M, Wijns W. The impact of myocardial blood flow quantitation with PET on the understanding of cardiac diseases. Eur Heart J 1996; 17:25–34.

20. Doucette JW, Corl PD, Payne HM, Flynn AE, Goto M, Nassi M. Validation of a Doppler guide wire for intravascular measurements of coronary artery flow velocity. Circulation 1992; 85:1899–1911.

21. Radvan J, Marwick T, Williams J, Camici P. Evaluation of the extent and timing of the coronary hyperemic response to dipyridamole. A study with transesophageal echocardiography and positron emission tomography with oxygen 15 water. J Am Soc Echocardiography. 1995; 8:864–873.

22. Kozàkovà M, Palombo C, Pratali L, Pittella G, Galetta F, L'Abbate A. Mechanisms of coronary flow reserve impairment in human hypertension. An integrated approach by transthoracic and transesophageal echocardiography. Hypertension 1997; 29:551–559.

23. Kozàkovà M, Palombo C, Galetta F, Pratali L, Giusti C, L'Abbate A. Structural and functional adaptation of coronary circulation in endurance athletes: a study b y transesophageal echo-doppler. Eur. Heart J 1996; 17 (abstracts suppl.):89.

24. Devereux RB, Reichek N. Echocardiographic determination of left ventricular mass in man: anatomic validation of the method. Circulation. 1977; 55:613–618.

25. de Simone G, Devereux RB, Daniels SR, Koren MJ, Meyer RA, Laragh JH. Effect of growth on variability of left ventricular mass: assessment of allometric signals in adults and children and their capacity to predict cardiovascular risk. J Am Coll Cardiol. 1995; 25:1056–1062.

26. Savage DD, Garrison RJ, Kannel WB, Levy D, AndersonSJ, Stokes J III, Feinleib M, Castelli WP. The spectrum of left ventricular hypertrophy in general population sample: The Framingham study. Circulation. 1987; 75 (Suppl. I):I-26–I-33.

27. Ganau A, Devereux RB, Roman MJ, de Simone G, Pickering TG, Saba PS, Vargiu P, Simongini I, Laragh JH. Patterns of left ventricular hypertrophy and geometric remodeling in essential hypertension. J Am Coll Cardiol. 1992; 19:1550–1558.

28. de Simone G, Devereux RB, Roman MJ, Ganau A, Saba PS, Alderman MH, Laragh JH. Assessment of left ventricular function by the midwall fractional shortening/end-systolic stress relation in human hypertension. J Am Coll Cardiol. 1994; 23:1444–1451.

29. Wilson JR, Reichek N, Hirshfeld J, Keller CA. Noninvasive assessment of load reduction in patients with asymptomatic aortic regurgitation. Am J Med. 1980; 68:664–674.

30. Reichek N, Wilson J, St.John Sutton M, Plappert TA, Goldberg S, Hirshfeld JW. Noninvasive determination of left ventricular end-systolic stress: Validation of the method and initial application. Circulation. 1982; 65:99–108.

31. Kozàkovà M, Palombo C, Galetta F., Bigalli G., Giusti C., L'Abbate A. Enhanced Flow-Mediated Coronary Dilation in Endurance Athelets: a Study by Means of Transesophageal Echo-Doppler. Circulation 1996; 94 (abstracts suppl.):I-305.

32. Parodi O, Neglia D, Palombo C, Sambuceti G, Giorgetti A, Marabotti C, Gallopin M, Simonetti I, and L'Abbate A. Comparative effects of enalapril and verapamil on myocardial blood flow in systemic hypertension. Circulation 1997; *in press.*

33. Bellina CR, Parodi O, Camici P, Salvadori PA, Taddei L, Fusani L, Guzzardi R, Klassen GA, L'Abbate A, Donato L. Simultaneous in vitro and in vivo validation of nitrogen-13-ammonia for the assessment of regional myocardial blood flow. J Nucl Med. 1990; 31:1335–43.

34. Gimelli A., Neglia D., Sambuceti G., Giorgetti A., Palombo C., Pedrinelli R., Parodi O. No Relationship Between Maximum Coronary Flow and Resistance and Left Ventricular Mass in Essential Hypertension. J Am Coll Cardiol 1996; 2 (supplement A):106A.

35. Palombo C., Neglia D., Sambuceti G., Marabotti C., L'Abbate A., Parodi O. Transient ECG Abnormalities During Increased Metabolic Demand and Dipyridamole Infusion Identify Different Patterns of Myocardial Perfusion in Hypertensive Patients. J Am Coll Cardiol 1993; 21:287A.

36. Opherk D, Zebe H, Weihe E, Mall AG, Durr Ch, Gravert B, Mehmel HC, Schwarz F, Kubler W. Reduced coronary dilator capacity and ultrastructural changes of the myocardium in patients with angina pectoris but normal coronary angiograms. Circulation. 1981; 63:1817–1822.

37. Sheridan DJ, McAinsh A, O'Gorman DJ. The coronary circulation in cardiac hypertrophy. J Cardiovasc Pharmacol. 1993; 22:S18–S28.

38. Marcus ML, Doty DB, Hiratzka LF, Wright CB, Eastman CL. A mechanism for angina pectoris in patients with aortic stenosis and normal coronary arteries. N Engl J Med. 1982; 307:1362–1367.

39. Cannon RO, Rosing DR, Maron BJ, Leon MB, Bonow RO, Watson RM, Epstein SE. Myocardial ischemia in patients with hypertrophic cardiomyopathy: contribution of inadequate vasodilator reserve and elevated left ventricular filling pressures. Circulation. 1985; 71:234–243.

40. Vogt M, Motz W, Strauer BE. Coronary haemodynamics in hypertensive heart disease. Eur Heart J. 1992; 13(suppl D):44–49.

41. Wangler RD, Peters KG, Marcus ML, Tomanek RJ. Effects of duration and severity of arterial hypertension and cardiac hypertrophy on coronary vasodilator reserve. Circ Res. 1982; 51:10–18.

42. Tomanek RJ, Schalk KA, Marcus ML, Harrison DG. Coronary angiogenesis during long-term hypertension and left ventricular hypertrophy in dogs. Circ Res. 1989; 65:352–359.

43. Tanaka M, Fujiwara H, Onodera T, Hamashima Y, Kawai C. Quantitative analysis of narrowings of intramyocardial small arteries in normal hearts, hypertensive hearts and hearts with hypertrophic cardiomyopathy. Circulation. 1987; 75:1130–1139.

44. Schwartzkopff B, Motz W, Frenzel H, Vogt M, Knauer S, Strauer BE. Structural and functional alterations of the intramyocardial coronary arterioles in patients with arterial hypertension. Circulation. 1993; 88:993–1003.

45. Antony I, Lerebours G, Nitenberg A. Loss of flow dependent coronary artery dilation in patients with hypertension. Circulation. 1995; 91:1624–1628.

46. Kuo L, Davis MJ, Chilian WH. Endothelium-dependent, flow-induced dilation of isolated coronary arterioles. Am J Physiol. 1990; 259:H1063–H1070.

47. Hintze TH, Vatner SF. Dipyridamole dilates large coronary arteries in conscious dogs. Circulation.1983; 68:1321–1327.

48. Drexler H, Zeiher AM, Wollschlager H, Meinertz T, Just H, Bonzel T. Flow-dependent coronary artery dilation in humans. Circulation. 1989; 80:466–474.

49. Brush JE, Faxon DP, Salmon S, Jacobs AK, Ryan TJ. Abnormal endothelium dependent coronary vasomotion in hypertensive patients. J Am Coll Cardiol. 1992; 19:809–815.

50. Treasure CB, Klein JL, Vita JA, Manoukian SV, Renwick GH, Selwyn AP, Ganz P, Alexander RW. Hypertension and left ventricular hypertrophy are associated with impaired endothelium-mediated relaxation in human coronary resistance vessels. Circulation. 1993; 87:86–93.

51. Chilian WM, Eastham CL, Layne SM, Marcus ML. Small vessel phenomena in the coronary microcirculation: phasic intramyocardial perfusion and microvascular dynamics. Prog Cardiovasc Dis 1988; 31:17–18.

52. Marcus ML, Chilian WM, Kanatsuka H, Dellsperger KC, Eastham CL, Lamping KG. Understanding the coronary circulation through studies at the microvascular level. Circulation 1990; 82:1–7.

53. Chilian WM, Layne SM, Eastham CL, Marcus ML. Heterogeneous microvascular coronary a-adrenergic vasoconstriction. Circ Res 1989; 64:376–388.

54. Camici P, Chiriatti G, Lorenzoni R, Bellina RC, Gistri R, Italiani G, Parodi O, Salvadori PA, Nista N, Papi L, L'Abbate A. Coronary vasodilation is impaired in both hypertrophied and non hypertrophied myocardium of patients with hypertrophic cardiomyopathy: a study with nitrogen-13 ammonia and positron emission tomography. J Am Coll Cardiol. 1991; 17:879–886.

55. Folkow B, Hallback M, Noresson E. Vascular resistance and reactivity of the microcirculation in hypertension. Blood Vessels. 1978; 15:33–45.

56. Tanaka M, Fujiwara H, Onodera T, Hamashima Y, Kawai C. Quantitative analysis of narrowings of intramyocardial small arteries in normal hearts, hypertensive hearts and hearts with hypertrophic cardiomyopathy. Circulation. 1987; 75:1130–1139.

57. Brilla CG, Janicki JS, Weber KT. Impaired diastolic function and coronary reserve in genetic hypertension. Role of interstitial fibrosis and medial thickening of intramyocardial coronary arteries. Circ Res. 1991; 69:2107–115.

58. Jones CJH, Kuo L, Davis MJ, DeFily DV, Chilian WM. Role of nitric oxide in the coronary microvascular responses to adenosine and increased metabolic demand. Circulation. 1995; 91:1807–1813.

59. Kuo L, Chilian WM, Davis MJ. Interaction of pressure and flow-induced responses in porcine coronary resistance vessels. Am J Physiol. 1991; 261:H1706–H1715.

60. Folkow B. The fourth Volhard lecture. Cardiovascular structural adaptation: its role in the initiation and maintainance of primary hypertension. Clin Sci Mol Med. 1975; 48:205–211.

61. Weber KT, Brilla CG. Pathological hypertrophy and cardiac interstitium. Circulation; 83:1849–1865.

62. Gardin JM, Drayer JIM, Weber M. Doppler echocardiographic assessment of left ventricular systolic and diastolic function in mild hypertension. Hypertension. 1987; 9(suppl II):II-90–II-96.

63. Marabotti C, Genovesi Ebert A, Palombo C, Giaconi S, Michelassi C, Ghione S. Echo-Doppler assessment of left ventricular filling in borderline hypertension. Am J Hypertens. 1989; 2:891–897.

64. Vatner SF, Shannon R, Hittinger L. Reduced subendocardial coronary reserve. A potential mechanism for impaired diastolic function in the hypertrophied and failing heart. Circulation. 1990; 81(suppl III):III-8–III-14.

65. Bache RJ, Vrobel TR, Ring SW, Emery RW, Andersen RW. Regional myocardial blood flow during exercise in dogs with chronic left ventricular hypertrophy. Circ Res. 1981; 48:76–81.

66. Hittingher L, Mirsky I, Shen YT, Patrick TA, Bishop SP, Vatner SF. Hemodynamic mechanisms responsible for reduced subendocardial coronary reserve in dogs with severe left ventricular hypertrophy. Circulation. 1995; 92:978–986.

67. Houghton JL, Frank MJ, Carr AA, von Dohlen TW, Prisant ML. Relations among impaired coronary flow reserve, left ventricular hypertrophy and thallium perfusion defects in hypertensive patients without obstructive coronary artery. J Am Coll Cardiol. 1990; 15:43–51.

68. Weber KT, Janicki JS. The metabolic demand and oxygen supply of the heart: Physiological and clinical considerations. Am J Cardiol. 1979; 44:722–729.

69. Hittinger L, Patrick T, Ihara T, Hasebe N, Shen Y-T, Kalthof B, Shannon RP, Vatner SF. Exercise induces cardiac dysfunction in both moderate, compensated and severe hypertrophy. Circulation. 1994; 89:2219–2231.

70. Gunther S, Grossman W. Determination of ventricular function in pressure-overload hypertrophy in man. Circulation. 1979; 59:679–688.

71. Motz W, Strauer BE. Improvement of coronary flow reserve after long-term therapy with enalapril. Hypertension 1996; 27:1031–1038.

72. Palombo C, Neglia D, Bigalli G, Sambuceti G, Marabotti C, Parodi O. Antihypertensive therapy improves regional myocardial blood flow and reduces perfusion dyshomogeneity in patients with hypertension and no coronary artery disease. Circulation 1993; 88:I167.

73. Brilla CG, Janicki JS, Weber KT. Cardioreparative effects of lisinopril in rats with genetic hypertension and left ventricular hypertrophy. Circulation. 1991; 5:1771–1779.

74. Clozel JP, Kuhn H, Hefti F. Effects of chronic ACE-inhibition on cardiac hypertrophy and coronary vascular reserve in spontaneously hypertensive rats with developed hypertension. J Hypertens. 1989; 7:267–275.

75. Marban E, Koretsune Y. Cell calcium, oncogens and hypertrophy. Hypertension. 1990; 15:652–658.

76. Motz W, Strauer BE. Left ventricular function and collagen content after regression of hypertensive hypertrophy. Hypertension. 1989; 13:43–50.

77. Vogt M, Kreutz KU, Motz W, Strauer BE. Regression of hypertrophy with nitrendipine: effects on systolic and diastolic function. Z Kardiol. 1989; 78:469–477.

78. Frielingsdorf J, Seiler C, Kaufmann P, Vassalli G, Suter T, Hess OM. Normalization of abnormal coronary vasomotion by calcium antagonists in patients with hypertension. Circulation. 1996; 93:1380–1387.

79. Haskell WL, Sims C, Myll Y, Bortz WM, Goar FGS, Alderman EL. Coronary artery size and dilating capacity in ultradistance runners. Circulation 1993; 87:1076–1082.

80. Berdeux A, Ghalen B, Dubois-Randé JL, Vigué B, La Rochelle CD, Hittinger L, Giudicelli JF. Role of vascular endothelium in exercise-induced dilation of large epicardial coronary arteries in concious dogs. Circulation 1994; 89:2799–2808.

81. Pelliccia A, Sparato A, Granata J, Biffi A, Caselli G, Alabiso A. Coronary arteries in physiological hypertrophy: Echocardiographic evidence of increased proximal size in elite athletes. Int J Sports med 1990; 11:120–126.

82. Currens JH, White PD. Half century of running. Clinical, physiologic and autopsy findings in the case of Clearence De Mare "Mr. Marathoner". N Engl J Med 1961; 265:988–993.

83. Schwartz JS, Baran KW, Bache RJ. Effect of stenosis on exercise-induced dilation of large coronary arteries. Am Heart J 1990; 119:520–524.

84. Dodge JT, Brown G, Bolson EL, Dodge HT. Lumen diameter of normal human coronary arteries: Influence of age, sex, anatomic variation and left ventricular hypertrophy or dilation. Circulation 1992; 86:232–246.

85. Rogers PJ, Miller TD, Bauer BA, Brum JM, Bove AA, Vanhoutte PM. Exercise training and responsiveness of isolated coronary arteries. J Appl Physiol 1991; 71:2346–2351.

86. Muller JM, Myers PR, Langhlin MH. Vasodilator responses of coronary resistance arteries of exercise-trained pig. Circulation. 1994; 89:2308–2314.

87. Laughlin MH, Oltman CL, Muller JM, Myers PR, Parker JL. Adaptation of the coronary circulation to exercise training. In cardiovascular response to exercise, CL Fletcher (ed), Mount Kisco, N.Y., Futura Publishing Co., 1994; p 175–205.

88. Parker JL, Oltman CL, Muller JM, Myers PR, Adams RH, Laughlin MH. Effect of exercise training on regulation of tone in coronary arteries and arterioles. Med Sci Sport Exerc 1994; 26:1252–1261.

89. Laughlin MH. Effect of exercise training on coronary circulation: Introduction. Med Sci Sport Exerc 1994; 26:1226–1234.

90. Wang J, Wollin MS, Hintze TH. Chronic exercise enhances endothelium-mediated dilation of epicardial coronary artery in conscious dogs. Circ Res 1993; 73:829–838.

25

ENDOTHELIAL DYSFUNCTION IN HYPERTENSION

Stefano Taddei and Antonio Salvetti[*]

I Clinica Medica
University of Pisa
Pisa, Italy

INTRODUCTION

Endothelial cells play a key role in the local regulation of vascular tone because of their strategic anatomical position between the circulating blood and vascular smooth muscle cells (1). The endothelium produces and releases several vasodilator substances, of which the most important is nitric oxide (NO) (2,3), a labile substance derived from the conversion of L-arginine into citrulline (4) by the activity of the enzyme NO-synthase (5). Importantly, this process can be inhibited by L-arginine analogues such as N^G-mono-methyl-L-arginine (L-NMMA) (6). Moreover, endothelial cells produce prostacyclin (7) and a not yet identified endothelium-derived hyperpolarizing factor (EDHF) (8). These substances can be produced and released through the stimulation of endothelial cells by mechanical forces (shear stress) (9) or surface receptor activation by specific agonists (acetylcholine, bradykinin, adenosine diphosphate, substance P etc) (1). Also, endothelium-derived NO is not only A potent relaxing agent, but it can additionally inhibit platelet aggregation (10), smooth muscle cell proliferation (11) and monocyte migration (12), thereby exerting a complex protective effect on the vessel wall. Finally, endothelium can produce vasoconstrictor substances such as cyclooxygenase-dependent endothelium-derived contracting factors (EDCF) which are mainly prostanoids, such as prostaglandin H_2 and thromboxane A_2 (13,14), or superoxide anions (15).

ENDOTHELIAL DYSFUNCTION AND HUMAN HYPERTENSION

Convincing evidence has documented that endothelial dysfunction is associated with experimental hypertension (16). It has been demonstrated that in most conditions endothe-

---
[*] Address for correspondence: Prof. Antonio Salvetti, I Clinica Medica, University of Pisa, Via Roma, 67, 56100 Pisa, Italy. Tel: +39-50-553407, Fax: +39-50-553407.

Hypertension and the Heart, edited by Zanchetti et al.
Plenum Press, New York, 1997

lium-dependent relaxations are curtailed in animal models of hypertension, possibly by a dysfunction in the NO system or EDCF production (16,17).

In healthy subjects, injection of L-NMMA into the brachial artery at a systemically ineffective infusion rate causes an evident decrease in forearm blood flow, measured by strain-gauge venous plethysmography (18). This finding clearly shows that L-NMMA induces vasoconstriction by blockade of NO production, indicating that this EDRF has a significant role in the determination of vascular tone. As compared to normotensive subjects, forearm vasoconstriction to intrabrachial L-NMMA is decreased in essential hypertensive patients, suggesting that basal release of nitric oxide is impaired in essential hypertension (19). This evidence has been reinforced by further demonstration from different laboratories (20–22) and never contradicted.

In humans, endothelial cells can also be stimulated by specific agonists such as acetylcholine, substance P or bradykinin, which cause a dose-dependent vasodilation. Studies conducted in different laboratories have given evidence of a blunted response to acetylcholine, methacholine, bradykinin and substance P in the forearm vascular bed of patients with essential hypertension as compared to normotensive controls (20,21,23–37) (table 1). Since in these studies the response to sodium nitroprusside, a direct smooth muscle cell relaxant compound (38), was found to be similar in the normotensive and hypertensive study population, these findings indicate the presence of impaired endothelium-dependent vasodilation in human hypertension. Moreover the presence of endothelial dysfunction has been also documented in the skin microcirculation (39), in subcutaneous small arterioles from gluteal biopsy (40–42), in the renal circulation (43–45) and in epicardial coronary arteries (46–51) and coronary microcirculation (52–55) (table 1). Finally, impaired endothelium-dependent vasodilation to acetylcholine has been demonstrated in the forearm vasculature of patients with hypertension secondary to primary aldosteronism or renovascular disease (27).

However the presence of endothelial dysfunction in essential hypertension was not confirmed in two negative papers (table 2). First, Cockcroft et al. demonstrated no differ-

Table 1. Evidence indicating the presence of endothelial dysfunction in different vascular beds of essential hypertensive patients

Forearm circulation	Skin microcirculation
Linder L et al. *Circulation* 1990	Rossi M et al. *J Cardiovasc Pharmacol* 1997
Panza JA et al. *N Eng J Med* 1990	**Renal circulation**
Hirooka Y et al. *Hypertension* 1993	Higashi Y et al. *Hypertension* 1995
Taddei S et al. *Hypertension* 1993	Mimran A et al. *Hypertension* 1995
Panza JA et al. *Circulation* 1993	Higashi Y et al. *Hypertension* 1996
Panza JA et al. *JACC* 1993	**Epicardial coronary arteries**
Panza JA et al. *JACC* 1994	Brush JE et al. *JACC* 1992
Taddei S et al. *Hypertension* 1994	Antony I et al. *Hypertension* 1994 *
Creager MA et al. *Hypertension* 1994	Egashira K et al. *Hypertension* 1995
Panza JA et al. *Circulation* 1995	Antony I et al. *Circulation* 1995 *
Taddei S et al. *Circulation* 1995	Antony I et al. *Circulation* 1996 *
Taddei S et al. *Circulation* 1995	Frielingsdorf J et al. *Circulation* 1996 *
Taddei S et al. *Hypertension* 1996	**Coronary microcirculation**
Taddei S et al. *Hypertension* 1997	Treasure CB et al. *Circ Res* 1992
Subcutaneous small arteries	Treasure CB et al. *Circulation* 1993
Schiffrin EL et al. *Hypertension* 1995	Egashira K et al. *J Clin Invest* 1993
Schiffrin EL et al. *J Hypertens* 1995	Egashira K et al. *Hypertension* 1995
Rizzoni D et al. *J Hypertens* 1997	*flow mediated dilation

Table 2. Positive and negative studies in the forearm
circulation of patients with essential hypertension

Positive studies in human forearm circulation					
Author	Reference	n° of NT	n° of HT	Agonist	Max rate
Linder L et al	*Circulation* 1990	8	8	Acetylcholine	160 mg/min
Panza JA et al	*N Eng J Med* 1990	18	18	Acetylcholine	30 m/min
Hirooka Y et al	*Hypertension* 1993	14	12	Acetylcholine	24 mg/min
Taddei S et al	*Hypertension* 1993	12	12	Acetylcholine	150 mg/min
Panza JA et al	*Circulation* 1993	10	11	Acetylcholine	30 mg/min
Panza JA et al	*Circulation* 1993	12	14	Acetylcholine	30 mg/min
Panza JA et al	*JACC* 1993	15	15	Acetylcholine	30 mg/min
Panza JA et al	*JACC* 1994	8	8	Substance P	4 pmol/min
Taddei S et al	*Hypertension* 1994	13	13	Acetylcholine	150 mg/min
Creager MA et al	*Hypertension* 1994	15	21	Methacholine	10 mg/min
Panza JA et al	*Circulation* 1995	10	12	Bradykinin	400 mg/min
				Acetylcholine	30 mg/min
Taddei S et al	*Circulation* 1995	53	57	Acetylcholine	150 mg/min
Taddei S et al	*Circulation* 1995	18	27	Acetylcholine	150 mg/min
Taddei S et al	*Hypertension* 1996	73	73	Acetylcholine	150 mg/min
Taddei S et al	*Hypertension* 1997	43	47	Acetylcholine	150 mg/min
Negative studies in human forearm circulation					
Author	Reference	n° of NT	n° of HT	Agonist	Max rate
Cockcroft JR et al	*N Eng J Med* 1994	19	17	Carbachol	2.5 mg/min
		18	41	Acetylcholine	15 mg/min
Bruning TA et al	*Hypertension* 1995	8	8	Methacholine	300 ng/Kg/min

NT, normotensive subjects; HT, essential hypertensive patients.

ence in forearm vasodilation to acetylcholine between antihypertensive patients and normotensive controls (56). This discrepancy is probably caused by the low concentrations of
acetylcholine employed by these authors (table 2). In the papers by Linder et al. (24) and
Taddei et al. (27), the amount of vasodilation induced by acetylcholine at a concentration
similar to the maximal level employed by Cockcroft et al. (around 15 µg/min) was not statistically different between normotensive subjects and essential hypertensive patients (56)
(fig. 1). Only when the authors increased the infusion rate of the agonist (up to 60 and 150
µg/min respectively) did they detect an endothelium-dependent vasodilation with statistically significant blunting in essential hypertensive patients as compared to normotensive
subjects. This result is in line with experimental literature demonstrating that endothelial
dysfunction can be detected only in the presence of a high degree of stimulation. It is also
worth noting that in several papers Panza et al. confirmed a blunted response to acetylcholine, although employing infusion rates in the same range as Cockcroft et al. (table 3).
However in the experimental conditions adopted by Panza et al., a degree of vasodilation
to acetylcholine in normotensive subjects of 20.8±8.0 ml/100 ml forearm tissue/min was
reached, which is in the same range as that obtained by the above quoted authors, while
Cockcroft et al. obtained a vasodilating effect of 14.2±1.6 ml/100 forearm tissue/min in
normotensive controls. This finding further points out the need to induce adequate stimulation in order to detect a possible difference in response to endothelium-dependent
agonists between normotensive subjects and essential hypertensive patients. The second
negative paper on this issue, by Brunning et al. (57), evaluated endothelium-dependent
vasodilation by methacholine infusion at rates comparable to other authors and did not

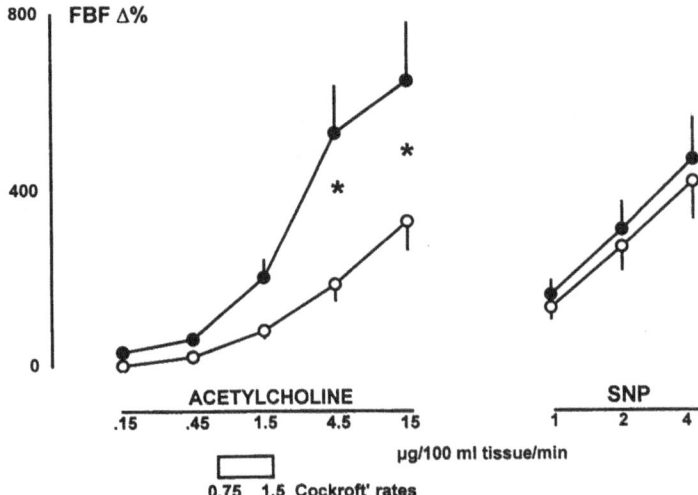

Figure 1. Line graphs show forearm blood flow (FBF) increase above basal induced by intra-arterial acetyl-choline (mg/100 ml forearm tissue/min) (left) and sodium nitroprusside (mg/100 ml forearm tissue/min) (right) in normotensive subjects (full circles) and essential hypertensive patients (open circles). Data are shown as means ± SEM and expressed as per cent increase above basal. Asterisks denote a significant difference between normoten-sive controls and hypertensive patients (p<0.05 or less). On the abscissa the acetylcholine infusion rates tested by Cockroft et al. in the study (ref.) not confirming the presence of endothelial dysfunction in essential hypertension are reported.

reproduce a difference in vascular response between hypertensive patients and normoten-sive controls. This study is flawed not only on account of the very low numerosity of the study population (8 hypertensives vs 8 normotensives) but also because the manner of pre-senting the data (only percent decrease in peripheral vascular resistances) does not allow in-depth analysis of the results and therefore impedes comparison of important parameters — such as maximal degree of forearm blood increase induced by the agonists — with those reported in other papers. We can therefore conclude that at the present time the evi-

Table 3. Difference in maximal vasodilation to acetylcholine in positive and negative studies on endothelial dysfunction in human hypertension

Positive studies in human forearm circulation				
Author	Reference	n°	Agonist	Max VD
Linder L et al	*Circulation* 1990	NT = 8	Acetylcholine	20.6±5.2
		HT = 8	160 mg/min	14.5±3.1
Panza JA et al	*N Eng J Med* 1990	NT = 18	Acetylcholine	20.8±8.0
		HT = 18	30 mg/min	9.1±5.0
Taddei S et al	*Hypertension* 1996	NT = 73	Acetylcholine	23.1±2.8
		HT = 73	150 mg/min	16.6±2.0
Negative studies in human forearm circulation				
Author	Reference	n°	Agonist	Max VD
Cockcroft JR et al	*N Eng J Med* 1994	NT = 18	Acetylcholine	14.2±1.6
		HT = 41	15 mg/min	14.1±1.6

NT, normotensive subjects; HT, essential hypertensive patients; Max VD, maximal vasodilation to the agonist.

dence that agonist-induced endothelial dysfunction is present in essential hypertension is largely demonstrated and confirmed while the available negative reports are few and not sufficiently convincing to counteract this statement.

Further controversy arises from use of acetylcholine as the agonist most widely employed to evaluate endothelium-dependent vasodilation (1). Thus, although muscarinic receptors are located on the endothelial cell surface, acetylcholine cannot be considered a physiological mediator of endothelium-dependent vasodilator since endogenous acetylcholine, which is released by nerve endings, is rapidly destroyed by cholinesterase and therefore cannot reach endothelial cells. However the presence of endothelial dysfunction in human hypertension has been confirmed by the utilization of stimuli such as bradykinin (34), substance P (31) or shear stress (47,49–51), which are also active endogenously. Another important issue concerns whether the degree of vasodilation reached by the previously mentioned endothelium-dependent agonists could be representative of blood flow modifications observed in physiological conditions. This argument can be addressed by comparing the flow response to acetylcholine or bradykinin and the ability of the forearm vascular bed to dilate under ischemia, which is the stimulus able to evoke the maximum degree of vasodilation in any vascular bed (fig. 2). It can be observed that the response to acetylcholine or bradykinin reaches around 25–30 ml/100 ml forearm tissue/min in normotensive subjects and 15–20 ml/100 ml forearm tissue/min in essential hypertensive patients, while the maximum vasodilation to ischemia reaches around 50 or 40 ml/100 ml forearm tissue/min in normotensive subjects and essential hypertensive patients respectively (fig. 2). It is evident from these data that the degree of vasodilation explored by testing endothelial function is within the mean ability of the vascular district to dilate and therefore in a physiologically functional range. Finally, another controversial point is represented by the mechanism through which acetylcholine causes vasodilation, and in particular whether the effect of the compound is totally endothelium-dependent. To resolve this issue it would be crucial to evaluate the vascular response to acetylcholine in the absence and presence of endothelium. This possibility is not ethically possible in humans

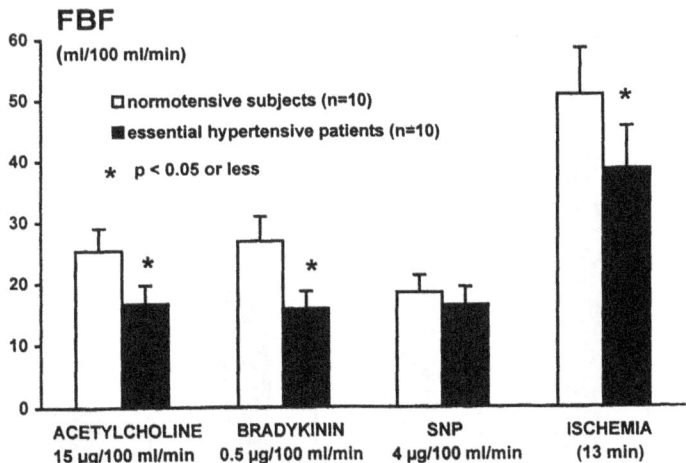

Figure 2. Bars indicate forearm blood flow increase above basal induced by acetylcholine, bradykinin, sodium nitroprusside and ischemia in normotensive controls and essential hypertensive patients. Data are shown as means ± SEM and expressed as absolute values. Asterisks denote a significant difference between normotensive controls and hypertensive patients (p<0.05 or less).

but similar information can be obtained from studies in epicardial coronary arteries. In segment of these vessels without angiographically evident atherosclerosis, intraarterial acetylcholine infusion induces relaxation. In contrast, in atherosclerotic segments, which are characterized by disruption of endothelial cells, intraarterial acetylcholine administration causes paradoxical vasoconstriction because of the stimulation of muscarinic receptors on muscle cells (58,59). These findings indirectly confirm that, at least in epicardial coronary arteries, the vasodilating effect of acetylcholine is endothelium-mediated. Moreover, the biochemical mechanism through which acetylcholine causes vasodilation has been specifically evaluated in the forearm circulation of healthy subjects. Vallance et al tested the effect of L-NMMA on vasodilation to acetylcholine, demonstrating that at a concentration of 4 pmol/min (corresponding to around 100 µg/100 ml forearm tissue/min) the compound was able to blunt the relaxing response to acetylcholine (18). The demonstration that L-NMMA reduced but did not abolish the vasodilating effect of acetylcholine raised the possibility that part of the effect of the compound is endothelium-independent. However this criticism does not take into account that L-NMMA is a competitive antagonist for NO-synthase and therefore its local concentration must be sufficient high to completely block the enzyme. In the paper by Vallance et al, a single dose of L-NMMA was tested. Therefore it is not possible to know what degree of antagonism was reached. To test this specific issue, we designed a study where we tested the effect of L-NMMA at increasing doses on the vasodilating response to acetylcholine in normotensive subjects. By increasing L-NMMA from 10 to 1000 µg/100 ml forearm tissue/min we obtained a dose-dependent inhibition of acetylcholine-induced vasodilation (evaluated at the highest infusion rates [4.5 and 15 µg / 100 ml forearm tissue / min] employed in our experimental conditions) ranging from around 20% to 90% (fig 3). Thus this study clearly demonstrates that in the forearm circulation of healthy humans the vasodilating effect of acetylcholine is exclusively NO-dependent. This finding is reinforced by the evidence that alternative mechanisms through which acetylcholine could induce vasodilation have been previously excluded in humans. In certain vessels from different animal species, acetylcholine can

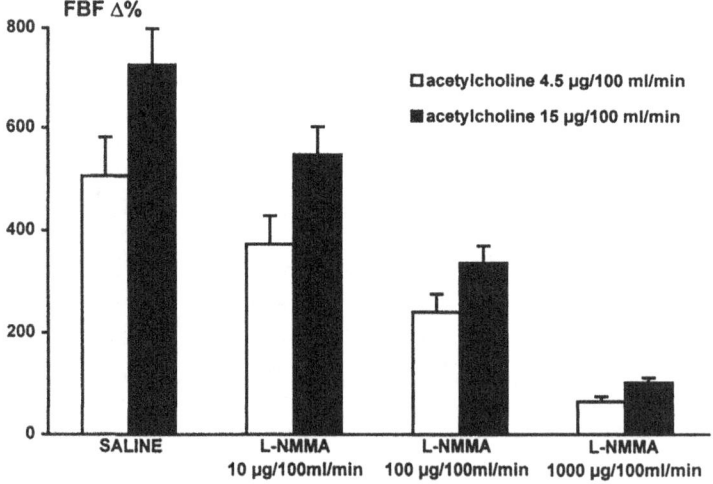

Figure 3. Bars indicate forearm vasodilation induced by intra-arterial acetylcholine under control conditions (saline infusion) and in presence of N^G-monomethyl-L-arginine (L-NMMA) at increasing infusion rates (µg/100 ml/min) in normotensive subjects. Data are shown as means ± SEM and expressed as percent increase above basal.

evoke relaxation through α-adrenolitic properties, by inducing prostacyclin or EDHF production. In healthy humans these possibilities have been excluded by the demonstration that neither phentolamine, an α-adrenoceptor antagonist (24), indomethacin (27) or acetyl salicylic acid (24), inhibitors of cyclooxygenase, or ouabain (35), an antagonist for EDHF, affect the vasodilating effect of acetylcholine.

MECHANISMS RESPONSIBLE FOR ENDOTHELIAL DYSFUNCTION IN ESSENTIAL HYPERTENSION

However, in our opinion, the degree of vasodilation to an endothelium-dependent agonist is not the best marker to evaluate the possible presence of endothelial dysfunction in any given study population. What is probably more important is to look at the mechanisms involved in endothelium-dependent vasodilation, since identification of the different pathways activated in the presence of essential hypertension, or other cardiovascular risk factors, not only better defines a dysfunctioning endothelium, but also allows to understand the clinical relevance of this vascular alteration. As previously stated, in healthy controls L-NMMA causes inhibition of the vasodilating action to acetylcholine (18,20,21). In contrast, in essential hypertensive patients L-NMMA does not change the response to acetylcholine (20,21,30,35), indicating the presence of a dysfunction in the NO-system. But this alteration is not the only one that can be identified in essential hypertension. In the same patients, but not in healthy controls, intrabrachial indomethacin can increase the vasodilating response to acetylcholine (27), confirming the experimental evidence that in primary hypertension EDCFs participate in the impaired endothelium-dependent vasodilation. Moreover, when the effect of L-NMMA on response to acetylcholine was retested in the presence of indomethacin, its inhibitory activity was restored, indicating that cyclooxygenase-derived EDCFs can at least partially impair the NO-system (60). On the basis of the experimental literature, the most likely candidates as the cause of NO breakdown are superoxide anions (61). In line with this possibility, preliminary observations (62) showed that intrabrachial administration of vitamin C, a superoxide anion scavenger, increased the vasodilating response to acetylcholine in the forearm vasculature of essential hypertensive patients, but not of normotensive controls. The effect of vitamin C on vasodilation to acetylcholine was specific since, in the same study population, the compound did not change the vascular response to sodium nitroprusside. Finally to test whether cyclooxygenase was the possible source of superoxide anions, we studied the effect of vitamin C in the presence of indomethacin, observing that cyclooxygenase inhibition prevented the facilitating effect of the superoxide anion scavenger on vasodilation to acetylcholine. Taken together these findings support the hypothesis that cyclooxygenase-dependent superoxide anion production could be one of the mechanisms responsible for endothelial dysfunction in essential hypertension (fig. 4).

CLINICAL SIGNIFICANCE OF ENDOTHELIAL DYSFUNCTION IN ESSENTIAL HYPERTENSION

It is evident that demonstration of a mere reduction in the ability of endothelial cells to dilate has a much lower pathophysiological significance than the demonstration that this alteration is caused by a defect in the L-arginine-NO pathway, mainly induced by the

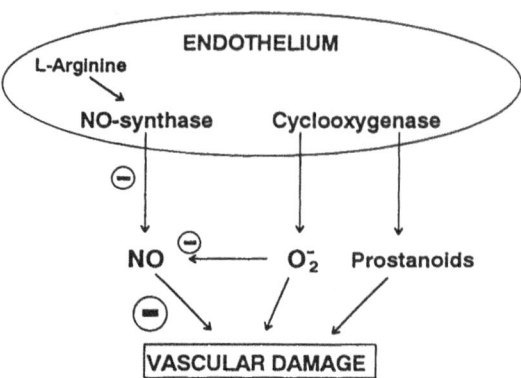

Figure 4. Mechanisms responsible for endothelial dysfunction in essential hypertension: a primary alteration in the L-arginine-NO pathway which leads to a decrease in NO production and/or effectiveness (left); production of cyclooxygenase dependent superoxide anions, which cause NO breakdown, and vasoconstrictor prostanoids.

production of oxygen free radicals. Thus if we consider the biological effects of NO, we can observe that it not only causes vasodilation, but also inhibits platelet aggregation (10), smooth muscle cell proliferation (11) and monocyte migration (12). Moreover EDCFs not only cause vasoconstriction but can also facilitate platelet aggregation or smooth muscle cell proliferation, either by a direct effect or indirectly by NO break-down. It is therefore conceivable that endothelial dysfunction could be the common pathogenetic mechanism inducing the development of atherosclerosis in the presence of hypertension. This possibility is in agreement with the evidence (63) that in never treated essential hypertensive patients maximum forearm blood flow response to acetylcholine, but not to sodium nitroprusside, was inversely ($r=-0.54$; $p<0.001$) related to intima-media thickening (IMT) of carotid arteries and unrelated either to left ventricular mass index or minimal forearm vascular resistances, an integrated index of vascular structural alterations. These data indicate that endothelial dysfunction is unrelated either to cardiac or microvascular structural changes induced by hypertension, while it is correlated with carotid artery IMT, an index of atherosclerotic vascular damage (64). Such a finding confirms that endothelial dysfunction could be involved in the pathogenesis of atherosclerosis in essential hypertensive patients (fig. 4). In line with this hypothesis is the demonstration that impaired endothelium-dependent vasodilation is not characteristic of essential hypertension only, but is also associated with different cardiovascular risk factors such as aging (33,37,65), post-menopause (66), hypercholesterolemia (67,68), diabetes mellitus (69,70) and smoking (71,72). Endothelial dysfunction is also detectable in the presence of coronary atherosclerosis (59). In addition the simultaneous presence of two cardiovascular risk factors, such as hypercholesterolemia and smoking (73) or aging and hypertension (33), induces a further deterioration of endothelium-dependent vasodilation. Endothelial function is thus impaired in the presence of various cardiovascular risk factors and deteriorates even further with their combination. Moreover, similarly to phenomena observed in essential hypertension, in hypercholesterolemic or diabetic patients and smokers, oxidative stress is one of the mechanisms identified as responsible for impaired endothelium-dependent vasodilation. Taken together, these findings suggest a link between endothelial dysfunction and cardiovascular damage. This possibility does not derive from a simplistic vision identifying endothelial dysfunction as the pathogenetic mechanism by the impaired ability of endothelium to dilate, but from a complex relationship between different mechanisms leading to vascular protection or damage. It is tempting to speculate that progressive impairment of the NO-pathway and the parallel production of EDCFs cause an unfavourable imbalance of the two systems causing vascular atherosclerosis.

CONCLUSIONS

Convincing evidence indicates that human essential hypertension is associated with blunted basal production of NO and impaired agonist-evoked endothelium-dependent vasodilation, which is probably the marker of a generalized endothelial dysfunction. Impaired endothelium-dependent vasodilation is characterized by production of factors such as superoxide anions, which can impair the beneficial and protective effects of NO on the vessel wall. Therefore endothelial dysfunction could be one of the promoters of athero sclerotic lesions and consequently of some of the cardiovascular complications associated with essential hypertension.

REFERENCES

1. Luscher TF, Vanhoutte PM: The endothelium: modulator of cardiovascular function. Boca Raton, Fla, CRC Press, 1990.
2. Furchgott RF, Zawadzki JV: The obligatory role of endothelial cells in the relaxation of arterial smooth muscle by acetylcholine. Nature 1980; 288:373–376.
3. Palmer RMJ, Ferrige AG, Moncada S: Nitric oxide release accounts for the biological activity of endothelium-derived relaxing factor. Nature 1987; 327:524–6.
4. Palmer RMJ, Ashton DS, Moncada S: Vascular endothelial cells synthesize nitric oxide from L-arginine. Nature 1988; 333:664–6.
5. Bredt DS, Hwang PM, Glatt CE, Lowenstein C, Reed RR, Snyder SH: Cloned and expressed nitric oxide synthase structurally resembles cytochrome P-450 reductase. Nature 1991; 351:714.
6. Rees DD, Palmer RMJ, Hodson HF, Moncada S: A specific inhibitor of nitric oxide formation from L-arginine attenuates endothelium-dependent relaxation. Br J Pharmacol 1989; 96:418–424.
7. Moncada S, Vane JR: Pharmacology and endogenous roles of prostaglandin endoperoxides, thromboxane A_2 and prostacyclin. Pharmacol Rev 1979; 30:293–331.
8. Feletou M, Vanhoutte PM: Endothelium-dependent hyperpolarization of canine coronary smooth muscle. Br J Pharmacol 1988; 93:515.
9. Rubanyi GM, Romero JC, Vanhoutte PM: Flow-induced release of endothelium-derived relaxing factor. Am J Physiol 1986; 250:H1145–H1149.
10. Radomski MW, Palmer RMJ, Moncada S: The anti-aggregating properties of vascular endothelium: Interactions between prostacyclin and nitric oxide. Br J Pharmacol 1987; 92:639–646. New York: Raven Press, 1989:1–13.
11. Scott-Burden T, Vanhoutte PM: The endothelium as a regulator of vascular smooth muscle proliferation. Circulation 1993; 87:V-51–V-55.
12. Kubes P, Suzuki M, Granger DN: Nitric oxide: an endogenous modulator of leucocyte adhesion. Proc Natl Acad Sci USA, 1991; 88; 4651–4655.
13. Miller VM, Vanhoutte PM: Endothelium-dependent contractions to arachidonic acid are mediated by products of cyclooxygenase. Am J Physiol 1985; 248:H432–H437.
14. Altiere RJ, Kiritsy-Roy JA, Catravas JD: Acetylcholine-induced contractions in isolated rabbit pulmonary arteries: Role of thromboxane A_2. J Pharmacol Exp Ther 1986; 236:535–541.
15. Katusic ZS, Vanhoutte PM: Superoxide anion is an endothelium-derived contracting factor. Am J Physiol 1989; 257:H33–H37.
16. Vanhoutte PM: Endothelium and control of vascular function. State of the art lecture. Hypertension 1989; 13:658–667.
17. Lüscher TF: Imbalance of endothelium-derived relaxing and contracting factors: a new concept in hypertension? Am J Hypertens 1990; 3:317.

18. Vallance P, Collier J, Moncada S: Effects of endothelium-derived nitric oxide on peripheral arteriolar tone in man. Lancet 1989; ii:997–1000.

19. Calver A, Collier J, Moncada S, Vallance P: Effect of local intra-arterial N^G-monomethyl-L-arginine in patients with hypertension: the nitric oxide dilator mechanism appears abnormal. J Hypertens 1992; 10: 1025–1031.

20. Panza JA, Casino PR, Kilcoyne CM, Quyyumi AA: Role of endothelium-derived nitric oxide in the abnormal endothelium-dependent vascular relaxation of patients with essential hypertension. Circulation 1993; 87: 1468–74.

21. Taddei S, Virdis A, Mattei P, Natali A, Ferrannini E, Salvetti A: Effect of insulin on acetylcholine-induced vasodilation in normotensive subjects and patients with essential hypertension. Circulation 1995; 92:2911–2918.

22. Lyons D, Webster J, Benjamin N: The effect of antihypertensive therapy on responsiveness to local intra-arterial N^G-monomethyl-L-arginine in patients with essential hypertension. J Hypertens 1994; 12:1047–1052.

23. Panza JA, Garcìa CE, Kilcoyne CM, Quyyumi AA, Cannon RO: Impaired endothelium-dependent vasodilation in patients with essential hypertension. Evidence that nitric oxide abnormality is not localized to a single signal transduction pathway. Circulation 1995; 91:1732–1738.

24. Linder L, Kiowski W, Buhler FR, Luscher TF: Indirect evidence for the release of endothelium-derived relaxing factor in the human forearm circulation in vivo: Blunted response in essential hypertension. Circulation 1990; 81:1762–1767.

25. Panza JA, Quyyumi AA, Brush JE Jr, Epstein SE: Abnormal endothelium dependent vascular relaxation in patients with essential hypertension. N Engl J Med 1990; 323:22–7.

26. Hirooka Y, Imaizumi T, Masaki H et al.: Captopril improves impaired endothelium-dependent vasodilation in hypertensive patients. Hypertension 1992; 20:175–180.

27. Taddei S, Virdis A, Mattei P, Salvetti A: Vasodilation to acetylcholine in primary and secondary forms of human hypertension. Hypertension 1993; 21:929–33.

28. Panza JA, Casino PR, Badar DM, Quyyumi AA: Effect of increased availability of endothelium-derived nitric oxide precursor on endothelium-dependent vascular relaxation in normal subjects and in patients with essential hypertension. Circulation 1993; 87:1475–1481.

29. Panza JA, Quyyumi AA, Callahan TS, Epstein SE: Effect of antihypertensive treatment on endothelium-dependent vascular relaxation in patients with essential hypertension. J Am Coll Cardiol 1993; 21:1145–1151.

30. Taddei S, Mattei P, Virdis A, Sudano I, Ghiadoni L, Salvetti A: Effect of potassium on vasodilation to acetylcholine in essential hypertension. Hypertension 1994; 23:485–490.

31. Panza JA, Casino PR, Kilcoyne CM, Quyyumi AA: Impaired endothelium-dependent vasodilation in patients with essential hypertension: evidence that the abnormality is not at the muscarinic receptor level. J Am Coll Cardiol 1994; 23:1610–1616.

32. Creager MA, Roddy MA: Effect of captopril and enalapril on endothelial function in hypertensive patients. Hypertension 1994; 24:499–505.

33. Taddei S, Virdis A, Mattei P, Ghiadoni L, Gennari A, Basile Fasolo C, Sudano I, Salvetti A: Aging and endothelial function in normotensive subjects and essential hypertensive patients. Circulation, 1995; 91: 1981–1987.

34. Panza JA, Garcia CE, Kilcoyne CM, Quyyumi A, Cannon III RO: Impaired endothelium-dependent vasodilation in patients with essential hypertension. Evidence that nitric oxide abnormality is not localised to a single signal transduction pathway. Circulation 1995; 91:1732–1738.

35. Taddei S, Virdis A, Mattei P, Natali A, Ferrannini E, Salvetti A: Effect of insulin on acetylcholine-induced vasodilation in normotensive subjects and patients with essential hypertension. Circulation 1995; 92:2911–2918.

36. Taddei S, Virdis A, Ghiadoni L et al.: Menopause is associated with endothelial dysfunction in women. Hypertension 1996; 28:576–582.

37. Taddei S, Virdis A, Mattei P, Ghiadoni L, Basile Fasolo C, Sudano I, Salvetti A: Hypertension causes premature aging of endothelial function in humans. Hypertension 1997; 29:736–743.

38. Schultz KD, Schultz K, Schultz G: Sodium nitroprusside and other smooth muscle relaxants increase cyclic GMP levels in rat ductus deferens. Nature 1977; 265:750–751.

39. Rossi M, Taddei S, Fabbri A, Tintori G, Credidio L, Virdis A, Ghiadoni L, Salvetti A, Giusti C: Cutaneous vasodilation to acetylcholine in patients with essential hypertension. J Cardiovasc Pharmacol 1997; in press.

40. Schiffrin EL, Deng LY: Comparison of effects of angiotensin I-converting enzyme inhibition and β-blockade for 2 years on function of small arteries from hypertensive patients. Hypertension 1995; 25[part 2]:699–703.

41. Schiffrin LE, Deng LY: Structure and function of resistance arteries of hypertensive patients treated with a β-blocker or a calcium channel antagonist. J Hypertens 1995; 14:1247–1255.

42. Rizzoni D, Muiesan ML, Porteri E, Castellano M, Zulli R, Bettoni G, Salvetti M, Monteduro C, Agabiti-Rosei E: Effects of long-term antihypertensive treatment with lisinopril on resistance arteries in hypertensive patients with left ventricular hypertrophy. J Hypertens 1997; 15:197–204.

43. Higashi Y, Oshima T, Ozono R, Watanabe M, Natsuura H, Kajiyama G: Effects of L-arginine infusion on renal hemodynamics in patients with mild essential hypertension. Hypertension 1995; 25[part 2]:898–902.

44. Mimran A, Ribstein J, DuCailar G: Contrasting effect of antihypertensive treatment on the renal response to L-arginine. Hypertension 1995; 26[part 1]:937–941.

45. Higashi Y, Oshima T, Ozono R, Watanabe M, Natsuura H, Kajiyama G: Renal response to L-arginine in salt-sensitive patients with essential hypertension. Hypertension 1996; 27[part 2]:643–648.

46. Brush JE, Faxon DP, Salmon S, Jacobs AK, Ryan TJ: Abnormal endothelium-dependent coronary vasomotion in hypertensive patients. J Am Coll Cardiol 1992; 92:809–815.

47. Antony I, Aptecar E, Lerebours G, Nitenberg A: Coronary artery constriction caused by the cold pressor test in human hypertension. Hypertension 1994; 24:212–219.

48. Egashira K, Suzuki S, Hirooka YA, Sugimachi M. Imaizumi T, Takeshita A: Impaired endothelium-dependent vasodilation of large epicardial and resistance coronary arteries in patients with essential hypertension. Different responses to acetylcholine and substance P. Hypertension 1995; 25:201–206.

49. Antony I, Lerebours G, Nitenberg A: Loss of flow-dependent coronary artery dilatation in patients with hypertension. Circulation 1995; 91:1624–1628.

50. Antony I, Lerebours G, Nitenberg A: Angiotensin-converting enzyme inhibition restores flow-dependent and cold pressor test-induced dilations in coronary arteries of hypertensive patients. Circulation 1996; 94: 3115–3122.

51. Frielingsdorf J, Seiler C, Kaufmann P, Vassalli G, Suter T, Hess OM: Normalization of abnormal coronary vasomotion by calcium antagonists in patients with hypertension. Circulation 1996; 93:1380–1387.

52. Treasure CB, Manoukian SV, Klein JL et al.: Epicardial coronary artery responses to acetylcholine are impaired in hypertensive patients. Circ Res 1992; 71,6–781.

53. Treasure CB, Klein JL, Vita JA, Manoukian SV, Renwick GH, Selwyn AP, Ganz P, Alexander RW: Hypertension and left ventricular hypertrophy are associated with impaired endothelium-mediated relaxation in human coronary resistance vessels. Circulation 1993; 87:86–93.

54. Egashira K, Inou T, Hirooka YA, Yamada A, Maruoka Y: Impaired coronary blood flow response to acetylcholine in patients with coronary risk factors and proximal atherosclerotic lesions. J Clin Invest 1993; 91: 29–37.

55. Egashira K, Suzuki S, Hirooka YA, Kai H, Sugimachi M, Imaizumi T, Takeshita A: Impaired endothelium-dependent vasodilation of large epicardial and resistance coronary arteries in patients with essential hypertension. Different responses to acetylcholine and substance P. Hypertension 1995; 25:201–206.

56. Cockroft JR, Chowienczyk PJ, Benjamin N, Ritter JM: Preserved endothelium-dependent vasodilation in patients with essential hypertension. N Engl J Med 1994; 330:1036–1040.

57. Brunning TA, Chang PC, Hendriks GC, Vermeij P, Pfaffendorf M, van Zwieten PA: In vivo characterization of muscarinic receptor subtypes that mediate vasodilation in patients with essential hypertension. Hypertension 1995; 26:70–77.

58. Hodgson JMcB, Marshall JJ: Direct vasoconstriction and endothelium-dependent vasodilation. Mechanisms of acetylcholine effects on coronary flow and arterial diameter in patients with nonstenotic coronary arteries. Circulation 1989; 79:1043–1051.

59. Yasue H, Matsuyama K, Matsuyama K, Okumura K, Morikami Y, Ogawa H: Responses of angiographically normal human coronary arteries to intracoronary injection of acetylcholine by age and segment. Possible role of early coronary atherosclerosis. Circulation 1990; 81:482–490.

60. Taddei S, Virdis A, Ghiadoni L, Magagna A, Salvetti A: Cyclooxygenase inhibition restores nitric oxide activity in essential hypertension. Hypertension 1997; in press.

61. Kontos HA, Kontos MC: Role of products of univalent reduction of oxygen in hypertensive vascular injury. In Hypertension: Pathophysiology, Diagnosis, and Management. Second Edition, edited by J.H. Laragh and B.M. Brenner, Raven Press, Ltd., New York 1995. pp 685–696.

62. Virdis A, Taddei S, Ghiadoni L, Salvetti A: Effect of vitamin C on vasodilation to acetylcholine in the forearm of essential hypertensive patients. Hypertension, 1996; 28:695(abs).

63. Virdis A, Taddei S, Ghiadoni L et al.: Endothelial function and common carotid wall thickening in untreated essential hypertensive patients. J Hypertens 1996; 14(suppl1):S48(abs).

64. Crouse III JR, Craven TE, Hagaman AP, Bond G: Association of coronary disease with segment specific intimal-medial thickening of the extracranial carotid artery. Circulation 1995; 92:1141–1147.

65. Zeiher AM, Drexter H, Saurbier B, Just H: Endothelium-mediated coronary blood flow modulation in humans. Effects of age, atherosclerosis, hypercholesterolemia, and hypertension. J Clin Invest 1993; 92:652–62.

66. Taddei S, Virdis A, Ghiadoni L, Mattei P, Sudano I, Bernini G, Pinto S, Salvetti A: Menopause is associated with endothelial dysfunction in women. Hypertension 1996; 28:576–582.

67. Creager MA, Cooke JP, Mendelsohn ME et al.: Impaired vasodilation of forearm resistance vessels in hypercholesterolemic humans. J Clin Invest 1990; 86:228–234.

68. Casino PR, Kilcoyne CM, Quyyumi AA, Hoeg JM, Panza JA: The role of nitric-oxide in endothelium-dependent vasodilation of hypercholesterolemic patients. Circulation 1993; 88:2541–2547.
69. Johnstone MT, Creager SJ, Scales KM, Cusco JA, Lee BK, Creager MA: Impaired endothelium-dependent vasodilation in patients with insulin-dependent diabetes mellitus. Circulation 1993; 88:2510–2516.
70. Ting HH, Timini FK, Boles KS, Creager SJ, Ganz P, Creager MA: Vitamin C improves endothelium-dependent vasodilation in patients with non-insulin-dependent diabetes mellitus. J Clin Invest 1996; 97: 22–28.
71. Kiowski W, Linder L, Stoschitzky K et al.: Diminished vascular response to inhibition of endothelium-derived nitric oxide and enhanced vasoconstriction to exogenously administered endothelin-1 in clinically healthy smokers. Circulation 1994; 90:27–34.
72. Celermajer DS, Adams MR, Clarkson P et al.: Passive smoking and impaired endothelium-dependent arterial dilatation in healthy young adults. N Engl J Med 1996; 334:150–154.
73. Heitzer T, Ylä-Herttauala S, Luoma J et al.: Cigarette smoking potentiates endothelial dysfunction of forearm resistance vessels in patients with hypercholesterolemia. Role of oxidized LDL. Circulation 1996; 93: 1346–1353.

ENDOTHELIAL DYSFUNCTION IN HYPERTENSIVES

An Uncertain Association

P. A. van Zwieten[*]

Departments of Pharmacotherapy, Cardiology, and Cardiopulmonary Surgery
Academic Medical Center
University of Amsterdam
P.O. Box 22700
1100 DE Amsterdam
The Netherlands

1. INTRODUCTION

The experimental evidence for endothelial dysfunction associated with hypertensive disease appears impressive at first sight, and the relationship between both phenomena has been zealously defended by its protagonists (1–3).

The following observations and arguments appear to be supportive of a relevant role of endothelial dysfunction in hypertensive disease:

a. In various animal models, the blockade of NO-synthesis by NO-synthase inhibitors, such as L-NAME and related agents causes hypertension and, in the long-term, the detrimental sequelae of this disorder (even including enhanced atherosclerosis) (4,5).

b. In salt-sensitive Dahl rats, the hypertensive action of salt overload is counteracted by treatment with L-arginine, the natural basis of the L-arginine–NO-pathway.

c. Several studies using human forearm plethysmography have shown that the endothelium-dependent vasodilator effect of acetylcholine (ACh) is attenuated in hypertensive patients and even in the non-hypertensive offspring of hypertensive parents (7–10). Furthermore, the vasoconstrictor response to L-arginine-antagonists proved diminished in hypertensives, whereas L-arginine itself enhanced the vasodilator effect of ACh.

* Address for correspondence: Prof. Dr. P. A. van Zwieten, Universiteit van Amsterdam, Academisch Medisch Centrum, Afd. Farmacotherapie/Cardiologie, Meibergdreef 15, 1105 AZ Amsterdam. Tel: 020-566 4977/4976, Fax: 020-696 8704

Hypertension and the Heart, edited by Zanchetti et al.
Plenum Press, New York, 1997

247

d. Measurements of whole-body NO-production indicated that in patients with essential hypertension, the synthesis of NO is diminished under basal conditions (11). The methodology used in this investigation did not allow to decide whether the impaired synthesis is primary or secondary to a rise in blood pressure.

However, the hypothesis of endothelial dysfunction as an important and specific mechanism in hypertensive disease and its complications is challenged more and more by experimental data and methodological disputes, and the debate on this issue is ongoing since a few years. In this connection, it appears mandatory not only to listen to the protagonists but also to critically evaluate the data that challenge the role of the endothelium in hypertension.

2. ARGUMENTS AGAINST THE OCCURRENCE OF GENERALIZED ENDOTHELIAL DYSFUNCTION IN HYPERTENSIVE DISEASE

2.1. Isolated Tissues and Animal Models

Several experiments in isolated blood vessels and animal models do not support the hypothesis that hypertensive disease is associated with functionally damaged endothelium. This subject was reviewed by Angus (12), who concluded that the numerous results obtained were at best controversial.

Several studies in isolated vessels taken from hypertensive animals have been performed. As described in the review by Angus (12), the results are controversial, and most of the studies used isolated conduit arteries (such as the aorta), which are not primarily relevant in connection with elevated blood pressure. Accordingly, the data obtained in isolated resistance vessels from hypertensive animals are so far not consistent and do not clearly point towards a generalized endothelial dysfunction associated with hypertensive disease.

As an example, we mention the studies by our own group in the isolated perfused mesenteric vascular bed of normotensive and spontaneously hypertensive rats (SHR) (13). In this study, an endothelium-dependent vasodilator response was evoked by methacholine (MCh). MCh was preferred over acetylcholine (ACh), since it is a stable compound which is not degraded by esterases. MCh displays the same receptor profile as ACh, that is non-selective agonism towards the various muscarinic-receptor subtypes (M_1, M_2, M_3, M_4). The vasodilator response to MCh was counteracted by different types of the (moderately) selective muscarinic-receptor angatonists. This pharmacological analysis indicated that the vasodilator effect of MCh is predominantly mediated by the endothelial M_3-receptor. The dilator response to MCh was also found in preparations obtained from SHR, and it proved exactly the same as that in the mesenteric vascular bed of normotensive animals. In both types of preparations, the receptor (M_3) was involved, as concluded from the analysis with selective muscarinic receptor antagonists (13).

A few data have been published on studies performed with isolated vessels obtained from hypertensive humans. In a recent study by Thybo et al. (14), subcutaneous resistance arteries taken from hypertensives were compared with those of appropriately matched control persons. Both the endothelium-dependent responses to acetylcholine and the endothelium-independent vasodilator action of sodium nitroprusside proved identical in both types of preparations. Consequently, these data do not support the hypothesis of a generalized abnormality in the endothelium-dependent or -independent relaxation in hypertensives.

2.2. Studies in the Human Forearm Vascular Bed

Venous occlusion plethysmography allows the determination or calculation of blood flow and vascular resistance in a human vascular bed in situ, and this methodology has proved most useful for quantitative pharmacodynamic studies. It should be realized that the various effects of drugs in this vascular bed predominantly involve resistance vessels.

We already mentioned that several investigators observed an attenuated vasodilator response to ACh in the forearm vascular bed of hypertensive patients (1–3). However, these findings have been challenged by others, who observed that endothelial function is preserved in this vascular bed in hypertensives.

A recent study by Laurent et al. (15) indicated that the mechanism of flow dilatation of the brachial artery, which is endothelium-dependent, is not impaired in subjects with essential hypertension. Comparable findings were obtained at the site of the femoral artery (16).

An extensive and well-designed study by Cockroft et al. (17) clearly shows that both endothelium-dependent (acetylcholine, carbachol) and endothelium-independent (Na-nitroprusside) vasodilatation are fully preserved in subjects with essential hypertension.

Our own group investigated the muscarinic-receptor-mediated vasodilatation in the human forearm vascular bed in hypertensives and appropriately matched normotensives (18,19). As in the aforementioned experiments in an isolated vessel preparation (13), methacholine (MCh) was used as the (non-selective) muscarinic-receptor agonist. These experiments clearly showed that endothelium-dependent, MCh-induced vasodilatation in the forearm vascular bed is predominantly mediated by muscarinic receptors of the M_3-subtype. As in the isolated vessel experiments, this conclusion was drawn from an analysis with selective muscarinic-receptor antagonists (18,19). Interestingly, the methacholine-induced vasodilator effect of methacholine and also that of Na-nitroprusside was fully preserved in hypertensives. Futhermore, the quantitative characteristics of the dose-response curves of methacholine in hypertensives were identical to those obtained in the age- and sex-matched normotensive control subjects (18,19). In addition, the influence of muscarinic-receptor antagonists (more or less selective for particular muscarinic-receptor subtypes) on M_3-receptor-mediated vasodilatation was identical in hypertensive and normotensive subjects, as visualized in Fig. 1 (19).

3. ATTEMPTS TO EXPLAIN THE DISCREPANCIES

There exists an obvious discrepancy between the various experimental findings obtained in investigations aiming at the clarification of the role of the endothelium in hypertensive disease. Much of this discrepancy may be attributed to differences in methodology, choice of tissues, preparations, subjects, et cetera.

A few points deserve to be mentioned here:

a. Evidence in favour of endothelial dysfunction in isolated vessels and animal models has been largely restricted to large conduit arteries, such as the aorta (12), and very few studies have been performed in resistance arteries, which are highly relevant in the regulation of blood pressure.

b. Several questions remain to be clarified with respect to the numerous studies in the human forearm vascular bed. Forearm plethysmography is frequently performed (also by our own group), because this vascular bed is readily accessible

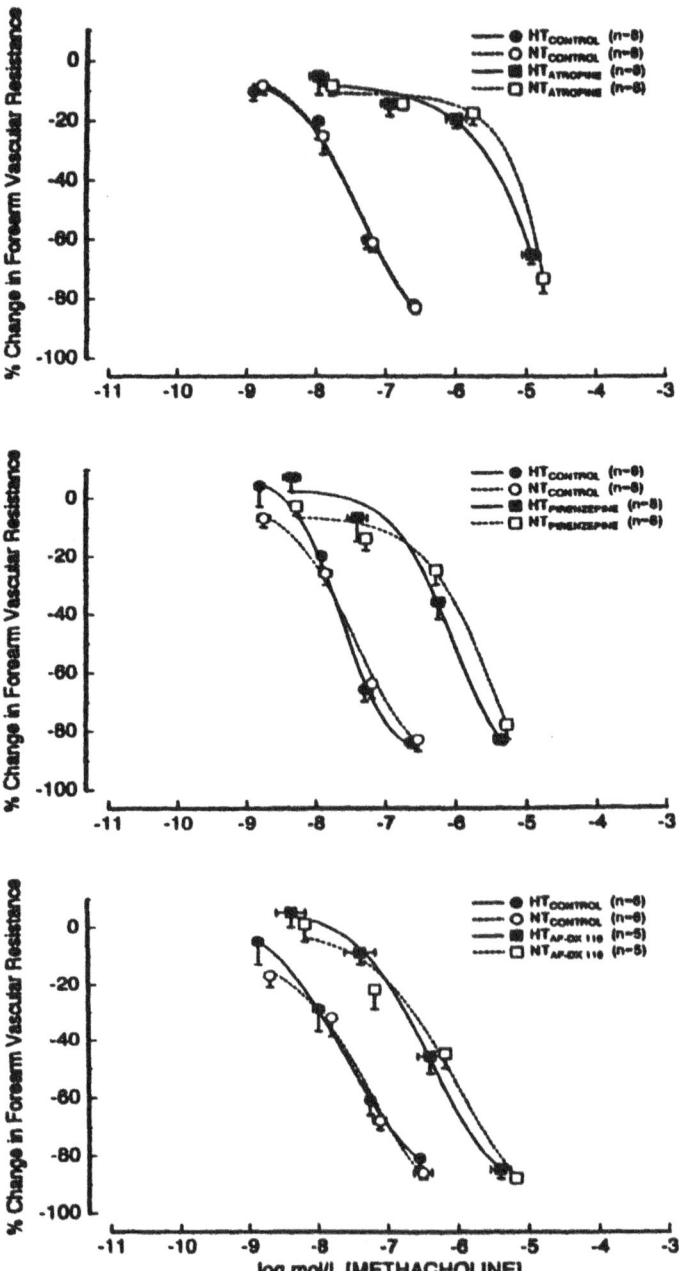

Figure 1. Line graphs show concentration-response curves in hypertensive patients (HT) and normotensive control subjects (NT) for the vasodilator response to methacholine in the presence of vehicle (control) and during simultaneous administration of the different muscarinic receptor antagonists. Top, atropine (50 ng per minute IA; middle, pirenzepine (500 ng/kg per minute IA); bottom, AF-DX 116 (4000 ng/kg per minute IA). Forearm vascular resistance is expressed as percent change relative to baseline. Values are mean ± SEM. Note the rank order for potency of the three antagonists in shifting the concentration-response curve of methacholine: atropine (nonselective) > pirenzepine ($M_1 > M_3 > M_2$) > AF-DX 116 ($M_2 > M_1 > M_3$). The curves obtained in hypertensive patients and normotensive control subjects coincide in all three series of experiments. From reference 19, with permission.

in humans, in contrast to several other circuits which may be much more relevant. Secondly, it is customary to study endothelial function by means of ACh, which is highly sensitive to biodegradation by esterases in the blood and in the vascular system. Accordingly, differences in esterase activity may play an important role (17). We already mentioned that for this reason we ourselves (18,19) prefer MCh as the agonist because of its insensitivity towards degradation by esterases. Furthermore, differences in the length of the forearm may be expected to influence the experimental results (17). Finally, it is uncertain whether this particular vascular bed is suitable for studies in hypertension, where splanchnic resistance vessels are probably the most important ones.

  c. The common denominator "hypertension" covers several subgroups of patients with different backgrounds, and there is no doubt that hypertension should be considered a heterogeneous disease. For this reason, it may well be that important discrepancies are brought about by the fact that rather different subgroups of patients have been investigated in the various studies. Identification of various subgroups of hypertensive patients would probably be helpful to explain some of the discrepancies. Unfortunately, it is so far unclear which criteria for the differentiation and identification of such subgroups have to be applied.

4. CONCLUSIONS AND PERSPECTIVES

Protagonists of an important role of endothelial dysfunction should take notice of the fact that several investigations have now been performed which speak against such a role. It particularly draws the attention to the fact that endothelial dysfunction has not convincingly been demonstrated to play a decisive role in hypertension. A great deal of the discrepancies is probably caused by methodological problems and diversities, whereas the heterogeneity of hypertensive disease may also play an important role.

A further issue that deserves our attention is the question how specific endothelial dysfunction, if it indeed occurs, may be in the pathophysiology of hypertension. The endothelium and its vasodilator function are known to deteriorate with increasing age and also in largely differing diseases, such as diabetes mellitus or hyperlipidaemia. It therefore remains doubtful whether endothelial dysfunction in hypertensive disease, if it indeed occurs, is a specific phenomenon or just the reflection of non-specific vascular damage. The uncertainty with respect to the morphological and functional deterioration in hypertensives as well as its lack of selectivity for this disease imply that endothelial dysfunction cannot be put forward as a generally accepted, functionally relevant process associated with hypertension.

REFERENCES

1. Vanhoutte PM, Boulanger CM. Endothelium-dependent responses in hypertension. Hypertens Res 1995; 18:87–98.
2. Nava E, Lüscher TF. Endothelium-derived vasoactive factors in hypertension: Nitric oxide and endothelin. J Hypertens 1995;13 (suppl 2):S39–S48.
3. Lüscher TF. The endothelium in hypertension: Bystander, target or mediator? J Hypertens 1994;12(suppl 10): S105–S116.
4. Ribeiro MO, Antunes E, de Nucci G, Lovisolo SM, Zatz R. Chronic inhibition of nitric oxide synthesis. A new model of arterial hypertension. Hypertension 1992;20:298–303.

5. Baylis C, Mitruka B, Deng A. Chronic blockade of nitric oxide synthesis in the rat produces systemic hypertension and glomerular damage. J Clin Invest 1992;90:278–281.

6. Chen PY, Sanders PW. L-arginine abrogates salt-sensitive hypertension in Dahl/Rapp rats. J Clin Invest 1991;88:1559–1567.

7. Linder L, Kiowski W, Bühler FR, Lüscher TF. Indirect evidence for the release of endothelium-derived relaxing factor in the human forearm circulation *in vivo*: Blunted response in essential hypertension. Circulation 1990;81:1762–1767.

8. Taddei S, Virdis A, Mattei P, Salvetti A. Vasodilatation to acetylcholine in primary and secondary forms of human hypertension. Hypertension 1993;21:929–933.

9. Panza JA, Casino PR, Kilcoyne CM, Quyyumi AA. Impaired endothelium-dependent vasodilatation in patients with essential hypertension: Evidence that the abnormality is not at the muscarinic receptor level. J Am Coll Cardiol 1994;23:1610–1616.

10. Panza JA, Garcia CE, Kilcoyne CM, Quyyumi AA, Cannon RO. Impaired endothelium-dependent vasodilatation in patients with essential hypertension: Evidence that nitric oxide abnormality is not localized to a single transduction pathway. Circulation 1995;91:1732–1738.

11. Forte P, Copland M, Smith LM, Milne E, Sutherland J, Benjamin N. Basal nitric oxide synthesis in essential hypertension. Lancet 1997;349:837–842.

12. Angus JA, Lew MJ. Interpretation of the acetylcholine test of endothelial cell dysfunction. J Hypertens 1992;10(suppl 7):S179–S186.

13. Hendriks MGC, Pfaffendorf M, van Zwieten PA. Characterization of the muscarinic receptors in the mesenteric vascular bed of spontaneously hypertensive rats. J Hypertens 1993;11:1329–1335.

14. Thybo NK, Mulvany MJ, Jastrup B, Nielsen H, Aalkjaer C. Some pharmacological and elastic characteristics of isolated small arteries from patients with essential hypertension. J Hypertens 1996;14:993–998.

15. Laurent S, Lacolley P, Brunel P, Laloux B, Safar ME. Flow-dependent vasodilation of brachial artery in essential hypertension. Am J Physiol 1990;258:H1004–H1011.

16. Girerd X, Arcaro G, Laurent S, Laloux B, Safar M. Study of flow-dependent vasodilation of the femoral artery in hypertensive and normotensive subjects. (In French.) Arch Mal Coeur Vaiss 1991;85:1075–1079.

17. Cockroft JR, Chowienczyck PJ, Ritter JM. Preserved endothelium-dependent vasodilation in patients with essential hypertension. N Engl J Med 1994;330:1036–1040.

18. Bruning TA, Hendriks MGC, Chang PC, Kuypers EA, van Zwieten PA. *In vivo* characterization of vasodilating muscarinic-receptor subtypes in humans. Circ Res 1994;74:912–919.

19. Bruning TA, Chang PC, Hendriks MGC, Vermeij P, Pfaffendorf M, van Zwieten PA. *In vivo* characterization of muscarinic receptor subtypes that mediate vasodilatation in patients with essential hypertension. Hypertension 1995;26:70–77.

27

HYPERTENSION, LEFT VENTRICULAR HYPERTROPHY, AND CORONARY FLOW RESERVE

Edward D. Frohlich*

Vice President for Academic Affairs
Alton Ochsner Medical Foundation
1516 Jefferson Highway
New Orleans, Louisiana 70121

The increased independent risk for premature cardiovascular mortality related to left ventricular hypertrophy (LVH) may be attributed to a number of underlying pathophysiological alterations[1]. Among the postulated mechanisms are: an intrinsic pathological defect inherent with the hypertrophied myocardium, *per se*; impaired ventricular pumping ability that may exacerbate decompensation; co-existent diseases of the left ventricle (e.g., occlusive epicardial artery atherosclerosis, exogenous obesity, diabetes mellitus); increased myocardial irritability that predisposes to sudden cardiac death; co-existing pharmacological therapy; and impaired coronary hemodynamics including coronary blood flow reserve. A number of current investigations are focusing on the possibility that reduced coronary blood flow and flow reserve predispose the hypertensive patient with LVH to premature mortality. Those factors that may participate in potentially lethal ischemia include: reduced basal coronary blood flow and coronary flow reserve; increased coronary vascular resistance and minimal coronary vascular resistance; reduced vasodilating capability of the hypertensive coronary arterioles (e.g., from reduced endothelial synthesis of nitric oxide and other substances); and altered blood viscosity in the coronary microcirculation.

METHODOLOGICAL APPROACHES

Prior Studies from This Laboratory

Our earlier studies had been directed to a number of factors that might participate in the altered systemic and coronary hemodynamics associated with hypertension and hypertensive LVH[2–9], non-hemodynamic factors that might participate in the development of

* Telephone: (504) 842-3700, Fax: (504) 842-3258

Hypertension and the Heart, edited by Zanchetti et al.
Plenum Press, New York, 1997

LVH and its reversal with antihypertensive pharmacological drugs[10–19], impaired left ventricular pumping ability associated with some, but not all, of those agents (which need not be drug class-specific)[20–26]. To accomplish these goals we first adapted electromagnetic[27] and radioactive microsphere flowmetry techniques for the rat[9–10]. Whereas the microspheres could be employed in anesthetized as well as in unanesthetized and unrestrained rats, the former procedure requires general anesthesia and an open-chest preparation.

Cardiovascular Mass

Moreover, since it was necessary to assess various physiological indices in rats with LVH and following pharmacological reversal of LVH, it was necessary to establish an experimental model that would permit a reproducible demonstration of pharmacologically-induced reversal of LVH within a short enough period of time so that hemodynamic factors were less likely to participate predominately in that reversal process. This was necessary since, given long enough time, all antihypertensive agents will reduce left ventricular mass (including diuretics) and direct-acting smooth muscle vasodilators[28–30]. To accomplish this, we developed a protocol involving 16 to 20 week old male spontaneously hypertensive rats (SHR) that were treated with antihypertensive agents for only three weeks[11,12]. These studies demonstrated that the centrally-active adrenergic inhibitors[22,23,20], beta-adrenergic receptor blockers[26,31], calcium antagonists[13,26], and angiotensin converting enzyme (ACE) inhibitors[18,19,21–23] reduced left ventricular mass within the three week treatment period. In contrast, the direct-acting smooth muscle relaxing vasodilators, alpha-adrenergic receptor inhibitors did not affect left ventricular mass[12,32]. These studies also demonstrated that, following the three week course of treatment, not all of the agents that reduced ventricular mass did so similarly, even within the same drug class. Thus, some agents reduced the mass of the hypertrophied left ventricle as well as in the non-hypertrophied right ventricle whereas others did not; some of the agents also reduced aortic mass whereas others did not; and some of the agents reduced left ventricular mass while at the time they increased right ventricular mass[20–25]. Most notably, the same findings were also obtained under similarly conducted short-term studies in patients with essential hypertension[30,32–39].

Left Ventricular Pump Performance

Pump performance of the left ventricle is maintained until the SHR is well over one and one-half years, very old for the rat, by assessing the ability of the heart to respond to a rapid infusion of blood over a one minute's time[3–5]. Question was raised, therefore, as to whether the ventricle can maintain its normal pump performance after pharmacologically-induced reduction of left ventricular mass[40]. For this reason, left ventricular pumping ability was assessed before and after reversal of LVH at the pharmacologically reduced afterload as well as when arterial pressure was abruptly increased by tightening a snare placed around the descending aorta[20–25]. These studies revealed that a centrally-acting adrenergic inhibitor was associated with an impaired left ventricular function curve[20], whereas, in general, the pump performance was well-maintained after reduction of left ventricular mass with ACE inhibitors, calcium antagonists, and a beta-adrenergic receptor blocker[22–26].

Coronary Hemodynamics

More recently, our efforts were directed to methods that permitted assessment of ventricular function in unanesthetized and unrestrained SHRs and their normotensive Wistar Kyoto controls. These rats were trained to exercise maximally on an electrically-driven treadmill or with specific pharmacological interventions in order to permit evaluation of changes in ventricular pump performance as well as evaluation of systemic and coronary hemodynamics[41]. To accomplish this, we implanted arterial and venous catheters for direct pressure measurements and injection of radioactive microspheres for determination of cardiac output and quantification of coronary (and other organ) blood flow(s) and blood flow reserve. The details of the techniques have been published[41–43]. Whereas the responses to maximal treadmill exercise were meaningful and reproducible, pharmacological interventions with either carbochrome or dipyridamole (neither papaverine nor adenosine were employed in these studies) provided a greater stimulus to augment coronary blood flow and achieve minimal coronary vascular resistance[41–44]. Accordingly, we have no doubt that these latter pharmacological interventions will be employed more in future experimental studies.

EXPERIMENTAL FINDINGS

Our initial studies with the ACE inhibitor quinapril demonstrated that even, in small doses that failed to reduce arterial pressure, left ventricular mass was reduced significantly[45]. However, when a full dose of that ACE inhibitor was employed, left ventricular mass was reduced; and this was associated with variable responses in the pumping ability of the left ventricle[22,23]. Furthermore, we found that when an ACE inhibitor was added to a calcium antagonist in doses designed to produce equivalent reductions in arterial pressure, the increased right ventricular mass produced by all calcium antagonist (resulting from collagen deposition) could be prevented even though no further reduction in collagen content of the left ventricular wall was not achieved[46,47].

In these forgoing studies, resting absolute coronary blood flow (ml/min) as well as relative coronary blood flow (ml/min/gm ventricle) were normal[7–9]. More recently, we determined the effect of low (10 mg per kg) and high (30 mg per kg) doses of the angiotensin II (type 1) receptor antagonist losartan on systemic and regional hemodynamics[42]. These studies demonstrated once again a structural/functional dissociation when left ventricular mass was reduced within the three week treatment period with losartan[42]. Thus, although both doses of losartan reduced left ventricular mass, only the higher dose significantly reduced arterial pressure. Moreover, although neither dose affected cardiac index, coronary or other blood flows at rest, significant increased cardiac index and coronary flow and decrease in coronary vascular resistance were achieved during maximal exercise. These changes with exercise, however, were not altered by losartan administration. Moreover, the increase in coronary blood flow and flow reserve induced by dipyridamole and the reduction in minimal coronary vascular resistance were markedly attenuated in the SHR (as compared with the WKY). However, the higher dose of losartan permitted a significantly greater increase in coronary flow reserve and a greater reduction in coronary vascular resistance in the SHR.

We then compared the above findings, obtained in the foregoing rats treated for only three weeks with those data obtained after the ACE inhibitor enalapril or the angiotensin II (type 1) receptor antagonist (losartan) (30 mg per kg per day of each) as well as after the combination of both agents (in one-half the dose, or 15 mg per kg per day of each agent) were administered for 12 weeks[43]. However, before that study was initiated, we had determined that treatment with either the ACE inhibitor enalapril or the angiotensin II (type 1) receptor antagonist losartan produced a significantly greater reduction in left ventricular mass after an additional nine weeks. Therefore, after 12 weeks of treatment, we

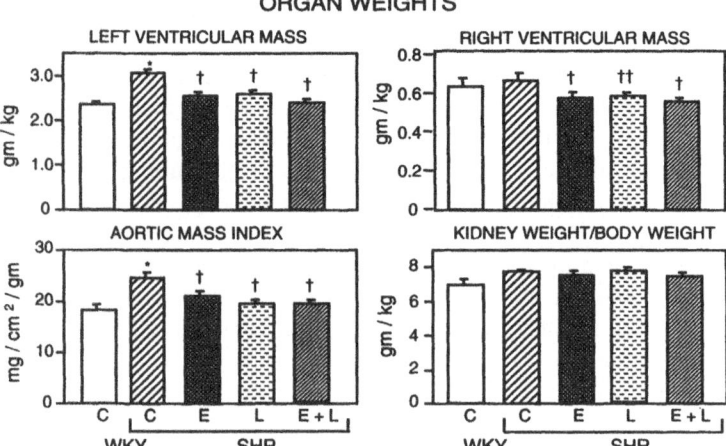

Figure 1. Changes in organ weights in response to 12 weeks of therapeutic intervention in control (tap-water treated) normotensive WKY rats (open bars) and in control tap-water (wide diagonal bars), enalapril (gray bars), losartan (dashed bars), and combination of enalapril and losartan (narrow diagonal bars) treated SHRs. H and HH represent significant changes (p<0.05 and 0.01, respectively) from the control SHR whereas * represents a significant change from the WKY control group at the p<0.05 level. Adapted from reference 43.

proceeded to determine the systemic and myocardial hemodynamic changes including cardiac index and organ blood flow(s) using radioactive microspheres at three times (baseline control, during maximal treadmill exercise, as well as with maximal coronary arterial dilation with dipyridamole). Each individual agent (enalapril and losarten) equally reduced mean arterial pressure (from approximately 160 to 118 mm Hg for each agent) in associa-

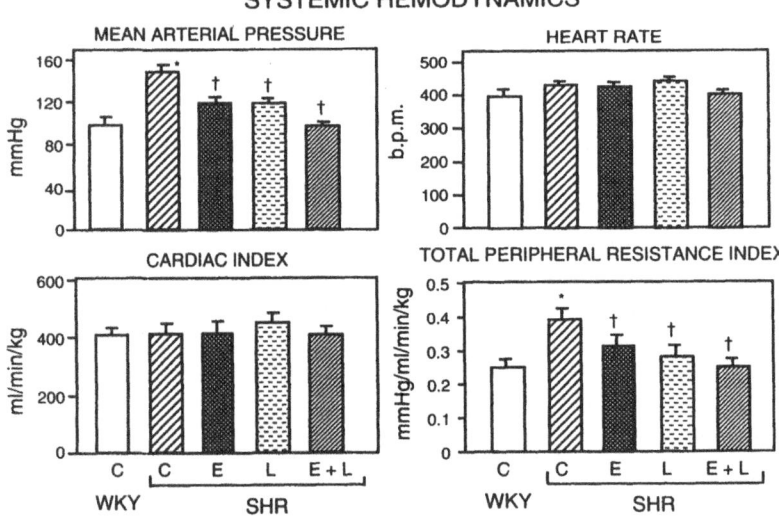

Figure 2. Changes in systemic hemodynamics in response to 12 weeks of therapeutic intervention in control (tap-water treated) normotensive WKY (open bars) and in control tap-water (wide diagonal bars), enalapril (gray bars), losartan (dashed bars), and combination of enalapril and losartan (narrow diagonal bars) treated SHRs. H represents significant changes (p<0.01 level) from the control SHR whereas * represents significant changes (p<0.01 level) from the control WKY rats. Adapted from reference 43.

tion with significant decreases in left as well as right ventricular and aortic mass is (but without changing renal weight). However, the combination of both agents (in one-half dose of each) reduced mean arterial pressure even more than each agent alone to 97 mmHg; and this was associated with a slightly further, but significant, reduction in left ventricular mass. However, right ventricular mass, aortic mass and renal mass were no different than after each agent was administered alone in twice the dosage (Figure 1)[43]. The changes in mean arterial pressure were also associated with proportionate changes in total peripheral resistance, heart rate and cardiac output remaining unchanged (Figure 2)[43].

It was of particular interest that the basal control (resting) cardiac index and coronary blood flows did not differ among each of the three treatment groups nor were they significantly different from the untreated SHRs or, for that matter, the normotensive WKY rats (Figure 3A)[43]. It was of further interest that whereas enalapril reduced minimal coronary vascular resistance, it improved neither coronary blood flow nor flow reserve (both with maximal exercise and dipyridamole) (Figure 3B)[43]. In contrast, losarten improved both coronary blood flow and flow reserve (with both types of interventions, physiological and pharmacological) (Figure 3A and 3B)[43]. Moreover, it was clear that the combination of both agents (in one-half dose of each) was more effective than either agent alone in improving coronary blood flow and flow reserve and in improving minimal coronary vascular resistance to the levels observed in the normotensive WKY rats (Figure 3A and 3B)[43].

DISCUSSION

The meta-analysis of the data obtained from the first 14 multicenter, controlled antihypertensive drug trials demonstrated the efficacy of the therapy in reducing the morbidity and mortality from stroke and coronary heart disease (CHD). While the reduction in deaths from CHD was highly significant ($p<0.001$), it was not to the degree that had been predicted (14 vs 20 to 25 percent)[48,49]. A subsequent meta-analysis of data from subsequent controlled, multicenter studies did, in fact, achieve the statistical significance that which was predicted (26 vs 20 to 25 percent) originally[50]. The major difference in these studies was in the dose of the thiazide diuretics that were employed (i.e., 25 to 50 vs 100 mg of hydrochlorothiazide or its equivalents) and the age of the subjects; the meta-analysis of the latter already involved primarily elderly patients with hypertension[50]. These findings tend to support the thesis that the diuretics, in the doses employed in the early multicenter trials, may have predisposed the treated patients to sudden cardiac death or cardiac arrest that could have been associated with hypokalemia[51]. This explanation contrasts with those earlier arguments raised editorially that suggested the CHD deaths in the studies included in earlier meta-analysis were attributable to myocardial infarction associated with relatively short-term alterations in lipid metabolism, associated with the diuretic[52]. It seems more reasonable, to my way of thinking, that in hypertensive patients with LVH, the mechanism for the greater percentage of CHD in the initial meta-analysis was related to sudden cardiac deaths from coronary insufficiency[53–58] or, perhaps, cardiac dysrhythmias secondary to hypokalemia. Indeed, an increased number of ventricular arrhythmias had been demonstrated in 24 and 48 hour Holter recordings in patients with hypertensive LVH[57,58]. It therefore, seems possible that hypokalemia may have been an important factor in those patients predisposed to cardiac dysrhythmia[59,60] although preexisting coronary insufficiency with hypertensive heart disease is a more likely explanation for the reduced actual percentage in CHD mortality (as compared with that which was predicted). In support of this concept are the data from the Multiple Risk Factor Interven-

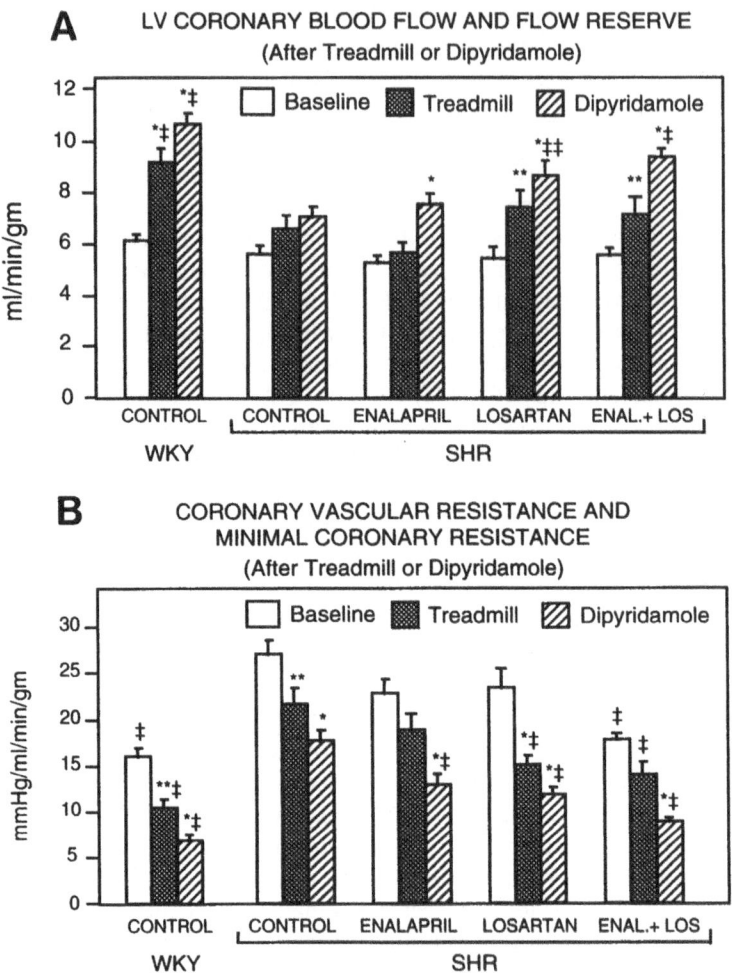

Figure 3. Left ventricular coronary blood flow and flow reserve (Figure 3A) and coronary vascular resistance and minimal coronary resistance (Figure 3B) at baseline, with maximal treadmill exercise, and with dipyridamole in control WKY and control, enalapril, losartan, and enalapril plus losartan treated SHR rats. 1* and ** or I represent significant differences at the p<0.01 and p<0.05 levels, respectively, for positive SHR.

tion Trial (MRFIT) which was included in the first meta-analysis. In that study, more patients of the special intervention (SI) group had electrocardiographic abnormalities than those patients included in the Usual Care (UC) treatment group[61].

Several early experimental studies in dogs with experimental LVH and hypertension have demonstrated a reduction in coronary blood flow and flow reserve[63–65]. These studies were supported by more recent clinical data in patients with hypertensive LVH using dipyridamole and other interventions designed to increase coronary flow and flow reserve[57,58]. The present findings in SHRs, also with a naturally developing hypertension, further demonstrate this thesis. Hence, whereas resting coronary blood flow may be normal in LVH of 20 week old mature adult SHR, the coronary blood flow reserve and the resting and minimal coronary vascular resistance were markedly impaired[41–44]. To date, our earlier studies with SHRs, treated with antihypertensive agents for three weeks did not seem to demonstrate improvement in the altered coronary hemodynamics[7-9]. Indeed, these improved coronary hemodynamics were not observed even when treatment with the ACE inhibitor enalapril was extended over a 12 week period[43]. By contrast, Scheler and associates, did demonstrate an increased coronary flow reserve in patients with essential hypertension who were treated for a more extensive time[58]. However, when we extended treatment to 12 weeks with losarten in the SHR of the present report, the coronary hemodynamics did improve; and this improvement was still more significant when both agents that interfere with the systemic and local myocardial renin-angiotensin systems were employed[43]. Others have also reported a synergistic response in pressure and left ventricular mass reduction when both enalapril and losarten were employed in patients with essential hypertension[66]. The explanation for this synergy is not available from present data, although the additional factor of increased local and systemic kinins generated through ACE inhibition has been postulated[67].

Finally, it is necessary to indicate that, to date, there have been no controlled studies reported that have demonstrated the increased risk associated with LVH in patients with hypertensive heart disease can be diminished by antihypertensive drug therapy. This is because in all extant published studies, it has not yet been possible to dissociate the risk reduction associated with reversal in left ventricular mass from the risk reduction associated with control of arterial pressure and the other effects of the antihypertensive employed including improved coronary hemodynamics and their possible antiarrhythmic effects[68]. Such studies will be difficult to develop using an appropriate control group of patients who are also treated, but it can be designed and, no doubt, it will be costly. The results of the present study strongly suggest that it is possible to assess coronary hemodynamics before, during and after such therapy is interposed and then discontinued; and this can now be assessed in patients using the same interventions (e.g., dipyridamole) to assess the reversibility of structural and functional hemodynamic alterations of the coronary circulation of patients with hypertension and LVH.

REFERENCES

1. Frohlich, ED: Left ventricular hypertrophy: An independent factor of risk. In: *Preventive Aspects of Coronary Heart Disease.* (Frohlich, ED, editor; Brest, AN, editor-in-chief) F.A. Davis Company, Philadelphia, pp. 85–94, 1990.
2. Pfeffer, MA, Frohlich, ED: Hemodynamic and myocardial function in young and old normotensive and spontaneously hypertensive rats. Circ Res. 32(I):28–38, 1973.
3. Pfeffer, MA, Pfeffer, JM, Frohlich, ED: Pumping ability of the hypertrophying left ventricle of the spontaneously hypertensive rat. Circ Res. 38:423–429, 1976.
4. Pfeffer, MA, Ferrell, BA, Pfeffer, JM, Weiss, AK, Fishbein, MC, Frohlich, ED: Ventricular morphology and pumping ability of exercised spontaneously hypertensive rats. Am J Physiol. 235:H193–H199, 1978.
5. Pfeffer, JM, Pfeffer, MA, Fishbein, MC, Frohlich, ED: Cardiac function and morphology with aging in the spontaneously hypertensive rat. Am J Physiol. 237:H461–H468, 1979.
6. Pfeffer, MA, Pfeffer, JM, Weiss, AK, Frohlich, ED: Development of SHR hypertension and cardiac hypertrophy during prolonged beta blockade. Am J Physiol. 232:H639–H644, 1977.
7. Nishiyama, K, Nishiyama, A, Frohlich, ED: Regional blood flow in normotensive and spontaneously hypertensive rats. Am J Physiol. 230:691–698, 1976.
8. Ishise, S, Pegram, BL, Yamamoto, J, Kitamura, Y, Frohlich, ED: Reference sample microsphere method: Cardiac output and blood flows in conscious rats. Am J Physiol. 239:H443–449, 1980.
9. Tsuchiya, M, Walsh, GM, Ferrone, RA, Ishise, S, Frohlich, ED: Application of combined Fick and radioactive microsphere methods for determination of systemic and regional hemodynamics in conscious rat. Japan Circ J. 44:400–402, 1980.

10. Frohlich, ED, Tarazi, RC: Is arterial pressure the sole factor responsible for hypertensive cardiac hypertrophy? Am J Cardiol. 44:959–963, 1979.

11. Ishise, S, Pegram, BL, Frohlich, ED: Disparate effects of methyldopa and clonidine on cardiac mass and haemodynamics in rats. Clin Sci. 59(VI):449s–452s, 1980.

12. Pegram, BL, Ishise, S, Frohlich, ED: Effect of methyldopa, clonidine, and hydralazine on cardiac mass and haemodynamics in Wistar-Kyoto and spontaneously hypertensive rats. Cardiovasc Res. 16:40–46, 1982.

13. Kobrin I, Sesoko S, Pegram BL, Frohlich ED: Reduced cardiac mass by nitrendipine is dissociated from systemic or regional haemodynamic changes in rats. Cardiovasc Res. 3:158–162, 1984.

14. Natsume, T, Gallo, A, Pegram, BL, Frohlich, ED: Hemodynamic effects of prolonged treatment with diltiazem in conscious normotensive and spontaneously hypertensive rats. Clin Exper Hyper. A7:1471–1479, 1985.

15. Tarazi, RC, Frohlich, ED: Is reversal of cardiac hypertrophy a desirable goal of antihypertensive therapy? Circulation. 75(I):113–117, 1987.

16. Frohlich, ED: State of the Art: The heart in hypertension: Unresolved conceptual challenges. Hypertension. 11(I):19–24, 1988.

17. Frohlich, ED: The First Irvine H. Page Lecture: The mosaic of hypertension: Past, present, and future. J Hypertens. 6(4):S2–S11, 1988.

18. Frohlich, ED, Iwata, T, Sasaki, O: Clinical and physiological significance of local tissue renin-angiotensin systems. Am J Med. 87:19S–23S, 1989.

19. Frohlich, ED: Overview of hemodynamic and non-hemodynamic factors associated with LVH. J Mol Cell Cardio. 21:3–10, 1989.

20. Sasaki, O, Kardon, MB, Pegram, BL, Frohlich, ED: Aortic distensibility and left ventricular pumping ability after methyldopa in Wistar-Kyoto and spontaneously hypertensive rats. J Vascular Med Biol. 1:59–66, 1989.

21. Natsume, T, Kardon, MB, Pegram, BL, Frohlich, ED: Ventricular performance in spontaneously hypertensive rats with reduced cardiac mass. Cardiovasc Drug Ther. 3:433–439, 1989.

22. Frohlich, ED, Sasaki, O: Dissociation of changes in cardiovascular mass and performance with angiotensin converting enzyme inhibitors in Wistar-Kyoto and spontaneously hypertensive rats. J Am Coll Cardiol. 16:1492–1499, 1990.

23. Frohlich ED, Horinaka S: Cardiac and aortic effects of angiotensin converting enzyme inhibitors. Hypertension. 18(II):2–7, 1991.

24. Frohlich ED: Regression of cardiac hypertrophy and left ventricular pumping ability post-regression. J Cardiovasc Pharmacol. 17(2):81–86, 1991.

25. Frohlich ED, Sasaki O, Chien Y, Arita M: Changes in cardiovascular mass, left ventricular pumping ability, and aortic distensibility after calcium antagonist in Wistar-Kyoto and spontaneously hypertensive rats. J Hypertens. 10:1369–1378, 1992.

26. Horinaka S, Frohlich ED: Cardiovascular mass and ventricular function after celiprolol in Wistar-Kyoto and spontaneously hypertensive rats. Cardiovasc Res. 16:396–400, 1992.

27. Pfeffer, MA, Frohlich, ED: Electromagnetic flowmetry in anesthetized rats. J Appl Physiol. 33:137–140, 1972.

28. Freis ED Regan RO: Relative effectiveness of chlorothiazide, reserpine, and hydralazine in spontaneously hypertensive rats. Clin Sci Mol Med. 51:635–637, 1976.

29. Pfeffer JM, Pfeffer MA, Fletcher P, Fishbein MC, Braunwald E: Favorable effects of therapy or cardiac performance in spontaneously hypertensive rats. Am J Physiol. 242(H):776–784, 1982.

30. Frohlich ED, Apstein C, Chobanian AV, Devereux RB, Dustan HP, Dzau V, Fauad-Tarazi F, Horan MJ, Marcus M, Massie B, Pfeffer MA, Re RN, Roccella EJ, Savage D, Shub C: The heart in hypertension. N Engl J Med. 327:998–1008, 1992.

31. Pfeffer, MA, Pfeffer, JM, Weiss, AK, Frohlich, ED: Development of SHR hypertension and cardiac hypertrophy during prolonged beta blockade. Am J Physiol. 232:H639–H644, 1977.

32. Pegram BL, Kobrin I, Natsume T, Gallo AJ, Frohlich ED: Systemic and regional hemodynamic effects of acute and prolonged treatment with urapidil or prazosin in normotensive and spontaneously hypertensive rats. Am J Med. 77(4A):64–73, 1984.

33. Dunn, FG, Oigman, W, Ventura, HO, Messerli, FH, Kobrin, I, Frohlich, E. D: Enalapril improves systemic and renal hemodynamics and allows regression of left ventricular mass in essential hypertension. Am J Cardiol. 53:105–108, 1984.

34. Dunn, FG, Oigman, W, Ventura, HO, Messerli, FH, Kobrin, I, Frohlich, ED: Systemic and renal effects of enalapril and its effects on cardiac mass. J Hypertens. 2(II):57–61, 1984.

35. Amodeo, C, Kobrin, I, Ventura, HO, Messerli, FH, Frohlich, ED: Immediate and short-term hemodynamic effects of diltiazem in patients with hypertension. Circulation. 73:108–113, 1986.

36. Dunn, FG, Ventura, HO, Messerli, FH, Kobrin, I, Frohlich, ED: Time course of regression of left ventricular hypertrophy in hypertensive patients treated with atenolol. Circulation. 76:254–258, 1987.

37. Grossman, E, Oren, S, Garavaglia, GE, Messerli, FH, Frohlich, ED: Systemic and regional hemodynamic and humoral effects of nitrendipine in essential hypertension. Circulation. 78:1394–1400, 1988.

38. Garavaglia, GE, Messerli, FH, Nunez, BD, Schmieder, RE, Frohlich, ED: Immediate and short-term cardiovascular effects of a new converting enzyme inhibitor (lisinopril) in essential hypertension. Am J Cardiol. 62:912–916, 1988.

39. Aristizabal D, Messerli FH, Frohlich ED: Disparate structural effects of left and right ventricles by angiotensin converting enzyme inhibitors and calcium antagonists. Am J Cardiol. 73:483–487, 1994.

40. Frohlich, ED: Clinical conference: Hypertensive cardiovascular disease. A pathophysiological assessment. Hypertension. 6:934–939, 1984.

41. Soria F, Frohlich ED, Aristizabal D, Kaneko K, Kardon MB, Hunter J, Pegram BL: Preserved cardiac performance with reduced left ventricular mass in conscious exercising spontaneously hypertensive rats. J Hypertens. 12:585–589, 1994.

42. Kaneko K, Susic D, Nunez E, Frohlich ED: Losartan reduces cardiac mass and improves coronary flow reserve in the spontaneously hypertensive rat. J Hypertens. 14:645–653, 1996.

43. Nunez, E, Hosoya K, Susic D, Frohlich ED: Enalapril and losartan reduced cardiac mass and improved coronary hemodynamics in SHR. Hypertension. 29:519–524, 1997.

44. Chien Y, Frohlich ED, Kardon MB, Hunter JM, Pegram BL: Coronary physiological flow reserve during treadmill exercise is preserved in spontaneously hypertensive rats (abstract). Circulation. 86(I):330, 1992.

45. Ando, K, Frohlich, ED, Chien Y, Pegram BL: Effects of quinapril on systemic and regional hemodynamics and cardiac mass in spontaneously hypertensive and Wistar-Kyoto rats. Journal of Vascular Medicine and Biology. 3:117–123, 1991.

46. Arita M, Horinaka S, Frohlich ED: Biochemical components and myocardial performance after reversal of left ventricular hypertrophy in spontaneously hypertensive rats. J Hypertens. 11:951–959, 1993.

47. Arita M, Horinaka S, Komatsu K, Frohlich ED: Reversal of left ventricular hypertrophy with different classes of drugs causes differing ventricular biochemical changes. J Hypertens. 11:S354–S355, 1993.

48. Collins C, Peto R, MacMahon S, Hebert H, Hebach NH, Eberlein KA, Godwin J, Olzibash N, Taylor JO, Hennekens CH: Blood pressure, stroke, and coronary heart disease. Part II. Short-term reductions in blood pressure overview of randomized drug trials in their epidemiological context. Lancet. 335:827–838, 1990.

49. MacMahon S, Peto R, Cutler, Collins R, Sorlie P, Neaton J, Abbott R, Godwin J, Dyer A, Stamler J: Blood pressure, stroke, and coronary heart disease. Part I. Prolonged differences in blood pressure: prospective observational studies corrected for the regression dilution bias. Lancet. 335:765–774, 1990.

50. Thijs L, Fagard R, Lijnen P, Staessen J, VanHoot R, Amery A: A meta-analysis of outcome trials in elderly hypertensives. J Hypertens. 10:1103–1109, 1992.

51. Siscovick DS, Raghunathan TE, Psaty BM, Koepsell TD, Wickland KG, Lin X, Cobb L, Rautaharju PM, Copass MK, Wagner EH: Diuretic therapy for hypertension N Engl J Med. 330:1852–1857, 1994.

52. Weinberger MH: Influence of an angiotensin converting enzyme inhibitor on diuretic induced metabolic effects in hypertension. Hypertension; 5:132–138, 1983.

53. Frohlich ED: Pathophysiology of systemic arterial hypertension. In: Hurst's The Heart Eighth Edition, (Schlant RC, Alexander RW, O'Rourke RA, Roberts R, Sonnenblick EH, editors). McGraw-Hill, Inc., New York, pp. 1391–1401, 1993.

54. Brush JE, Cannon RO, Schenke WH, Bonow RO, Leon MB, Maron BJ, Epstein SE: Angina due to coronary microvascular disease in hypertensive patients without left ventricular hypertrophy. N Engl J Med. 319:1302–1307, 1988.

55. Pegram BL, Ishise S, Frohlich ED: Effect of methyldopa, clonidine, and hydralazine on cardiac mass and haemodynamics in Wistar-Kyoto and spontaneously hypertensive rats. Cardiovasc Res. 16:40–46, 1982.

56. Treasure CB, Klein JC, Vita JA, Manoukianu SV, Renwick GH, Selwyn AP, Ganz P, Alexander RW: Hypertension and left ventricular hypertrophy are associated with impaired endothelium-mediated relaxation in human coronary artery resistance vessels. Circulation. 87:86–93, 1993.

57. Houghton JL, Frank MJ, Carr AA, vanDohlen TW, Prisant IM: Relations among impaired coronary flow reserve, left ventricular hypertrophy and Thallium perfusion defects in hypertensive patients without destructive coronary artery disease. J Am Coll Cardiol. 15:43–51, 1990.

58. Scheler S, Wolfgang M, Strauer BE: Mechanisms of angina pectoris in patients with systemic hypertension and normal epicardial arteries by arteriogram. Am J Cardiol. 73:478–482, 1994.

59. Messerli FH, Ventura HO, Elizardi DJ, Dunn FG, Frohlich ED: Hypertension and sudden death: Increased ventricular ectopic activity in left ventricular hypertrophy. Am J Med. 77:18–22, 1984.

60. Frohlich, ED: Cardiac hypertrophy in hypertension. N Engl J Med. 317:831–833, 1987.

61. Multiple Risk Factor Intervention Trial Research Group. Mortality rates after 10.5 years for participants in the Multiple Risk Factor Intervention Trial: Findings to a prior hypothesis of the trial. JAMA. 263:1795–1801, 1990.

62. Marcus ML, Koyanagi S, Harrison DG, Doty DB, Hiratzka LF, Eastham CL: Abnormalities in the coronary circulation that occur as a consequence of cardiac hypertrophy. Am J Med. 75(suppl 3A):62–66, 1983.

63. Marcus ML, Doty DB, Hiratzka LF, Wright CG, Eastham CL: Decreased coronary reserve: a mechanism for angina pectoris in patients with aortic stenosis and normal coronary arteries. N Engl J Med. 307:1362–1366, 1982.

64. Marcus ML, Mueller TM, Gascho JA, Kerber RE: Effects of cardiac hypertrophy secondary to hypertension on the coronary circulation. Am J Cardiol. 44:1023–1028, 1979.

65. Mueller TM, Marcus ML, Kerber RE, Young JA, Barnes RW, Abboud FM: Effect of renal hypertension and left ventricular hypertrophy on the coronary circulation in dogs. Circ Res. 42:543–549, 1978.

66. Azizi M, Guyene TT, Chatellier G, Wargon M, Menard J: Additive effects of losartan and enalapril on blood pressure and plasma active renin. Hypertension. 29:634–640, 1997.

67. Frohlich ED: Current clinical pathophysiological considerations in essential hypertension. Medical Clinics of North America. (In Press).

68. Frohlich, ED: Is reversal of left ventricular hypertrophy in hypertension beneficial? Hypertension. 18(I): 133–138, 1991.

28

HYPERTENSIVE HEART DISEASE, VENTRICULAR DYSRHYTHMIAS, AND SUDDEN DEATH

Franz H. Messerli* and Leszek Michalewicz

Department of Internal Medicine
Section on Hypertensive Diseases
Ochsner Clinic and Alton Ochsner Medical Foundation
New Orleans, Louisiana

Left ventricular hypertrophy (LVH) has been identified as one of the strongest pressure-independent risk factors for sudden death, acute myocardial infarction, congestive heart failure and other cardiovascular morbidity and mortality. [1,2,3] These findings clearly abolish the concept of LVH being a benign adaptive process serving to compensate for the increased hemodynamic burden. Fig. 1. Based on these epidemiologic observations, a patophysiologic or electrophysiologic chain of evidence linking hypertension, LVH, and sudden death has been put forward. Although it is unclear whether a reduction in LVH confers benefit over and above the benefit of lowering blood pressure alone, the effects various antihypertensive agents have on LVH come under scrutiny.

LVH AND VENTRICULAR ARRHYTHMIAS

As early as 1984, we reported that hypertensive patients with LVH have a significantly greater prevalence of premature ventricular contractions and complex ventricular arrhythmias than do patients without LVH or normotensive patients, [3] a finding that was later expanded to obese patients with eccentric LVH [4] and confirmed in large population-based studies. [5,6] Although it is still controversial whether these findings could explain at least in part the higher incidence of sudden cardiac death in these patients, a study from the Framingham cohort [7] indicated recently that in patients with LVH, the presence of asymptomatic ventricular arrhythmias was indeed associated with a nearly two-fold increase in mortality.

---

* Address correspondence to Dr. Messerli, Ochsner Clinic, 1514 Jefferson Highway, New Orleans, Louisiana 70121. Phone: (504) 842-4077, Fax (504) 842-4220.

Hypertension and the Heart, edited by Zanchetti et al.
Plenum Press, New York, 1997

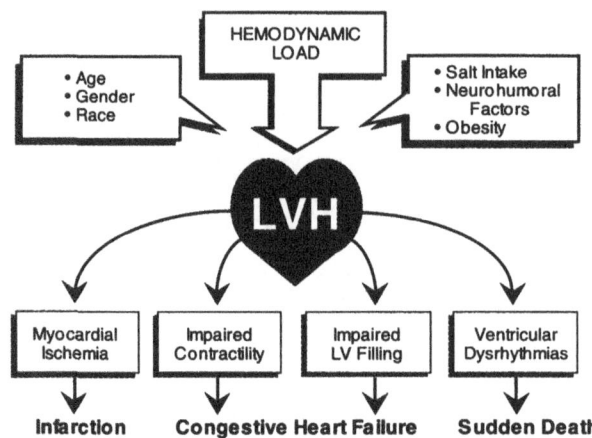

Figure 1. Risk factors in the development of left ventricular hypertrophy (LVH). (From Messerli FH, Soria F: Hypertension, left ventricular hypertrophy, ventricular ectopy, and sudden death. *Am J Med* 1992;93[Suppl 2A]: 21S–26S.)

In our study, ventricular ectopic activity was increased in patients with echocardiographically demonstrated LVH (475±852 PVC/24 h), as compared with normal patients (8.17±20.1 PVC/24 h) or hypertensive patients without LVH (10±22.1 PVC/h) (both p<0.01 versus hypertensive patients with LVH group). As of this writing, more than 15 independent studies have been published [3,9–27] (Table 1); all but one [17] found a higher percentage of patients with ventricular arrhythmias in the LVH group than in patients with normal hearts, although the correlation between pressure levels, LVH, and ventricular arrhythmias was rather weak. [18] The data regarding the association of LVH and atrial arrthythmias are sparse. Data from the Framingham cohort [28] support evidence of an increased prevalence of atrial fibrillation among patients with hypertensive cardiovascular disease as compared with control subjects, both in men (risk ratio 2.1) and in women (risk ratio 1.9). [28] Moreover, when different cardiovascular risk factors were taken into consideration, LVH was found to be a better predictor of atrial fibrillation than smoking, hypertension, or diabetes. [28]

ETIOLOGY OF VENTRICULAR ECTOPY IN HYPERTENSION

The mechanism by which LVH leads to increased arrhythmogenicity and ultimately to increased mortality remains unknown. A variety of factors associated with LVH are currently being considered as possible mechanisms:

1. LVH and hypertension without LVH are commonly associated with subendocardial ischemia. Microvascular angina has been reported to be common in hypertensive patients even in the absence of LVH. [29–34]
2. In the course of hypertensive cardiac hypertrophy, the coronary arteries fail to grow at a rate sufficient to compensate for the muscular hypertrophy. [33]
3. Hypertension by itself, irrespective of LVH, is a major risk factor for coronary artery disease. [35]
   All three of these mechanisms result in decreased coronary reserve and chronic ischemia, which is a well-recognized stimulus for arrhythmias of all types.

Table 1. LVH and Ventricular Ectopy

Author	Year	Criterion	Normal LV Mass		LV Hypertrophy	
			PVC/24h	% Patients with PVC	PVC/24h	% Patients with PVC
Messerli [9]	81	Lown>2	10	0%	475*	63%*
Loaldi [10]	83	PVC/h>10		17%		18%
Mc Lenachan [11]	87	couplets		16%		36%*
Aronow [12]	87	couplets		44%		75%*
Levy [13]	87	PVC/h>1		30%		35%*
Lavie [14]	88	Lown>2	24	0%	291*	35%*
Papademetriou [15]	89		65		346*	
Szlachcic [16]	89	PVC/h>30		29%		42%*
James [17]	89	couplets	742	56%	412*	24%*
Galinier [20]	91	Lown>2	23	4%	826*	50%*
Melina [21]	91		50		134*	
Ghali [22]	91	PVC/h>30		0%		15%
Novo [23]	92	PVC/h>30		8%		26%*
Nunez [25]	94	Lown>2		0%		46%*
Vardas [26]	94	Lown>1		25%		27.6%
Schillaci [27]	96	Lown>1		31%		54%*

LV = left ventricular; LVH = left ventricular hypertrophy; PVCs = premature ventricular contractions.
*p<0.05 vs patients with normal LV mass.

4. The irregular hypertrophy pattern [2,36] could, indeed, impede the homogeneous propagation of the electric impulse throughout the myocardium. Any disturbance of impulse propagation can give rise to reentry mechanisms and thereby lead to ectopic impulse formation. In current practice, the pattern of hypertrophy detected on echocardiography is considered to be related to the patient's prognosis and to the type of cardiovascular complications one may expect to encounter in the course of hypertension, although the exact mechanism is not understood [2,37] Thus, eccentric hypertrophy has been associated with more severe ventricular arrhythmias, [36] while concentric hypertrophy is more closely related to ischemic events resulting from abnormal coronary autoregulation. [38] Even the less frequently detected isolated septal hypertrophy is associated with an increased prevalence of atrial and ventricular arrhythmias, although its significance is unknown. [39]

5. The amount of fibrosis within the myocardium is also known to vary, depending primarily on the pathophysiologic mechanism accounting for hypertension in each patient. Increased fibrosis is a well-recognized factor accounting for non-homogeneous propagation of electrical impulses throughout the myocardium. Any disturbances of impulse propagation can give rise to reentry mechanisms and thereby lead to ventricular arrhythmias.

6. The hypertrophied cardiac myocyte has been documented to be electrophysiologically different from and more arrhythmogenic than the normal myocyte. [40] A number of structural changes that occur in hypertrophy have been related to the susceptibility of the hypertrophied myocardium for arrhythmias. Low resistance pathways through the intercalated discs of the hypertrophic myocardium undergo changes that serve to increase the surface of the gap region involved in cell-to-cell communication. [41] In addition, dilatation of the transverse tubule system (involved in the transmission of the surface action potential

to the sarcomere) [41] and increase in the number of mitochondrias (responsible for the cell energy status) have been detected. However, it has not as yet been shown whether these structural changes correlate with electrophysiologic abnormalities.

7. Excessive fluctuation in arterial pressure, as occurs in severe hypertension, may be arrhythmogenic [42–44] because it changes the loading conditions of the left ventricle. The cardiac myocyte is capable of reacting to a variety of external stimuli modifying its structural and functional behavior. [45] The stretch-activated channel in the cytoplasmic membrane detects external physical stimuli (ie, in the form of pressure changes), giving rise to a sequence of intracellular ionic events that affect the electrical stability of the cell. Both experimental and clinical studies have shown that mechanical stretching of the myocyte induces a decrease in the electric threshold, as was shown by James and Jones [44] who gradually increasing afterload by pharmacological means, demonstrated a positive correlation between this parameter and the rate of ventricular ectopic activity. Conversely, work from other laboratories has shown that acute reductions in afterload caused by electrically inactive drugs such as nitroprusside in patients with high basal rate of ventricular ectopy drastically diminishes the prevalence of arrhythmias. [43] Thus, this mechanism is regarded as one of the factors implicated in the genesis of ventricular arrhythmias of patients with LVH.

8. Excessive activity of the sympathetic nervous system and the renin-angiotensin system has been implicated in the pathogenesis of essential hypertension and may play a particularly important role in the development of LVH. Sympathetic stimulation has been well documented to exert a direct proarrhythmic effect. [46–49] Although the renin-angiotensin system has been implicated in the pathogenesis of LVH [50–51], the evidence that cellular angiotensin levels may exert direct arrhythmogenic effects is somewhat less conclusive.

It seems, therefore, that the arrhythmogenicity of LVH is multifactorial in origin. However, regardless of the exact or predominant electrophysiologic mechanism, it is clear that the hypertrophied myocardium provides fertile soil for the sprouting of ventricular ectopic beats.

VENTRICULAR ECTOPY AND SUDDEN DEATH

The fact that ventricular ectopy is common in patients with LVH does not prove that these irregular heartbeats herald ventricular fibrillation or other fatal electric events. Several electrophysiologic studies carried out in patients with LVH come to contradictory results [52–55]. Vester et al [54] documented enhanced arrhythmogenicity in a series of 40 hypertensive patients in whom coronary heart disease had been previously excluded. The authors found a significantly higher left ventricular mass index (158 ± 44 vs 222 ± 112 g/m^2) and lower ejection fraction (71 ± 17 vs 47 ± 18) in the group of patients in whom malignant arrhythmias (VT or VF) were induced by programmed electrical stimulation.

A not-very-well controlled study by Aronow et al [56], in a geriatric population followed for an average of 27 months, showed that hypertensive patients without documented coronary artery disease and with echocardiographic LVH were significantly more likely to develop new cardiac events than their counterparts without LVH (31% vs 10%). It stands to reason but remains unproven that, in a population documented to be at a very high risk of sudden cardiac death (such as patients with LVH), persons with the greatest degree of electric instability are likely to be at highest risk.

ANTIHYPERTENSIVE TREATMENT AND REDUCTION OF LVH

Of all antihypertensive drugs, ACE inhibitors are probably the most effective in reducing LVH. [57–60] Recently, Schmieder et al performed a meta-analysis that only considered randomized studies comparing the effects of two or more therapies by assessing LVH and structure with blindly read echocardiograms. [60] Out of more than 400 applications, only 39 clinical trials fulfilled these criteria. Similar to previous meta-analyses, the decrease in left ventricular mass was greater with active drug treatment than with placebo and was directly related to the pretreatment left ventricular mass, control of pressure and duration of treatment. When the analysis was adjusted for the study duration, ACE inhibitors were most efficient in reducing LVH, followed by calcium channel blockers, the diuretics and the beta blockers. [60] Fig. 2. Indeed, some reports suggest that ACE inhibitors may lower blood pressure more than one would expect from their unloading properties alone. The ability of ACE inhibitors at a dose that does not lower blood pressure to produce regression in LVH supports the hypothesis that the local cardiac angiotensin system is a significant determinant of heart structure and function. [61,62] As a class, calcium antagonists seem slightly less potent in reducing LVH than the ACE inhibitors, with heart rate lowering agents possibly having a greater effect than the dihydropyridines. A lesser effect on LVH is assigned to the beta-blockers, the postsynaptic alpha-blockers and the diuretics. However, recent findings in 690 men from the VA cooperative study showed hydrochlorothiazide to be as efficacious as captopril, and more efficacious than atenolol, diltiazem, prazosin or clonidine in reducing LVH. [63] It must be emphasized, however, that with a few exceptions [64–66] there are no prospective, randomized, controlled trials comparing the effects of various antihypertensive drugs on left ventricular mass. Also, there is uncertainty as to what a drug-induced reduction of LVH exactly means in terms of morbidity and mortality and there are no conclusive data that a reduction in LVH would confer a benefit that exceeded the one conferred by the reduction in arterial pressure per se. These drawbacks notwithstanding, it can be extrapolated that the combination of an ACE inhibitor with a calcium blocker ought to be particularly efficacious with regard to a reduction of LVH (Table 2). Because both of these drug classes have the potential to interfere with pathogenesis of LVH at a similar level, one can argue that this combination will reduce LVH more than one would expect from its blood pressure lowering effects alone.

Whether angiotensin receptor inhibitors, either in monotherapy or in combination, are as efficient as ACE inhibitors in reducing LVH remains undocumented at the present time. Most of the other commonly used combinations, such as diuretics plus beta-blockers, ACE inhibitors plus beta-blockers, as well as beta-blockers plus dihydropyridine calcium antagonists, are prone to reduce LVH in parallel with the fall in arterial pressure.

Figure 2. Percentage of change in left ventricular mass index with the 4 antihypertensive drug classes. Mean values and 95% confidence intervals adjusted for duration are given. ACE indicates angiotensin-converting enzyme. Asterisk indicates p < .01 between drug classes; dagger indicates p < .10 between drug classes. LVMI = left ventricular mass index. (From Schmieder RE, Martus P, Klingbeil A. Reversal of left ventricular hypertrophy in essential hypertension. A meta-analysis of randomized double-blind studies. JAMA 1996; 275:1507–1513.)

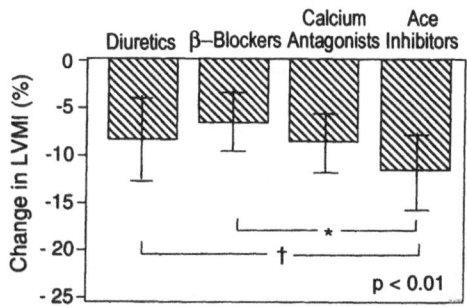

Table 2. Possible synergism resulting from a combination
of a calcium antagonist and an ACE inhibitor

	DHP-Calcium antagonist	HRL Calcium antagonist	ACE inhibitor
Kidneys			
↑ Renal blood flow	yes	yes	yes
↑ Efferent vasodilation	little	yes	yes
↑ Afferent vasodilation	yes	yes	yes
↓ Microproteinuria	little	yes	yes
"Renoprotection"	unknown	possible	yes
Vascular Tree			
↓ Endothelin mediated vasoconstriction	yes	yes	no
↑ Nitric oxide release	no	no	yes
↑ Arterial compliance	yes	yes	yes
↓ Vascular hypertrophy	yes	yes	yes
↓ Atherogenesis	yes	yes	yes
Heart			
↓ Left ventricular hypertrophy	yes	yes	yes
↑ Left ventricular filling	yes	yes	no
↑ Contractility, unloading	some	no	yes
↑ Coronary flow	yes	yes	some
Secondary "cardioprotection"	no	some	yes

ACE = Angiotensin converting enzyme, DHP = Dihydropyridine, HRL = Heart-rate-lowering, ↑ = increase, ↓ = decrease. From Messerli FH, Michalewicz L. Effects of combination therapy on the heart. J Hum Hypert 1997;11:29-33.

Drug classes that either stimulate the renin angiotensin system or the sympathetic nervous system, or both, are less likely to reduce LVH and more likely to induce arrhythmias than drug classes that do not stimulate these systems. The combination of an arteriolar vasodilator, such as hydralazine or minoxidil, with a diuretic should, therefore, probably not be used in an asymptomatic patient with left ventricular hypertrophy. Such a combination may also synergistically elicit hypokalemia, which could aggravate or trigger ventricular arrhythmias.

EFFECT OF REDUCTION OF LVH ON VENTRICULAR ECTOPY

The reduction of LVH in hypertensive patients has been shown to diminish the ventricular arrhythmias. [4,66] This "antiarrhythmic" effect seems to be nonspecific and independent of the drug used to reduce LVH. We have documented that a reduction of LVH as the result of 3 months' treatment with a calcium antagonist drastically diminished ventricular ectopy. [4] In contrast, in the very same study, the patient group treated with a diuretic exhibited neither a decrease in left ventricular mass nor in ventricular ectopy. One might argue, however, that calcium antagonists are electrophysiologically active drugs, and therefore the decrease in ventricular ectopy could be directly related to an antiarrhythmic effect of the drug on the ectopically firing myocardium. However González-Fernández et al [66], in an double-blinded study, showed that use of an ACE inhibitor led to a marked reduction in LVH and, at the same time, to a marked reduction in ventricular ectopy, whereas in the placebo group LVH progressed and there was no change in ventricular ectopy. Since a reduction in ventricular ectopy has been found with use of a calcium antagonist, an ACE inhibitor and a beta-blocker [67–70] it seems safe to assume that the decrease in ventricular ectopy associated with a reduction in LVH is not related to a direct antiarrhythmic effect of the drug only. That hemodynamic unloading and improvement of latent subendocardial ischemia were responsible for the reduction in arrhythmias seems unlikely in view of the fact that in our study and in others, despite their similar reduction of the hemodynamic burden, diuretics had no antiarrhythmic effect. However, the potential proarrhythmic effects of diuretics might have outweighed the beneficial hemodynamic effects induced by this class of agents. [71] Diuretics have been shown to increase ventricular ectopy, both at rest and during exercise [72,73]. This proarrhythmic effect may result from an intracellular electrolyte shift.

DECREASE IN LVH AND THE RISK OF SUDDEN CARDIAC DEATH

Studies of the effects of the reduction of LVH on cardiovascular morbidity and mortality are rare. Preliminary reports from Framingham [74] have documented that a decrease of LVH as assessed by electrocardiographic criteria does, indeed, lead to a decrease in the risk of sudden cardiac death, acute myocardial infarction, and congestive heart failure. The clinical outcome, as evaluated by the percentage of patients who developed a cardiovascular event (cardiac death, myocardial infarction, stroke, angina, or need for coronary revascularization) over a ten-year period, was drastically reduced in patients in whom the LVH was reversed versus those in whom LVH persisted at the end of follow-up (3% versus 25%; p<0.01). Similarly, a multicenter study in Eastern Europe [75] showed that patients in whom left ventricular mass decreased during antihypertensive therapy had much fewer morbid cardiovascular events than patients in whom left ventricular mass remained unchanged or increased. Although both of these studies provide encouraging results, they do not allow the firm conclusion that a reduction of LVH per se prolongs life. In order to sustain such a conclusion, a study would have to show that a reduction of LVH confers a clinical benefit over and above the reduction in blood pressure alone. Until such data are presented, we should remain cautious in making reduction of LVH the sole therapeutic goal.

CONCLUSIONS

LVH has been identified as a significant independent risk factor and a harbinger of sudden death, myocardial infarction, congestive heart failure, and other events leading to cardiovascular morbidity and mortality. LVH has been shown to be associated with electric instability leading to premature ventricular contractions and higher grade ventricular arrhythmias. LVH can be reduced by antihypertensive therapy and not all drugs seem to be equally effective. A reduction of LVH has been shown to diminish LVH associated arrhythmias. However, it remains unclear whether a reduction of LVH and/or LVH associated arrhythmias confers a clinical benefit that exceeds the one from the reduction in blood pressure per se.

REFERENCES

1. Kannel WB. Prevalence and natural history of electrocardiographic left ventricular hypertrophy. Am J Med 1983;75(Suppl 3A):4–11.
2. Koren MJ, Devereux RB, Casale PN, Savage DD, Laragh JH. Relation of left ventricular mass and geometry to morbidity and mortality in uncomplicated hypertension. Ann Intern Med 1991;114:345–352.

3. Messerli FH, Ventura HO, Elizardi DJ, Dunn FG, Frohlich ED. Hypertension and sudden death: increased ventricular ectopy activity in left ventricular hypertrophy. Am J Med 1984;77:18–22.

4. Messerli FH, Nunez BD, Nunez MM, Garavaglia GE, Schmieder RE, Ventura HO. Hypertension and sudden death: Disparate effects of calcium entry blocker and diuretic therapy on cardiac dysrhythmias. Arch Intern Med 1989;149(Suppl 6):1263–1267.

5. Levy D, Anderson KM, Savage DD, et al: Echocardiographically detected left ventricular hypertrophy: Prevalence and risk factors. The Framingham Heart Study. Ann Intern Med 1988;108:7–13.

6. McLenachan JM, Henderson E, Morris KI, et al: Ventricular arrhythmias in patients with hypertensive left ventricular hypertrophy. N Engl J Med 1987;317:787–792.

7. Bikkina M, Larson MG, Levy D: Asymptomatic ventricular arrhythmias and mortality risk in subjects with left ventricular hypertrophy. J Am Coll Cardiol 1993;22:1111–1116.

9. Messerli FH, Glade LB, Elizardi DG, Dreslinski GR, Dunn FG, Frohlich ED. Cardiac rhythm, arterial pressure, and urinary catecholamines in hypertension with and without left ventricular hypertension. Am J Cardiol 1981;47:480.

10. Loaldi A, Pepi M, Agostoni PG, et al. Cardiac rhythm in hypertension assessed through 24-hour ambulatory electrocardiographic monitoring effects of load manipulation with atenolol, verapamil, and nifedipine. Br Heart J 1983;50:118–126.

11. McLenachan JM, Henderson E, Morris KI, Dargie HJ. Ventricular arrhythmias in patients with hypertensive left ventricular hypertrophy. N Engl J Med 1987;317:787–792.

12. Aronow WS, Epstein S, Schwartz KS, Koenigsberg M. Correlation of complex ventricular arrhythmias detected by ambulatory electrocardiographic monitoring with echocardiographic left ventricular hypertrophy in persons older than 62 years in a long-term health care facility. Am J Cardiol 1987;60:730–732.

13. Levy D, Anderson KM, Savage DD, Balkus SA, Kannel WB, Castelli WP. Risk of ventricular arrhythmias in left ventricular hypertrophy: the Framingham Study. Am J Cardiol 1987;60:560–565.

14. Lavie CJ Jr, Nunez BD, Garavaglia GE, Messerli FH. Hypertensive concentric hypertrophy: When is ventricular ectopic activity increased? South Med J 1988;81:696–700.

15. Papademetriou V, Notargiacomo A, Heine D, Fletcher R, Freis E. Ventricular arrhythmias in patients with essential hypertension [Abstract]. J Am Coll Cardiol 1989;13:105A.

16. Szlachcic J, London M, Tubau JF, O'Kelly B, Mangano D. Incidence of serious ventricular arrhythmias during surgery in hypertensives with left ventricular hypertrophy [Abstract]. J Am Coll Cardiol 1989;13:105A.

17. James MA, Jones JV. Ventricular arrhythmia in untreated hypertensive patients compared with a matched normal population. J Hypertens 1989;7:409–415.

18. Ferrara N, Furgi G, Longobardi G, Nicolino A, Acanfora D, Leosco D, Rengo F. Relation between age, left ventricular mass and ventricular arrhythmias in patients with hypertension. J Hum Hypertens 1995;9(7):881–587.

19. Siegel D, Cheitlin MD, Blaek DM, Seeley D, Hearst N, Hulley SB. Risk of ventricular arrhythmias in hypertensive men with left ventricular hypertrophy. Am J Cardiol 1990;65:742–747.

20. Galinier M, Fermond B, Lambert V, et al. When is a search for ventricular arrhythmias necessary in hypertensive patients. J Hypertens 1991;9:874–875.

21. Melina D, Colivicchi F, Guerrera G, Santoliquido A. Rhythm of disturbances in essential hypertension [Letter]. J Human Hypertens 1991;5:233.

22. Ghali JK, Kadakia S, Cooper RS, Liao YL. Impact of left ventricular hypertrophy on ventricular arrhythmias in the absence of coronary artery disease. J Am Coll Cardiol 1991;17:1277–1282.

23. Novo S, Barbagallo M, Abrignani M, Alaimo G, Nardi E, Corrao S, Papadia C, Strano A. Cardiac arrhythmias as correlated with the circadian rhythm of arterial pressure in hypertensive subjects with and without left ventricular hypertrophy. Eur J Clin Pharmacol 1990;39(Suppl 1):49–51.

24. Messerli FH, Grodzicki T. Hypertension, left ventricular hypertrophy, ventricular arrhythmias and sudden death. Eur Heart J 1992;13(Suppl D):66–69.

25. Nunez BD, Lavie CJ, Messerli FH, Scmieder RE, Garavaglia GE, Nunez M. Comparision of diastolic left ventricular filling and cardiac dysrhythmias in hypertensive patients with and without isolated septal hypertrophy. Am J Cardiol 1994;74(6):585–589.

26. Vardas PE, Simandirakis EN, Parthenakis FI, Manios EG, Eleftherakis NG, Terzakis DE. Study of late potentials and ventricular arrhythmias in hypertensive patients with normal electrocardiograms. Pacing Clin Electrophysiol 1994;(4 Pt 1):577–584.

27. Schillaci G, Verdecchia P, Borgioni C, Ciucci A, Zampi I, Battistelli M, Gattobigio R, Sacchi N, Porcellati C. Association between persistent pressure overload and ventricular arrhythmias in essential hypertension. Hypertension 1996;2:284–289.

28. Kannel WB, Abbott RD, Savage DD, McNamara PM. Epidemiologic features of chronic atrial fibrillation. N Engl J Med 1982;306:1018–1022.

29. O'Gorman DJ, Sheridan DJ. Abnormalities of the coronary circulation associated with left ventricular hypertrophy. Clin Sci 1991;81:703–713.

30. Houghton JL, Prisant LM, Carr AA, von Dohlen TW, Frank MJ. Relationship of left ventricular mass to impairment of coronary vasodilator reserve in hypertensive heart disease. Am Heart J 1991;121(4 Pt 1): 1107–1112.

31. Lucarini AR, Picano E, Salveti A. Coronary microvascular disease in hypertensives. Clin Exp Hypertens 1992;A14:55–66.

32. Houghton JL, Carr AA, Prisant LM, et al. Morphologic, hemodymanic and coronary perfusion characteristics in severe left ventricular hypertrophy secondary to systemic hypertension and evidence for nonatherosclerotic myocardial ischemia. Am J Cardiol 1992;69:219–224.

33. Harrison DG, Marcus ML, Dellsperger KC, Lamping KG, Tomanek RJ. Pathophysiology of myocardial perfusion in hypertension. Circulation 1991;83(Suppl III):III-14–III-18.

34. Burke AP, Farb A, Liang YH, Smialek J, Virmani R. Effect of hypertension and cardiac hypertrophy on coronary artery morphology in sudden cardiac death. Circulation 1996;94(12):3138–3145.

35. Burke AP, Farb A, Malcom GT, Liang YH, Smialek J, Virmani R. Coronary risk factors and plaque morphology in men with coronary disease who died suddenly. N Engl J Med 1997;336(18):1276–1282.

36. Levy D, Anderson KM, Plehn J, Savage DD, Christiansen JC, Castelli WP. Echocardiographically determined left ventricular structural and functional correlates of complex or frequent ventricular arrhythmias on one-hour ambulatory electrocardiographic monitoring. Am J Cardiol 1987;59:836–840.

37. Palatini P, Maraglino G, Accurso V, Sturaro M, Toniolo G, Dovigo P, Baccillieri S. Impaired left ventricular filling in hypertensive left ventricular hypertrophy as a marker of the presence of an arrhythmogenic substrate. Br Heart J 1995;73(3):258–262.

38. Polese A, De Cesare N, Fabbiocchi N, Loaldi A, Montorsi P, Guazzi MD. Coronary autoregulation in hypertension: Correlation with left vetricular mass [Abstract]. J Am Coll Cardiol 1990;15:111A.

39. Nunez BD, Messerli FH, Garavaglia GE, Schmieder RE. Exagerrated atrial and ventricular excitability in hypertensive patients with isolated septal hypertrophy (ISH) (abstr). J AM Coll Cardiol 1987;9:225.

40. Toyoshima H, Park Y-D, Ishikawa Y, et al. Effects of ventricular hypertrophy on conduction velocity of activation front in the ventricular myocardium. Am J Cardiol 1982;49:1938–1945.

41. Leyton RA, Sonneblick EH. The ultrastructure of the failing heart. Am J Med Sci 1969;258:304–327.

42. Sideris DA, Kontoyannis DA, Miehalis L, Adraetas A, Moulopoulos SD. Acute changes in blood pressure as a cause of cardiac arrhythmias. Eur Heart J 1987;8:45–52.

43. Sideris DA, Toumanidis ST, Kostis EB, Diakos A, Moulopoulos SD. Arrhythmogenic effect of high blood pressure: Some observation on its mechanisms. Cardiovasc Res 1989;23:983–992.

44. James MA, Jones JV. Systolic wall stress and ventricular arrhythmia: The role of acute change in blood pressure in the isolated working rat heart. Clin Sci 1990;79:499–504.

45. Bustamante JO, Ruknudin A, Sachs F. Stretch-activated channels in heart cells: relevance to cardiac hypertrophy. J Cardiovasc Pharmacol 1991;17(Suppl 2):S110–S113.

46. Schwartz P, LaRovere MT, Vanoli E. Autonomic nervous system and sudden cardiac death. Experimental basis and clinical observations for post-myocardial infarction risk stratification. Circulation 1992; 85(Suppl I): I-77–I-91.

47. Anderson JL, Rodier HE, Green LS. Comparative effects of beta-adrenergic blocking drugs on experimental ventricular fibrillation threshold. Am J Cardiol 1983;51:1196–1202.

48. Palatini P, Julius S. Heart rate and cardiovascular risk. J Hypertens 1997;15(1):3–17.

49. Amerena J, Julius S. The role of the autonomic nervous system in hypertension. Hypertens Res 1995;18(2): 99–110.

50. Paul M, Ganten D. The molecular basis of cardiovascular hypertrophy: the role of the renin-angiotension system. J Cardiovasc Pharmacol 1992;19(Suppl 5):S51–S58.

51. Harrap SB, Mitchell GA, Casley DJ, Mirakian C, Doyle AE. Angiotensin II, sodium, and cardiovascular hypertrophy in spontaneously hypertensive rats. Hypertension 1993;21:50–55.

52. Kowey PR, Friechling TD, Sewter J, et al. Electrophysiological effects of left ventricular hypertrophy. Effect of calcium and potassium channel blockade. Circulation 1991;83:2067–2075.

53. Clementy J, Coste P, Dallocchio M, Bricaud H. Data of programmed ventricular stimulation in left ventricular hypertrophy of hypertensive origin [French]. Annales de Cardiologie et d' Angiologie 1989;38: 297–303.

54. Vester EG, Kuhls S, Ochiulet-Vester J, Vogt M, Strauer BE. Electrophysiological and therapeutic implication of cardiac arrhythmias in hypertension. Eur Heart J 1992;13(Suppl D):70–81.

55. Singh JP, Sleight P, Kardos A, Hart G. QT interval dynamics and heart rate variability preceding a case of cardiac arrest. Heart 1997;77(4):375–377.

56. Aronow WS, Epstein S, Koenigsberg M, Schwartz KS: Usefulness of echocardiographic left ventricular hypertrophy, ventricular tachycardia and complex ventricular arrhythmias in predicting ventricular fibrillation or sudden cardiac death in elderly patients. Am J Cardiol 1988;62(16):1124–1125.
57. Dahlöf B, Pennert K, Hansson L: Reversal of left ventricular hypertrophy in hypertensive patients. A meta-analysis of 109 treatment studies. Am J Hypertens 1992;5:95–110.
58. Böhlen L, Weidmann BL, de Courten M, et al: Antihypertensive drug effects on left ventricular hypertrophy: meta-analysis considering duration of treatment (abstract). J Hypertens 1994;12(Suppl 3):S140.
59. Cruickshank JM, Lewis J, Moore V, Dodd C: Reversibility of left ventricular hypertrophy by differing types of antihypertensive therapy. J Hum Hypertens 1992;6:85–90.
60. Schmieder RE, Martus P, Klingbeil A: Reversal of left ventricular hypertrophy in essential hypertension. JAMA 1996;275:1507–1513.
61. Pfeffer MA, Braunwald E, Moye LA, et al: Effect of captopril on mortality and morbidity in patients with LV dysfunction after myocardial infarction. Results of the survival and ventricular enlargement trial. The SAVE Investigators. N Engl J Med 1992;327:669–677.
62. Dzau VJ: Local expression and pathophysiological role of renin angiotensin in the blood vessels and heart, in Grobecker H, Heusch G, Strauer BE (eds): Angiotensin and Heart. New York, Springer Verlag, 1993, pp 1–14.
63. Gottdiener JS, Reda DJ, Massie BM, Materson BJ, Williams DW, Anderson RJ: Circulation 1997;95(8):2007–14.
64. Dahlöf B, Hansson L: Regression of left ventricular hypertrophy in previously untreated essential hypertension: different effects of enalapril and hydrochlorothiazide. J Hypertens 1992;10:1513–1524.
65. Dahlöf B, Hansson L: The influence of antihypertensive therapy on the structural arteriolar changes in essential hypertension: different effects of enalapril and hydrochlorothiazide. J Intern Med 1993;234:271–279.
66. Gonzáles-Fernández RA, Rivera M, Rodriguez PJ, et al: Prevalence of ectopic ventricular activity after left ventricular mass regression. Am J Hypertens 1993;6(suppl):308–313.
67. Corea L, Bentivoglio M, Verdecchia P. Echocardiographic left ventricular hypertrophy as related to arterial pressure and plasma norepinephrine concentration in arterial hypertension. Reversal by atenolol treatment. Hypertension 1983;5:837–843.
68. Rowlands DB, Glover DR, Stallard TJ, Littler WA. Control of blood pressure and reduction of echocardiographically assessed left ventricular mass with once-daily timolol. Br J Clin Pharmacol 1982;14:89–95.
69. Gong L, Zhang W, Zhu Y, Zhu J, Kong D, Page V, Ghadirian P, LeLorier J, Hamet P. J Hypertens 1996;14(10):1237–1245.
70. Goldstein S. Beta blockers in hypertensive and coronary heart disease. Arch Intern Med 1996;156(12):1267–1276.
71. Siscovick DS, Raghunathan TE, Psaty BM, Koepsell TD, Wicklund KG, Lin X, Cobb L, Rautaharju PM, Copass MK, Wagner EH: N Engl J Med 1994; 330(26):1852–7.
72. Caralis PV, Materson BJ, Perez-Stable E: Potassium and diuretic-induced ventricular arrhythmias in ambulatory hypertensive patients. Miner Electrolyte Metab 1984,10:148–154.
73. Hollifield JW. Potassium and magnesium abnormalities: diuretics and arrhythmias in hypertension. Am J Med 1984;77(Suppl 5A):28–32.
74. Levy D, Salomon M, D'Agostino RB, Belangerr AJ, Kannel WB. Prognostic implications of baseline electrocardiographic features and their serial changes in subjects with left ventricular hypertrophy. Circulation 1994;90(4):1786–1793.
75. Yurenev AP, Dyakonova HG, Novikov ID, et al. Management of essential hypertension in patients with different degrees of left ventricular hypertrophy. Multicenter trial. Am J Hypertens 1992;5(6 Pt 2):182S–189S.

29

HYPERTENSION AND HEART FAILURE

M. Gary Nicholls, A. Mark Richards, and Evan J. Begg

Department of Medicine
Christchurch Hospital
Christchurch, New Zealand

1. INTRODUCTION

Heart failure in Western countries presents major problems. Approximately 1–3% of the population, fewer in young and middle-life, and more in the later decades of life, are said to suffer from heart failure[1-3]. Evidence is that the prevalence rate is increasing with time[4,5]. Longevity, though improved by some treatments[6], notably angiotensin converting enzyme inhibitors, remains a matter of months once clinically severe hart failure is established[7]. Furthermore, functional status and wellbeing by most criteria are more adversely affected by heart failure than by various forms of arthritis or chronic lung disease, for example[8]. From an economic point of view, heart failure accounts for approximately 1–2% of total health care budgets in Western countries[3,9-11], and is likely to increase with time.

In view of the above, it is logical to consider measures which prevent, or at least delay, the onset of heart failure. The basis of prevention is accurate understanding of the major aetiologic factors for heart failure.

2. AETIOLOGY OF HEART FAILURE

The list of causes of heart failure is a long one[12,13]. Retrospective surveys of patients presenting to hospital with heart failure tend to report coronary artery disease as the most common cause, with hypertension accounting for less than 20% of cases[14,15]. Intuitively, however, it is likely that studying a hospital population with established heart failure may provide an underestimate of hypertension as an aetiologic factor. For example, blood pressure generally falls with the onset of heart failure, and a normal or even low blood pressure at the time of hospitalisation may mask sustained hypertension prior to the patient seeking medical attention. Likewise, blood pressure tends to fall after acute myocardial infarction which is, of course, one complication of hypertension. Again, the patient presenting to hospital with myocardial infarction with or without subsequent heart failure, may give little clue to previous hypertension. Silent myocardial infarction is relatively common in hypertensives[16], so patients ultimately presenting in heart failure may show lit-

Hypertension and the Heart, edited by Zanchetti et al.
Plenum Press, New York, 1997

273

tle evidence that sustained hypertension was an underlying aetiological factor. Since the mortality rate post-myocardial infarction is relatively high in patients who have been hypertensive[17], prior hypertension may again remain unsuspected in the patient presenting with myocardial infarction and progresses rapidly to heart failure then death.

Another point which tends to obscure the hypertension-heart failure link is that heart failure is usually a complication after many years, and often decades, of elevated blood pressure. Formal placebo-controlled antihypertensive drug trials lasting 2–5 years in young and middle aged hypertensive patients are ill equipped to demonstrate any protective effect of such drug treatment in so far as heart failure is concerned. Antihypertensive drug trials in the elderly, or of long duration in middle aged patients, will be required to demonstrate a protective effect in this regard. Finally, as mentioned later, reliance on clinical suspicion and non-specific tests for a diagnoses of heart failure in a hypertensive population, is likely to under-estimate the true prevalence of left ventricular dysfunction.

3. HYPERTENSION AND HEART FAILURE

Early studies, before the introduction of antihypertensive drug treatment, suggested that at least in Western countries, hypertension was the commonest cause of non-rheumatic heart failure[18–20]. Furthermore, the few long term observational studies of sizeable hypertensive populations receiving no, or limited, drug treatment, pointed to heart failure as a contributing factor or cause of death in most, or a sizeable minority of patients[18,21,22]. The study of men born in 1913 in Gothenburg, Sweden, indicated that 46% of patients presenting with overt congestive heart failure had prior hypertension, and 55% coronary heart disease with 79% having any one of these conditions[23]. For patients with so-called "latent" congestive heart failure, 52% were documented as having prior hypertension and 25% coronary heart disease[23]. From re-examination of these data in 1989 it was concluded, using multivariate regression analysis, that hypertension and smoking were the major independent risk factors for the development of congestive heart failure[24].

For middle-aged hypertensive men receiving antihypertensive therapy, the prevalence of congestive heart failure at the completion of the 10 year follow-up was 5.9%[25].

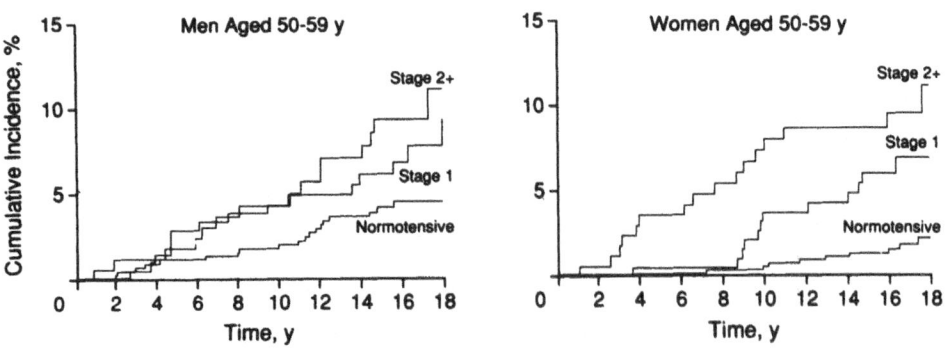

Figure 1.   Cumulative incidence of congestive heart failure in men and women aged 50 to 59 years according to hypertension status at baseline. Stage 1 hypertension was defined as systolic blood pressure of 140–159mmHg or diastolic pressure of 90–99mmHg in subjects not receiving antihypertensive treatment, and stage 2 or greater (stage 2+) was defined as systolic blood pressure greater than 160mmHg, diastolic pressure greater than 100mmHg, or the current use of antihypertensive treatment. From 26, with permission.

Pivotal to defining the link between hypertension and heart failure, is the Framingham Heart Study. As reported in 1996 and during a mean of 14.1 years' follow-up, there were 392 new cases of heart failure, 91% of which had antecedent hypertension. The incidence of heart failure was greater at increasing blood pressure levels (Figure 1) and increased as a function of age and duration of follow-up[26]. This "dose-response" relationship for level of blood pressure and risk of heart failure was probably first noted by Smirk[27], and is to be expected if the association is one of cause and effect. Multivariate analysis indicated that hypertension had a high population attributable risk for heart failure, accounting for 39% of cases in men and 59% in women[26]. Framingham data suggested, furthermore, that there has been no significant change in the frequency of hypertension as the attributable cause of heart failure during four decades of observation between 1948 and 1988[28]. That hypertension remains the prime aetiologic factor is supported by evidence from the Northern California Kaiser Permanente Medical Care Program which concluded that the higher rate of hospitalisation for congestive heart failure among African Americans compared with whites was explained by the greater prevalence of hypertension and diabetes in the former racial group[29]. Hypertension appeared to be the dominant identifiable pathogenetic factor for heart failure in both African Americans and whites. These data were collected over a median period of 9.5 years following at least one "multiphasic health check up" between the years 1978 and 1984[29].

The Framingham Study also reported a link between established or borderline isolated systolic hypertension and congestive heart failure[30,31]. Whilst this does not necessarily indicate cause and effect, the protective action of antihypertensive drug treatment in the Systolic Hypertension in the Elderly Program (SHEP)[32], leaves little doubt that indeed the epidemiological association is a biologically important one which can be modified by reducing arterial pressure.

The link between hypertension and heart failure has tended to concentrate on patients presenting with systolic left ventricular dysfunction. Improved understanding and diagnosis of diastolic left ventricular dysfunction might reveal an even closer linkage overall between hypertension and heart failure. Available evidence, summarised in 1995, suggests that somewhere between 11–83% of patients with diastolic heart failure had previous hypertension[33]. This wide range of estimates indicates the need for accurate prospective population studies focussing on diastolic left ventricular dysfunction.

If hypertension is an important aetiologic factor for the development of heart failure, one would anticipate a description of plausible pathophysiologic links between the two. In fact, numerous authors have addressed how hypertension can lead to heart failure either through direct effects on the myocardium causing systolic and/or diastolic dysfunction, or through abnormalities of the coronary circulation[34-37]. Other chapters in this publication address this issue in depth.

As mentioned in passing above, the association between hypertension and heart failure, as determined from epidemiologic studies, need not necessarily be through cause and effect. The case would be very much stronger if antihypertensive drug treatment, from formal placebo-controlled, randomised and blinded studies revealed that reducing arterial pressure protected from, or delayed the onset of, heart failure. A majority of antihypertensive drug trials are ill equipped to address this topic, since follow-up treatment has been in the region of 2–5 years, whereas, at least for young and middle-aged hypertensive patients, one would not anticipate the onset of heart failure for a matter of decades. Studies in elderly hypertensives are more likely to be fruitful in this regard since the long term effects of untreated hypertension may be revealed in the course of such formal trials. Likewise, controlled trials in patients with severe grades of hypertension would be better placed than trials in mild to moderate hypertension. In fact, evidence from the major trials over the last 20 years is that antihypertensive treatment reduces the incidence of heart failure by approximately 50%[38], and this protective effect is, as predicted, most readily seen in patients with severe grades of hypertension, as in the Veterans Administration Co-operative Study[39,40] and in elderly hypertensives studied, for example, in the Swedish Trial in Old Persons with Hypertension (STOP)[41] and SHEP[32].

Our current understanding of the causal link between hypertension and heart failure is less than ideal, since the clinical diagnosis of heart failure is frequently inaccurate. The prevalence of heart failure, whether defined by a reduced left ventricular ejection fraction or by abnormalities in left ventricular diastolic function, might be seriously miscalculated where classical clinical symptoms and signs, or non-specific tests such as chest radiology and electrocardiography, are used as the sole diagnostic indices[42-46]. Echocardiography or radionuclide ventriculography, and/or measurements of circulatory levels of cardiac natriuretic peptides are likely to uncover patients with impaired left ventricular function before the classical clinical symptoms and signs are established[42-48].

4. PREVENTING HEART FAILURE: SHOULD WE DELAY TREATING PATIENTS WITH HYPERTENSION?

If long-sustained hypertension is the prime cause of heart failure in Western populations, should antihypertensive drug treatment be withheld for years and even decades until an estimated 5 year risk of a major cardiovascular event is 10% or more, as is proposed by the New Zealand Guidelines[49]? In fact, it is surprising that most guidelines for the management of hypertension make little mention of heart failure, concentrating instead on coronary heart disease and stroke as end-points to be prevented by antihypertensive drug therapy. Discussion is needed as to whether the time frame, when considering risks of hypertensive complications, should be approximately 5 years, or whether, in the case of young and middle-aged patients this should be extended to take into account the possibility of heart failure many years, even decades, later. This is worthy of consideration by individual patients with their informed physician. It is also relevant to the fiscal aspects of treating hypertension. Commentators viewing the costs of antihypertensive drug treatment, like those involved in drawing up guidelines, have tended to ignore heart failure as a complication of hypertension and therefore down-played the potential for cost savings by delaying or preventing the onset of heart failure[50]. In our view, the economics of treating hypertension need to consider the long-term view, and take account of heart failure and its prevention, along with vascular dementia, end-stage renal failure etc, rather than concentrating mostly or exclusively on stroke and coronary heart disease. In this regard, we echo the sentiments of the World Hypertension League[51].

Hypertension, of course, is one aetiologic risk factor for coronary artery disease which causes or contributes to the development of heart failure in a sizeable minority of patients in Western countries[26]. Any programme aimed at preventing or delaying the onset of heart failure should logically, therefore, take account of coronary risk factors in addition to hypertension.

5. OVERVIEW

Heart failure has emerged as a major and increasing burden in regard to morbidity and mortality in Western societies, and the costs of treating established heart failure are enormous. The study of hospitalised patients with heart failure in regard to aetiology gives an inaccurate perspective. Long-term prospective studies, and particularly the Framingham Study, indicate that hypertension is the most important single aetiologic factor. Furthermore, an overview of antihypertensive drug trials indicates that drug treatment of hypertension reduces the incidence of heart failure by approximately 50%. The time profile for the development of heart failure in hypertensive patients is a long one, and guidelines for the treatment of hypertension which concentrate on short-term antihypertensive studies in middle-aged patients have down-played or simply ignored the vital association between hypertension and heart failure.

Rather than concentrating just on the short-term risks of stroke and coronary heart disease, such recommendations need to consider also the longer-term potential for developing heart failure with its bleak profile of morbidity, mortality and drain on the economy. At the very least, patients need to be informed of the long-term risks of heart failure if their hypertension remains untreated, and the demonstrable protective effect of antihypertensive therapy. In this regard, and particularly in early or middle-life, decisions on antihypertensive drug treatment based on a 5 year time horizon are unacceptable in our view. As noted by Zanchetti, patients aged 45 years with a blood pressure of 150/100mmHg have a shortened life expectancy (by 11.5 years in men, 8.5 years in women) compared with normotensives, yet they have a mean life expectancy of 20.5 and 28.5 years respectively[52]. One goal of the physician must be to ensure patients have the option of achieving their full life span.

REFERENCES

1. Massie BM, Shah NB. The heart failure epidemic: magnitude of the problem and potential mitigating approaches. Current Opinion in Cardiology 1996;11:221–226.
2. Eriksson H. Heart failure: a growing public health problem. J Int Med 1995;237:135–141.
3. Doughty R, Yee T, Sharpe N, MacMahon S. Hospital admissions and deaths due to congestive heart failure in New Zealand, 1988–91. NZ Med J 1995;108:473–475.
4. Ghali JK, Cooper R, Ford E. Trends in hospitalization rates for heart failure in the United States, 1973–1986. Evidence for increasing population prevalence. Arch Intern Med 1990;150:769–773.
5. Reitsma JB, Mosterd A, de Craen AJM, Koster RW, van Capelle FJL, Grobbee DE. Increase in hospital admission rates for heart failure in the Netherlands, 1980–1993. Heart 1996;76:388–392.
6. Stevenson WG, Steven son LW, Middlekauff HR, Fonarow GC, Hamilton MA, Woo MA, Saxon LA, Natterson PD, Steimle A, Walden JA, Tillisch JH. Improving survival for patients with advanced heart failure: a study of 737 consecutive patients. JACC 1995;26:1417–1423.
7. Ho KKL, Anderson KM, Kannel WB, Grossman W, Levy D. Survival after the onset of congestive heart failure in Framingham Heart Study subjects. Circulation 1993;88:107–115.
8. Stewart AL, Greenfield S, Hays RD, Wells K, Rogers WH, Berry SD, McGlynn EA, Ware JE. Functional status and well-being of patients with chronic conditions. JAMA 1989;262:907–913.
9. McMurray J, Hart W, Rhodes G. An evaluation of the cost of heart failure to the National Health Service in the UK. Br J Med Economics 1993;6:99–110.
10. Launois B, Reboul-Marty J, Battais K, Lefebvre P. Le coût de la sévérite de la maladie: le cas de l'insuffisance-cardiaque. J d'Economie Médicale 1990;8:395–412.
11. O'Connell JB, Bristow MR. Economic impact of heart failure in the United States: time for a different approach. J Heart Lung Transplant 1994;13:S107–S112.
12. Sander GE, Giles TD. Specific heart muscle disease. Current Opinion in Cardiology 1991;6:401–410.
13. Dec GW, Fuster V. Idiopathic dilated cardiomyopathy. N Engl J Med 1994;331:1564–1575.
14. Teerlink JR, Goldhaber SZ, Pfeffer MA. An overview of contemporary etiologies of congestive heart failure. Am Heart J 1991;121:1852–1853.
15. Andersson B, Waagstein F. Spectrum and outcome of congestive heart failure in a hospitalized population. Am Heart J 1993;126:632–640.
16. Kannel WB, Dannenberg AL, Abbott RD. Unrecognised myocardial infarction and hypertension: the Framingham study. Am Heart J 1985;109:581–585.

17. Rabkin SW, Mathewson FA, Tate RB. Prognosis after acute myocardial infarction: relation to blood pressure values before infarction in a prospective cardiovascular study. Am J Cardiol 1977;40:604–610.
18. Nicholls MG. Hypertension, hypertrophy, heart failure. Heart (suppl.3) 1996;76:92–97.
19. Clawson BJ. Incidence of types of heart disease among 30,265 autopsies, with special reference to age and sex. Am Heart J 1941;22:607–624.
20. Wartman WB, Hellerstein HK. The incidence of heart disease in 2,000 consecutive autopsies. Annals Intern Med 1943;28:41–65.
21. Perera GA. Hypertensive vascular disease: description and natural history. J Chron Dis 1955;1:33–42.
22. Bechgaard P. A 40 years' follow-up study of 1000 untreated hypertensive patients. Clin Sci Mol Med 1976;51:673s–675s.
23. Eriksson H, Svärdsudd K, Caidahl K, Bjurö T, LarssonB, Welin L, Ohlson L-O, Wilhelmsen L. Early heart failure in the population. The study of men born in 1913. Acta Med Scand 1988;223:197–209.
24. Eriksson H, Svärdsudd K, Larsson B, Ohlson LO, Tibblin G, Welin L, Wilhelmsen L. Risk factors for heart failure in the general population: the study of men born in 1913. European Heart J 1989;10:647–656.
25. Samuelsson O, Wilhelmsen L, Pennert K, Berglund G. Angina pectoris, intermittent claudication and congestive heart failure in middle-aged male hypertensives. Acta Med Scand 1987;221:23–32.
26. Levy D, Larson MG, Vasan RS, Kannel WB, Ho KKL. The progression from hypertension to congestive heart failure. JAMA 1996;275:1557–1562.
27. Smirk FH. Congestive heart failure. *In*: Smirk FH, Editor. High Arterial Pressure. Oxford, Blackwell 1957: p86–88.
28. Ho KKL, Anderson KM, Kannel WB, Grossman W, Levy D. Survival after the onset of congestive heart failure in Framingham Heart Study subjects. Circulation 1993;88:107–115.
29. Alexander M, Grumbach K, Selby J, Brown AF, Washington E. Hospitalization for congestive heart failure. JAMA 1995;274:1037–1042.
30. Kannel WB, Dawber TR, McGee DL. Perspectives on systolic hypertension. Circulation 1980;61:1179–1182.
31. Sagie A, Larson MG, Levy D. The natural history of borderline isolated systolic hypertension. N Engl J Med 1993;329:1912–1917.
32. SHEP Cooperative Research Group. Prevention of stroke by antihypertensive drug treatment in older persons with isolated systolic hypertension. Final results of the Systolic Hypertension in the Elderly Program (SHEP). JAMA 1991;265:3255–3264.
33. Vasan RS, Benjamin EJ, Levy D. Prevalence, clinical features and prognosis of diastolic heart failure: an epidemiologic perspective. J Am Coll Cardiol 1995;26:1565–1574.
34. Vatner SF. Reduced subendocardial myocardial perfusion as one mechanism for congestive heart failure. Am J Cardiol 1988;62:94E–98E.
35. Vogt M, Strauer BE. Systolic ventricular dysfunction and heart failure due to coronary microangiopathy in hypertensive heart disease. Am J Cardiol 1995;76:48D–53D.
36. Westerhof N, O'Rourke MF. Haemodynamic basis for the development of left ventricular failure in systolic hypertension and for its logical therapy. J Hypertens 1995;13:943–952.
37. Vasan RS, Levy D. The role of hypertension in the pathogenesis of heart failure. Arch Intern Med 1996;156:1789–1796.
38. Moser M, Hebert PR. Prevention of disease progression, left ventricular hypertrophy and congestive heart failure in hypertension treatment trials. J Am Coll Cardiol 1996;27:1214–1218.
39. Veterans Administration Cooperative Study Group on Antihypertensive Agents. Effects of treatment on morbidity in hypertension. Results in patients with diastolic blood pressures averaging 115–129mmHg. JAMA 1967;202:1028–1034.
40. Veterans Administration Cooperative Study Group on Antihypertensive Agents. Results in patients with diastolic blood pressures averaging 90–114mmHg. JAMA 1970;213:1143–1152.
41. Dahlöf B, Lindholm LH, Hansson L, Schersten B, Ekbom T, Wester P-O. Morbidity and mortality in the Swedish Trial in Old Patients with Hypertension (STOP-Hypertension). The Lancet 1991;338:1281–1285.
42. Barnett DB. Heart failure. Diagnosis of symptomless left ventricular dysfunction. The Lancet 1993;341:1124–1125.
43. Remes J, Miettinen H, Reunanen A, Pyörälä. Validity of clinical diagnosis of heart failure in primary health care. European Heart J 1991;12:315–321.
44. Wheeldon NM, MacDonald TM, Flucker CJ, McKendrick AD, McDevitt DG, Struthers AD. Echocardiography in chronic heart failure in the community. Q J Med 1993;86:17–23.
45. Clarke KW, Gray D, Hampton JR. Evidence of inadequate investigation and treatment of patients with heart failure. Br Heart J 1994;71:584–587.
46. Francis CM, Caruana L, Kearney P, Love M, Sutherland GR, Starkey IR, Shaw TRD, McMurray JJV. Open access echocardiography in management of heart failure in the community. BMJ 1995;310:634–636.

47. Hillis GS, Al-Mohammad A, Wood M, Jennings KP. Changing patterns of investigation and treatment of cardiac failure in hospital. Heart 1996;76:427–429.

48. Struthers AD. Prospects for using a blood sample in the diagnosis of heart failure. QJ Med 1995;88:303–306.

49. Guidelines for the management of mildly raised blood pressure in New Zealand. Core Services Committee, PO Box 5013, Wellington, New Zealand.

50. Johannesson M. Economic evaluation of hypertension treatment — methods and empirical results. *In*: Textbook of Hypertension. Ed. JD Swales. Blackwell Scientific Publications, p.1292–1303.

51. World Hypertension League. Update/Le Point. Economics of hypertension control. Bulletin of the WHO 1995;73:417–424.

52. Zanchetti A. Presidential Lecture. Antihypertensive therapy: pride and prejudice. J Hypertens 1995;13: 1522–1528.

SPEAKERS

Prof. Enrico Agabiti Rosei
Istituto di Patologia Medica
Ospedale Civile
P.le Spedali Civili, 1
25123 Brescia
Italy
Tel. 0039 (30) 3995248 (direct);
  0039 (30) 396044
Fax 0039 (30) 3384348

Dr. Christian G. Brilla
Associate Professor of Medicine
Molekular-kardiologisches Labor
Klinikum
Der Philipps-Universität
Karl-von-Frisch-Str. 1
35033 Marburg
Germany
Tel. 0049 (6421) 286.462 (direct);
  0049 (6421) 285032/5033 (lab.)
Fax 0049 (6421) 288.954 (direct);
  0049 (6421) 288.964 (lab.)

Prof. Antonio Coca
Unidad de Hipertension Arterial
Hospital Clinico y Provincial
Servicio de Medicina Interna General
Facultad de Medicina
Universitad de Barcelona
Villarroel, 170
08036 Barcelona
Spain
Tel. 0034 (3) 227.54.00 (ext 2240)
Fax 0034 (3) 227.54.54

Dott. Cesare Cuspidi
Istituto di Clinica Medica Generale e
  Terapia Medica
Centro di Fisiologia Clinica e Ipertensione
Padiglione "Sacco"
Ospedale Maggiore di Milano
Via Francesco Sforza, 35, 20122 Milano
Tel. 0039 (2) 55033518 (direct)
Fax 0039 (2) 5457666

Prof. Richard B. Devereux
Department of Medicine
Division of Cardiology
The New York Hospital — Cornell
  Medical Center
Box 222, 525 East 68th Street
New York, New York 10021, U.S.A.
Tel. 001 (212) 746.4655
Fax 001 (212) 746.8451

Dr. Anna F. Dominiczak
Department of Medicine & Therapeutics
Western Infirmary, University of Glasgow
Glasgow G11 6NT, U.K.
Tel. 0044 (141) 211.2688
Fax 0044 (141) 211.1763

Dr. Edward D. Frohlich
Vice President for Academic Affairs
Alton Ochsner Medical Foundation
1516 Jefferson Highway
New Orleans, Louisiana 70121, U.S.A.
Tel. 001 (504) 842.3700
Fax 001 (504) 842.3258

Dott. Guido Grassi
Centro di Fisiologia Clinica e Ipertensione
Istituto Clinica Medica Generale e Terapia
  Medica
Policlinico
Via Francesco Sforza, 35
20122 Milano, Italy
Tel. 0039 (2) 55033557 (direct);
  0039 (2) 55184606
Fax 0039 (2) 5457666

Dr. Jacques-Antoine Haefliger
Department of Internal Medicine B
Laboratory of Molecular Biology 19-135
Centre Hospitalier Universitaire Vaudois
C.H.U.V. — 1011 Lausanne
Switzerland
Tel. 0041 (21) 314.0927
Fax 0041 (21) 314.0630

Prof. Lennart Hansson
Division of Clinical Hypertension Research
Department of Geriatrics
University of Uppsala
P.O. Box 609
75125 Uppsala, Sweden
Tel. 0046 (18) 101.384
Fax 0046 (18) 177.973

Prof. Federico Lombardi
Cardiologia
Istituto di Scienze Biomediche
Ospedale San Paolo
Università di Milano
Via A. di Rudinì, 8
20142 Milano, Italy
Tel. 0039 (2) 8184461
Fax 0039 (2) 89129973

Dr. Manuel Luque Otero
Unidad de Hipertension
Hospital Universitario San Carlos
Universidad Complutense
Avda Martin Lagos s/n
28040 Madrid, Spain
Tel. 0034 (1) 3303.458 (direct);
  0034 (1) 3303.000
Fax 0034 (1) 734.3848 (direct);
  0034 (1) 533.0264

Prof. Fabio Magrini
Centro di Fiiologia Clinica e Ipertensione
Istituto di Clinica Medica Generale e
  Terapia Medica
Padiglione "Sacco", Policlinico
Via Francesco Sforza, 35
20122 Milano, Italy
Tel. 0039 (2) 55033523 (direct);
  0039 (2) 55195252
Fax 0039 (2) 5457666

Prof. Jean-Michel Mallion
Chef de Service
Médecine Interne et Cardiologie
Hypertension Artérielle
CHU Centre Hospitalier Universitaire de
  Grenoble
Hôpital A. Michallon
Rez-de-chaussée haut, B.P. 217
38043 Grenoble Cedex 09, France
Tel. 0033 (76) 76.76.54.40
Fax 0033 (76) 76.55.59

Prof. Franz H. Messerli
Department of Hypertension
Ochsner Clinic
1514 Jefferson Highway
New Orleans, Louisiana 70121, USA
Tel. 001 (504) 842.3144; 001 (504) 842.4077;
Fax 001 (504) 842.4220

Dr. Ludwig Neyses
Klinikum der Bayerischen
Julius-Maximilians-Universität Würzburg
Medizinische Universitätsklinik
Luitpoldkrankenhaus
Josef Schneider-Straße 2
97080 Würzburg, Germany
Tel. 0049 (931) 201.2774
Fax 0049 (931) 201.2291

Prof. M. Gary Nicholls
Department of Medicine
The Christchurch School of Medicine
Christchurch Hospital, P.O. Box 4345
Christchurch, New Zealand
Tel. 0064 (3) 3640.825; 0064 (3) 3640.640;
  0064 (3) 3640.80825
Fax 0064 (3) 3640.935

Dr. Carlo Palombo
CNR, Istituto del Consiglio Nazionale
  delle Ricerche
Istituto di Fisiologia Clinica
Via Paolo Savi, 8, 56126 Pisa, Italy
Tel. 0039 (50) 583111
Fax 0039 (50) 592391;
  0039(50) 553461

Prof. Achille Cesare Pessina
Direttore, Clinica Medica I
Istituto di Medicina Clinica
Dipartimento di Medicina Clinica e
  Sperimentale
Università degli Studi di Padova
Policlinico Universitario
Via Giustiniani, 2, 35126 Padova, Italy
Tel. 0039 (49) 8212279; 0039 (49) 8752701;
Fax 0039 (49) 8754179

Dr. Mary J. Roman
Division of Cardiology
Cornell University Medical College
525 East 68th Street
New York, New York 10021, U.S.A.
Tel. 001 (212) 746.4685
Fax 001 (212) 746.8451

Dr. Luis M. Ruilope
Servicio de Hipertensión
Hospital 12 de Octubre
Carretera de Andalucia Km 5.400
28041 Madrid, Spain
Tel. 0034 (1) 3908.284 (direct);
  0034 (1) 3908.000
Tel. and Fax 0034 (1) 507.284.8566
Fax 0034 (1) 576.5644
Secretary Mrs. Marybell

Prof. Antonio Salvetti
Cattedra Medicina Interna
Università degli Studi di Pisa
Istituto di Clinica Medica I
Centro Ipertensione
Via Roma, 67, 56100 Pisa, Italy
Tel. 0039 (50) 502586;
  0039 (50) 592409
Tel. and Fax 050/553407 (direct)
Secretary Mrs. Donatella

Dr. Roland E. Schmieder
Medizinische Klinik IV
Universität Erlangen-Nürnberg Süd
Breslaüer Str. 201
90471 Nürnberg, Germany
Tel. 0049 (911) 398.5124;
  0049 (911) 398.3119
Fax 0049 (911) 398.3183

Prof. B.E. Strauer
Direktor der Medizinischen
Med. Klinik and Policlinic B
Heinrich Heine University
Moorenstraße 5
40225 Düsseldorf, Germany
Tel. 0049 (211) 811.8801
Fax 0049 (211) 811.8812

Dr. Yao Sun
Department of Internal Medicine
University of Missouri-Columbia
Division of Cardiology
MA432 Medical Science Building
1 Hospital Drive
Columbia, Missouri 65212
U.S.A.
Tel. 001 (314) 882.8580
Fax 001 (314) 884.4691

Dr. Laurence Tiret
Scientific Director
Epidémiologie Cardio-Vasculaire
INSERM U258, Hôpital Broussais
96, rue Didot
75674 Paris Cedex 14
France
Tel. 0033 (1) 4395.9563;
  0033 (1) 4395.9567
Fax 0033 (1) 4593.4269

Prof. Thomas Unger
Direktor
Klinikum der Christian-Albrechts-
  Universität zu Kiel
Institut für Pharmacologische
Hospitalstraße 4
D-24105 Kiel, Germany
Tel. 0049 (431) 597.3500/01
Fax 0049 (431) 597.3522

Prof. P.A. van Zwieten
Departments of Pharmacotherapy,
   Cardiology and Cardiopulmonary Surgery
Academic Medical Center
University of Amsterdam
P.O. Box 22700, Meibergdreef 15
1105 de Amsterdam, The Netherlands
Tel. 0031 (20) 566.4977
Fax 0031 (20) 696.8704

Prof. Malcom J. West
Department of Medicine
University of Queensland
Level B1, Pathology Building
Prince Charles Hospital
Chermside, Queensland 4032
Australia
Tel. 0061 (7) 3350.8381
Fax 0061 (7) 3359.2173

INDEX

Acetylcholine, 237, 239, 240, 249, 250
Adenosine, 226
Adrenalectomy, 66
Adrenergic nervous
    system, 105, 155
    tone, 93
Aging process and the cardiovascular system, 13, 14,
    17, 21, 242
Aldosterone, 36, 119
    and myocardial growth, 97
    excess of, 64
Alpha-blockers, 195
Ambulatory blood pressure, 95, 103
Angina, 2, 211, 264, 269
Angiogenesis, 167
Angiotensin
    I receptor antagonists, 43, 59, 161, 163, 167
    II, 25, 30, 35, 36, 55, 58, 79, 93, 118, 124, 162, 163,
        173, 196
    receptors, 58, 118
Angiotensin-converting enzyme (ACE), 124
    and kininase II, 159
    binding, 58
    expression, 162
    gene, 111, 120, 137
    gene I/D polymorphism, 111, 120
    gene polymorphism and cardiac hypertrophy, 118
    genotype, 114, 117, 120
    inihibitors, 43, 58, 130, 139, 140, 152, 160–164,
        168, 190–192, 194–196, 204, 228, 254, 259,
        267, 273
        and the heart, 268
        and the kidney, 268
        and the vascular tree, 268
        sympatholitic effects, 200
Antihypertensive treatment, 130, 189, 191, 192, 217,
    228, 254
Aortic coarctation, 21
Arrhythmias, 159, 162, 193, 199, 257, 263–266, 268
Arterial function
    and aging, 14
    and baroreceptors, 178
    and estrogens, 84
    and hypertension, 15

Arterial vessels
    compliance, 6, 13, 18, 125, 128, 155
    pressure waveform, 21
    stiffness, 13
Atherosclerosis, 6, 126, 128, 129, 139, 151, 215, 216,
    227, 253
Athletes, 151, 219, 229; see also Exercise
Atrial natriuretic peptides, 103, 104, 106

Baroreceptors, 177, 178
Beta-blockers, 8, 139, 152, 190–192, 194–196, 200,
    211, 254, 267
Blood pressure, 92
    ambulatory values, 139
    dipper profile, 98
    non-dipper profile, 98
Blood viscosity, 253
Bradykinins, 159–161, 164, 167, 168, 236, 239

Calcium antagonists, 152, 190–192, 194–196, 200,
    204, 211, 223, 228, 254
Captopril, 161
    and thrombolysis study (CATS), 112
Cardiac failure, 168
Cardiac fibroblasts, 27, 35, 36
Cardiac function, 4
Cardiac kinins, 160
Cardiac index, 107
Cardiac mass, 119
Cardiac myocytes, 71, 86, 87, 199, 209
Cardiac output, 4, 17, 64, 107
Cardiomyopathy, 113
Cardiopulmonary receptors, 176–178
Cardiovascular Health Study, 10
Cardiovascular morbidity, 2, 8, 63, 95, 99, 190, 192,
    200, 215, 257, 263, 267, 269
Cardiovascular mortality, 2, 8, 63, 99, 190, 192, 200,
    215, 253, 257, 263, 267, 269
Cardiovascular risk factors, 2, 136, 140, 189, 191, 200,
    202, 215, 253, 263, 269, 276
Carotid artery, 6, 124–128
    intima-media thickening, 155
    structure, 154
    ultrasonography, 6

Catecholamines, 93, 97
Chymase like substances, 124
Collagen, 36, 38, 208, 211
  gene expression, 56
  increase and hypertension, 208
  volume fraction, 52
Combination therapy, 195, 268
Congestive heart failure, 91, 162, 199, 263, 269, 273,
    274, 276, 277
Conn adenoma, 65
Connexin, 71, 72, 79, 80
  channel, 73, 74
Coronary artery, 151–153, 185, 209, 212, 216, 227
  arteriogram, 211
  autoregulation, 227–228, 265
  blood flow, 7, 25, 161, 162, 167, 168, 208–210, 218,
    222, 223, 229, 255, 258, 275
  disease, 91, 257, 273, 274
  flow reserve, 5, 145, 146, 151, 155, 156, 207, 210–
    212, 216, 217, 219, 223, 224, 253, 264
  flow velocity, 228
  hemodynamics, 253, 254, 259
  obstruction, 1
  reserve, 227
  risk development in young adults (CARDIA) study,
    112
  vascular resistances, 208, 212, 215, 226, 227, 255
  stenoses, 2

Diabetes mellitus, 136, 137, 242, 250, 253, 264
  Control and Complication Trial, 138
Diastolic dysfunction, 53, 146, 207, 209, 211, 212,
    228, 275
Diastolic function, 145, 154, 199, 210
Diastolic transmitral flow velocity, 65
Dipyridamole, effects on coronary circulation, 221,
    256, 259
Diuretics, 8, 139, 152, 190–192, 194–196, 257, 269
DNA
  binding, 42, 83
  estrogen promoter, 84
  changes, 1, 63, 112, 202, 219, 224, 226

Echocardiography, 1, 8, 45, 104, 106, 145–147, 152,
    177, 189, 190, 195, 202, 216
  backscatter analysis, 50
  criteria (American Society), 95
  dipyridamole-atropine, 219, 220–224
  Gray Scale Analysis, 50
  pulsed Doppler, 150
  right ventricular, 149
  transesophageal echo doppler, 217, 219, 226,
    227
Ejection fraction, 266
Electrocardiography in cardiac hypertrophy criteria,
    9, 145, 147, 189
Electron microscopy, 74
Enalapril, 59, 139, 211, 223, 224, 255, 259

Endothelial cells, 167, 235
  derived contracting factors, 235
  dysfunction, 136, 140, 227, 228, 236, 238, 239, 241, 250
  function, 159
  hyperplasia, 209
Endothelin I, 58
Endothelium
  and acetylcholine, 239, 247, 248
  and methacoline, 237, 248
  and hypertension, 247, 248, 235
Erythrocytes
  Na^+-H^+ exchange, 97
  Na^+-Li^+ countertransport, 97
Estrogens, 83
  and lipid metabolism, 83, 84
  and myocardium, 85
  receptors, 85
Exercise, 148, 93, 199, 229, 255, 256
  training, 147, 153
Experimental animal models
  of aortic coarctation, 21, 257
  of myocardial infarction, 55

Fibrosis, 199, 208, 210, 211, 227, 229, 265
Flowmetry, 254
Forearm blood flow
  effect of acetylcholine, 238, 240
  effect of L-NMMA, 235
  plethysmography, 249
  vascular resistances, 242
Framingham Heart Study, 9, 10, 92, 111, 118

Gap junction channels, 72, 74
Gender, 2, 148
Gene, 30, 83
  α-actin, 27
  expression, 86
  hypertrophic program, 86
Genetic factors, 93
Genetic polymorphisms, 117
Genotype, 112
Growth
  effects of calcium on, 196
  factors, 40, 167, 209, 210

Heart rate variability, 181–186
  and domain analysis, 184, 185
Hydralazine, 23
Hydrochlorothiazide, 23, 267
Hyperaldosteronism, 40
  primary, 63, 64, 65
Hypercholesterolemia, 242
Hypertension, 123, 146, 191, 207, 211, 216, 222, 238,
    250, 253, 264, 266, 273, 275, 276, 277
  and arterial compliance, 14
  and arterial stiffness, 13
  and heart rate variability, 181
  and cardiovascular mortality, 215

Hypertension (*cont.*)
  and coronary flow reserve, 226, 229
  effects on the heart, 4, 78
  Optimal Treatment study (HOT), 147
  renovascular, 38, 63, 64, 66
  spontaneously hypertensive rats, 40, 86, 159, 163,
      175, 200, 257

Insulin
  and cardiac hypertrophy, 173
  resistance, 98, 138, 140
  sensitivity, 137
Ischemic heart disease, 199
  and heart rate variability, 181

Kallicrein-kinin-system, 160
Kininase II, 159
Kinins, 163, 168
  and ACEI, 160, 168

L-Arginine, 26
Left ventricle
  function, 150, 202, 212, 254, 274
  geometry, 146
  hypertophy
    concentric, 4, 6, 17, 65, 92, 106, 107, 126, 146,
        147, 155, 229
    eccentric, 4, 17, 65, 92, 107, 108, 146, 147, 155
    in athletes, 145
    prognosis, 2, 7, 129
    regression, 1, 8, 9, 152, 155, 185, 191202, 203
  mass, 1, 2, 17, 64, 66, 103, 118, 146, 153, 176, 185,
      189, 191, 192, 199, 202, 254, 267. 269
  index, 203, 266
  remodelling, 4, 107, 108, 126, 146
  performance, 254
  stress, 199
  structure, 17, 18
  wall thickness, 2, 18, 64, 66, 104, 148
  weight, 31
Lipid metabolism, 84
L-NAME, 25, 26, 247
Losartan, 23, 25, 59, 255, 259

Meta-analysis, 189, 190, 191, 194, 195, 200
Microalbuminuria, 135, 138
Microcirculation, 236
Microneurography, 174–176
Multicenter isradipine/diuretic atherosclerosis study
    (MIDAS), 130
Multiple Risk Factor Intervention Trial (MRFIT), 257
Muscarinic receptors, 240, 248
Myocardial ATP, 150
Myocardial collagen, 45
Myocardial fibrosis, 35, 38, 45, 51, 52, 129
Myocardial growth, 97
Myocardial infarction, 2, 56, 112, 263, 269, 273, 274
Myocardial ischemia, 160, 210, 211, 212, 215
Myocardial mass, 208, 228

Myocardial oxygen
  consumption, 207, 215, 218, 227
  demand, 152
  supply, 212
Myocardial perfusion, 224
Myocardial remodelling, 208, 228
Myosin chains, 27, 193

Nitric oxide, 25, 228, 235, 241, 247
N-monometil-L-arginina (LNMMA), 235, 240, 241
Non-pharmacological treatment of hypertensin, 192, 193
Norepinephrine, 93, 174–177

Pacing, 222, 224
Penn Convention criteria, 95
Perindopril, 23, 25, 59, 163, 164
Peripheral vascular resistances, 17, 106–108
Peterson's elastic modulus, 14, 125
PGE $_2$, 36
PGH$_2$, 235
Phospholipase C, 97
Plasma renin activity, 176, 177
Positron emission tomography, 217, 218, 221, 223,
    224, 226, 227
Pressure overload, 92, 150, 173, 207
Proto-oncogenes, 25, 86, 210
Pulmonary circulation, 149

Quantitative autoradiography, 58
Quantitative trait loci, 30
Quinapril, 255

Radionucleotide angiography, 150
Ramipril, 161, 163, 164, 167
Renal circulation, 236
Renal damage, 136, 276
Renal insufficiency, 137
Renin-angiotensin system, 30, 35, 64, 93, 94, 17, 118,
    124, 155, 164, 266
  and cardiac remodelling, 210
  gene polymorphism, 111
Resistance arteries, 128

Salt
  intake, 94, 97, 105, 106
  sensitivity, 91, 140
  urinary excretion, 96
Septal wall thickness, 96
Smoking, 242
Spectral analysis, 183
Stroke, 2, 257, 269
  prone rats, 23, 163
Studies of left ventricular dysfunction (SOLVD), 111
Sudden death, 3, 91, 193, 263, 266, 269
Survival and ventricular enlargement study (SAVE),
    111
Swedish trial in old person with hypertension (STOP),
    276
Sympathetic nerve traffic, 174, 186, 266

Sympathetic nervous system activation, 176, 181, 182, 184
   and cerebral circulation, 174
   and heart, 174
   and hypertension, 174, 175
   and kidney, 174
   and vagal balance, 182, 185
   overactivity, 173
Systolic dysfunction, 275
Systolic hypertension in the elderly program study
     (SHEP), 275, 276

Thyroid hormones, 173
Tissue characterization, 49
Tissue chymase, 119
Tissue echoreflectivity, 49, 53
Treatment of mild hypertensive study (THOMS),
     9, 147, 193, 194, 200
Tromboxane A$_2$, 235

Ultrasounds, 45, 46, 119, 154; *see also*
     Echocardiography

Vagal modulation, 182, 186
Vascular hypertrophy, 125, 127, 128, 130
Vascular stiffness, 17
Vascular structure, 5, 212
Vasomotor tone, 124
Vasodilators, 195, 249
Veteran Administration study, 194, 201, 267, 276
Video densitometry, 50
Volume overload, 92, 103, 173

Wall
  thickness, 17, 21
  stress, 5

Young's modulus, 14

The manufacturer's authorised representative in the EU is Springer
Nature Customer Service Centre GmbH, Europaplatz 3, 69115 Heidelberg,
Germany. If you have any concerns regarding our products, please
contact ProductSafety@springernature.com

Printed and bound by CPI Group (UK) Ltd, Croydon, CR0 4YY
24/04/2026
02096348-0017